Second Edition

The Brigham Intensive Review *of* Internal Medicine

QUESTION & ANSWER COMPANION

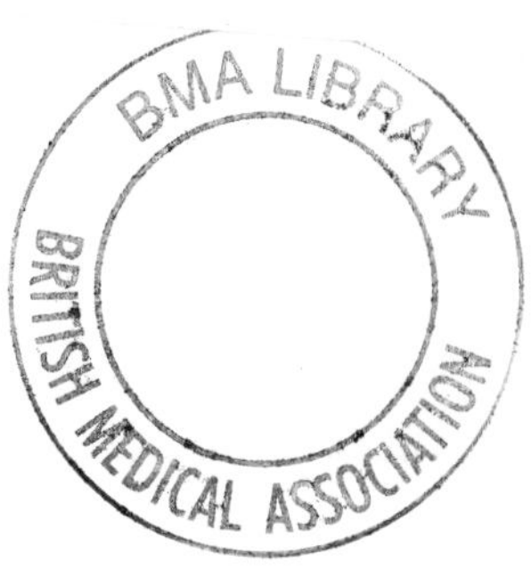

Ajay K. Singh, MBBS, FRCP, MBA
Senior Associate Dean
Global and Continuing Education
Harvard Medical School
Physician, Renal Division
Brigham and Women's Hospital
Boston, MA

Sarah P. Hammond, MD
Assistant Professor of Medicine
Harvard Medical School
Division of Infectious Diseases
Department of Medicine
Brigham and Women's Hospital
Boston, MA

Joseph Loscalzo, MD, PhD
Hersey Professor of the Theory and Practice of Physic
Harvard Medical School
Chairman, Department of Medicine
Physician-in-Chief

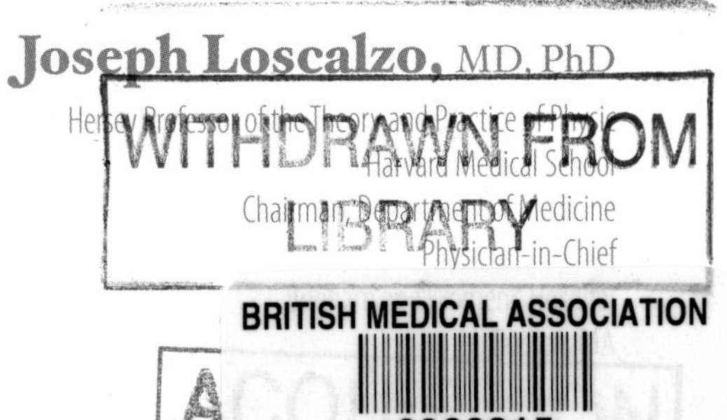

ELSEVIER

ELSEVIER

1600 John F. Kennedy Blvd.
Ste 1800
Philadelphia, PA 19103-2899

THE BRIGHAM INTENSIVE REVIEW OF INTERNAL MEDICINE
QUESTION & ANSWER COMPANION, SECOND EDITION ISBN: 978-0-323-48043-7

Library of Congress Cataloging-in-Publication Data

Names: Singh, Ajay, 1960- editor. | Loscalzo, Joseph, editor.
Title: The Brigham intensive review of internal medicine question & answer companion / [edited by] Ajay K. Singh, Joseph Loscalzo.
Description: Second edition. | Philadelphia, PA : Elsevier, [2019] | Includes index.
Identifiers: LCCN 2017042502 | ISBN 9780323480437 (pbk. : alk. paper)
Subjects: | MESH: Internal Medicine--methods | Physical Examination--methods | Problems and Exercises
Classification: LCC RC46 | NLM WB 18.2 | DDC 616--dc23 LC record available at https://lccn.loc.gov/2017042502

Executive Content Strategist: Kate Dimock
Senior Content Development Specialist: Joan Ryan
Publishing Services Manager: Catherine Jackson
Book Production Specialist: Kristine Feeherty
Design Direction: Patrick Ferguson

Printed in China
Last digit is the print number: 9 8 7 6 5 4 3 2 1

Contributors

Amy Bessnow, MD
Instructor in Medicine
Harvard Medical School
Department of Medicine
Brigham and Women's Hospital
Dana-Farber Cancer Institute
Boston, MA
Hematology and Oncology

Robert Burakoff, MD, MPH
Vice Chair for Ambulatory Services
Department of Medicine
Weill Cornell Medical College
New York, NY;
Site Chief
Division of Gastroenterology and Endoscopy
New York–Presbyterian Lower Manhattan Hospital
New York, NY;
Visiting Scientist
Harvard Medical School
Boston, MA
Gastroenterology

Elizabeth Gay, MD
Member of the Faculty of Medicine
Harvard Medical School
Division of Pulmonary and Critical Care Medicine
Department of Medicine
Brigham and Women's Hospital
Boston, MA
Pulmonary and Critical Care Medicine

Sarah P. Hammond, MD
Assistant Professor of Medicine
Harvard Medical School
Division of Infectious Diseases
Department of Medicine
Brigham and Women's Hospital
Boston, MA
Infectious Diseases
General Internal Medicine

Ole-Petter R. Hamnvik, MB BCh BAO, MMSc
Assistant Professor of Medicine
Harvard Medical School
Division of Endocrinology, Diabetes, and Hypertension
Department of Medicine
Brigham and Women's Hospital
Boston, MA
Endocrinology

Galen V. Henderson, MD
Assistant Professor of Medicine
Harvard Medical School
Department of Neurology
Brigham and Women's Hospital
Boston, MA
General Internal Medicine

Jennifer A. Johnson, MD
Assistant Professor of Medicine
Harvard Medical School
Division of Infectious Diseases
Department of Medicine
Brigham and Women's Hospital
Boston, MA
Infectious Diseases

Ann S. LaCasce, MD
Associate Professor of Medicine
Harvard Medical School
Department of Medical Oncology
Dana-Farber Cancer Institute
Department of Medicine
Brigham and Women's Hospital
Boston, MA
Hematology and Oncology

Ernest I. Mandel, MD
Instructor in Medicine
Harvard Medical School
Division of Renal Medicine
Department of Medicine
Brigham and Women's Hospital
Boston, MA
Nephrology and Hypertension

Muthoka L. Mutinga, MD
Assistant Professor of Medicine
Harvard Medical School
Division of Gastroenterology, Hepatology, and Endoscopy
Department of Medicine
Brigham and Women's Hospital
Boston, MA
Gastroenterology

Anju Nohria, MD, MSc
Assistant Professor of Medicine
Harvard Medical School
Division of Cardiovascular Medicine
Department of Medicine
Brigham and Women's Hospital
Boston, MA
Cardiovascular Disease

Molly Perencevich, MD
Instructor in Medicine
Harvard Medical School
Division of Gastroenterology, Hepatology, and Endoscopy
Department of Medicine
Brigham and Women's Hospital
Boston, MA
Gastroenterology

Megan Prochaska, MD
Research Fellow in Medicine
Harvard Medical School
Department of Medicine
Brigham and Women's Hospital
Boston, MA
Nephrology and Hypertension

Scott L. Schissel, MD
Instructor in Medicine
Harvard Medical School
Chief, Department of Medicine
Brigham and Women's Faulkner Hospital
Division of Pulmonary and Critical Care Medicine
Brigham and Women's Hospital
Boston, MA
Pulmonary and Critical Care Medicine

Lori Wiviott Tishler, MD
Assistant Professor of Medicine
Harvard Medical School
Division of General Internal Medicine and Primary Care
Department of Medicine
Brigham and Women's Hospital
Boston, MA
General Internal Medicine

Derrick J. Todd, MD, PhD
Instructor of Medicine
Harvard Medical School
Division of Rheumatology, Immunology, and Allergy
Department of Medicine
Brigham and Women's Hospital
Boston, MA
Rheumatology

Preface

Preparing for the American Board of Internal Medicine (ABIM) certifying or recertifying examination requires knowledge and clinical experience that can be evaluated by successfully answering questions in a test format. In this Question and Answer book, our goal is to provide the reader with 450 questions across 9 subspecialties in internal medicine. These questions test knowledge on topics relevant to the ABIM boards. As a companion to the *Brigham Intensive Review of Internal Medicine,* now in its third edition, this book is focused on how one applies knowledge to answer board questions successfully. The annotated answers are detailed, and they review the steps in critical thinking required to get to the correct answer.

The authors who have contributed questions and annotated answers to this book are some of our most senior physicians in the department. We sincerely thank them for their efforts and commitment to this project. We asked them to put themselves "in the head" of the ABIM to identify the topics that might be addressed in the board examination. We believe this book will be a valuable study tool to gauge one's knowledge in preparation for the examination.

We wish to thank Stephanie Tran and Michelle Deraney for supporting us in the development of this book. Without them this book would not have been possible. Our thanks also go to our families who have supported all of our academic activities, including this important project.

Ajay K. Singh, MBBS, FRCP, MBA
Joseph Loscalzo, MD, PhD
Sarah P. Hammond, MD

Contents

1 Infectious Diseases

SARAH P. HAMMOND AND JENNIFER A. JOHNSON

1. A 28-year-old woman who has lived her entire life in Providence, Rhode Island, presents 3 days after returning from a 2-week trip to Thailand complaining of fever to 102°F, muscle aches, and severe retroorbital headache. She has no gastrointestinal symptoms. She traveled only to the towns of Bangkok, Chiang Mai, and Phuket. She attended a travel clinic before traveling and was told there was no malaria in these towns, so she did not take prophylaxis. She denied contact with bodies of fresh water. Examination is unremarkable other than temperature of 101.8°F. Remarkable laboratory findings include a leukocyte count of 2200 cells/μL^3, hematocrit of 37%, and platelets of 62,000 cells/μL^3. Chemistries are normal. A peripheral blood smear for parasites is sent and is negative.

   Which of the following is the most likely diagnosis in this traveler?
   A. Leptospirosis
   B. Malaria
   C. Typhoid
   D. Hepatitis A
   E. Dengue

2. A 55-year-old male smoker with severe chronic obstructive pulmonary disease (COPD) is hospitalized in the medical intensive care unit. He now requires intubation and mechanical ventilation for hypercarbic respiratory failure after failing noninvasive ventilation.

   To reduce this patient's risk for developing ventilator-associated pneumonia, you recommend:
   A. Elevation of the head of the bed to 15 degrees to prevent aspiration
   B. Suctioning of subglottic secretions
   C. Twenty-four hours of prophylactic systemic antibiotics, especially if the intubation was emergent
   D. Daily changing of the ventilatory circuit
   E. Nasotracheal intubation rather than orotracheal intubation

3. A 47-year-old woman with a history of renal transplantation presents with 4 days of profuse nonbloody diarrhea, abdominal pain, and high fevers. She received her kidney transplant 10 years ago from a living unrelated donor for polycystic kidney disease and has had no episodes of rejection since. Her donor was cytomegalovirus (CMV) immunoglobulin G (IgG) negative, and she was CMV IgG positive before transplant. Her chronic medications for transplant include tacrolimus, low-dose prednisone, and mycophenolate mofetil and have not changed in several years. She is a third-grade teacher and has recently been taking care of the class pets, which include two goldfish and a hamster. On presentation she has a fever to 102.1°F and has diffuse tenderness of the abdomen without rebound.

   The most likely cause of her present illness is:
   A. Salmonellosis
   B. Medication-induced diarrhea related to the cumulative effects of mycophenolate
   C. Cytomegalovirus colitis
   D. Norovirus gastroenteritis
   E. Irritable bowel syndrome

4. A 24-year-old man with ulcerative colitis presents in January for a first primary care clinic visit with you as his new primary care physician. He was diagnosed with ulcerative colitis involving the entire colon 10 months ago and initially was treated with corticosteroids and mesalamine. In the last 3 months he has been doing well on mesalamine and azathioprine, which are his only medications. He works as a paralegal and hopes to attend law school in the next few years. He lives with his girlfriend of 2 years with whom he is monogamous. He uses condoms for birth control. He is feeling well today. Physical examination is unremarkable; he is afebrile and well appearing. You review his immunization history—he has not received any vaccines within the past 6 years; his last vaccination was the conjugate meningococcal vaccine at age 18.

   In addition to vaccinating for influenza and human papillomavirus, he should also receive which of the following vaccines?
   A. Tetanus, diphtheria (Td) vaccine
   B. Pneumococcal 13-valent conjugate (PCV13) vaccine
   C. *Haemophilus influenzae* B vaccine
   D. Pneumococcal 23-valent polysaccharide vaccine
   E. Meningococcus B vaccine

5. A 36-year-old man is found to have a positive tuberculosis interferon gamma release assay result as part of a workplace screening program. He is originally from Bangladesh and was vaccinated with the bacillus calmette-Guérin (BCG) vaccine during childhood. He immigrated to the United States 6 months ago. He reports feeling well. He has no fever, cough, or weight loss. Physical examination is normal.

The next best step in his management should be:

A. Sputum for smear microscopy and mycobacterial culture
B. Initiation of isoniazid prophylaxis to prevent reactivation of latent tuberculosis infection
C. Chest x-ray to assess for active pulmonary disease
D. Perform a tuberculin skin test (purified protein derivative [PPD] test) to confirm the skin test result

6. A previously well 62-year-old man presents to the hospital with increasing weakness in his lower extremities. Examination reveals decreased reflexes symmetrically, which progresses proximally over the course of several hours. He is diagnosed with Guillain–Barré syndrome and admitted to the intensive care unit for treatment. On history, he reports several days of nausea, vomiting, and diarrhea approximately 2 months prior.

The most likely infectious cause of his gastrointestinal illness was:

A. *Campylobacter*
B. *Giardia*
C. *Salmonella*
D. *Cryptosporidium*
E. *Escherichia coli O157:H7*

7. A 24-year-old woman calls your office complaining of burning with urination, and increased urinary urgency and frequency. She reports no fever, nausea, vomiting, or flank pain. She has been in a monogamous relationship for 3 years, and she had one prior episode of cystitis, more than a year ago.

Which of the following agents is the best treatment for acute uncomplicated cystitis?

A. Cephalexin 500 mg twice daily for 7 days
B. Ciprofloxacin 250 mg twice daily for 3 days
C. Nitrofurantoin macrocrystals 100 mg twice daily for 5 days
D. Amoxicillin 500 mg three times daily for 7 days

8. A 65-year-old woman with recently diagnosed diffuse large B-cell lymphoma presents with malaise, nausea, and mild jaundice. She was diagnosed with diffuse large B-cell lymphoma after developing massive right cervical lymphadenopathy and daily fevers 7 months ago. She was profoundly anemic when she presented and required a blood transfusion at that time. Pretreatment work up revealed the following: HIV antibody/antigen negative, hepatitis A IgG positive, hepatitis B surface antigen negative, hepatitis B core IgG positive, hepatitis B DNA not detected, hepatitis C IgG negative. She was treated with six cycles of rituximab, cyclophosphamide, doxorubicin, vincristine, and prednisone (R-CHOP), which ended several weeks ago and achieved complete remission based on positron emission tomography (PET) CT imaging. Basic laboratory findings when she presents now are notable for aspartate aminotransferase (AST) 527 U/L, alanine aminotransferase (ALT) 495 U/L, total bilirubin 3.5 mg/dL, with a normal international normalized ratio (INR). Her past history is notable for immigrating to the United States from rural Vietnam 2 years ago. She had a PPD skin test at the time she immigrated and she was treated for latent tuberculosis with a 9-month course of isoniazid that finished before the diagnosis of lymphoma.

A likely cause of her abnormal liver function tests and malaise is:

A. Hepatitis C infection resulting from blood transfusion
B. Recurrence of her lymphoma
C. Acute hepatitis A infection
D. Delayed isoniazid toxicity
E. Reactivation of hepatitis B infection

9. A 34-year-old teacher presents to her primary care physician with 1 week of severe cough. Her symptoms began 2 weeks prior with a mild fever and rhinorrhea. She has been experiencing posttussive emesis every couple of hours. She takes levothyroxine for hypothyroidism but otherwise has no chronic illnesses. Whooping cough is suspected, and a polymerase chain reaction (PCR) of a respiratory specimen is sent to test for *Bordetella pertussis.*

The best management is:

A. Treat with codeine-containing cough syrup for symptom control and wait for confirmation of *B. pertussis* infection.
B. It is too late to treat for *B. pertussis* with antibiotics; reassure her that the cough will improve in the next 2–4 weeks and administer the TDaP vaccine now.
C. Start empiric azithromycin for a 5-day course.
D. Start empiric levofloxacin for a 7-day course.
E. It is too late to treat for *B. pertussis* with antibiotics; administer immunoglobulin to provide passive immunity.

10. A 57-year-old man from lower Delaware presents to an urgent care center after being bitten by a tick. He reports that he spent many hours in his garden over the weekend and was bitten by many insects. He returned to his work as an accountant after the weekend and has been mostly spending time inside since then. This morning, a Tuesday, he noticed an engorged tick at his waist line, which he removed. At the moment he feels well other than worrying about getting sick from this tick. He has had no fevers, rashes, joint pains, or headache. He brought the removed tick with him, and it appears to be an engorged deer tick.

The best management plan is:

A. Ceftriaxone 250 mg intramuscular × 1
B. Amoxicillin 500 mg by mouth three times a day for 14 days
C. Check Lyme disease serologies, and treat with antibiotics if the serology is positive.
D. Doxycycline 100 mg by mouth twice a day for 14 days
E. Doxycycline 200 mg by mouth × 1

11. A 53-year-old woman with well-controlled non–insulin-dependent diabetes and obesity develops an area of swelling and pain on the right thigh. Over about 3 days, the area becomes fluctuant and she develops a large area of erythema around it. She presents to the emergency room, where she is found to have a low-grade fever but is otherwise stable. The collection, which measures 2.5 cm in diameter, is lanced, producing a small amount of purulent material, which is drained and swabbed for culture. The culture of the wound later grows *Staphylococcus aureus*.

In addition to excellent wound care, which of the following antibiotics would be the best choices for outpatient treatment of this skin and soft tissue infection?

A. Levofloxacin
B. Clarithromycin
C. Trimethoprim-sulfamethoxazole
D. Penicillin
E. Rifampin

12. A 26-year-old graduate student presents for evaluation after being bitten on the right shin by her neighbor's playful Labrador puppy. Her past medical history is notable for undergoing splenectomy for treatment of idiopathic thrombocytopenic purpura at age 24, which was curative. She takes no medications and has no allergies. On examination she has normal vital signs and appears well. On the right shin are two puncture marks, which are still bleeding slightly. There is no purulence and no surrounding erythema of the skin.

The most appropriate management is:

A. Sequester the puppy and treat the patient with human rabies immunoglobulin.
B. Oral trimethoprim-sulfamethoxazole
C. No therapy is necessary.
D. Intravenous ceftriaxone
E. Oral amoxicillin-clavulanate

13. A 67-year-old female is recovering following an elective total hip arthroplasty. On postoperative day 5, she complains of worsening diarrhea and abdominal pain. Her white blood cell count has risen from 9000 to 21,000 cells/μL. Testing of the stool reveals a positive glutamate dehydrogenase antigen and a positive toxin A/B assay confirming the diagnosis of *Clostridium difficile*. The team notes that this is the third patient with *C. difficile* infection on their unit in the past 2 weeks.

To help reduce further horizontal transmission, you recommend:

A. Identification and treatment of asymptomatic carriers
B. Strict adherence to standard precautions, including hand hygiene with an alcohol hand rub
C. Use of a chlorine-containing cleaning agent to address environmental contamination
D. Contact precautions for any patient suspected of having *C. difficile* infection until 48 hours of therapy have been given
E. Prophylactic metronidazole for all patients on the unit

14. A 67-year-old woman with end-stage renal disease is admitted from hemodialysis with hypoxia, fever, hypotension, and cough. She is diagnosed with multifocal pneumonia. Her course is complicated by respiratory failure requiring ongoing mechanical ventilation. She is treated with levofloxacin, piperacillin-tazobactam, and vancomycin, and her respiratory status improves over the first 2 days of admission. Her medical history is notable for type 2 diabetes, hypertension, and end-stage renal disease. She has been on hemodialysis for the last 7 weeks through a tunneled catheter while a fistula in the right upper extremity matures. On hospital day 4 she redevelops daily fevers as high as 102.5°F and hemodynamic instability that persists for 2 days. On hospital day 6, blood cultures are reported as growing yeast.

The best management in addition to repeating blood cultures is:

A. Start intravenous fluconazole 800 mg daily.
B. Remove the tunneled dialysis catheter, stop unnecessary antibiotics, and observe.
C. Start intravenous isavuconazonium.
D. Start intravenous caspofungin.
E. Start intravenous liposomal amphotericin.

15. A 43-year-old woman calls to report that she is very concerned because she found a large lump under her left arm. She has no personal or family history of malignancy. She has no other complaints. On examination, her vital signs are normal. She has one tender 2 × 3 cm mobile mass under her left arm, with overlying erythema. She works at an urban animal shelter. At home she has two recently adopted kittens, one of whom was ill about 2 months earlier. She tried to force-feed the kitten antibiotics and was scratched repeatedly.

Among cat-associated zoonoses, the most likely pathogen in this case is:

A. *Bartonella henselae*
B. *Toxocara cati*
C. *Toxoplasma gondii*
D. *Yersinia pestis*
E. *Pasteurella multocida*

16. A 26-year-old woman presents for a new primary care provider visit. She has no health complaints, and her medical history is notable only for appendectomy at age 23. She immigrated to the United States from Vietnam 7 years ago. She recently finished her undergraduate degree and will start a new job as a first-grade teacher in a few weeks. She is sexually active with her boyfriend of 1 month and reports using condoms for birth control. She has a history of occasionally smoking marijuana but has not done so for over 3 years.

In addition to giving influenza and tetanus/diphtheria/acellular pertussis vaccines, screening for hepatitis B infection is ordered. Which detail in the patient's history indicates that she should be screened for hepatitis B?

A. New sexual partner
B. Woman of childbearing age
C. History of marijuana use
D. Country of birth
E. New profession as a teacher

17. A 45-year-old woman was diagnosed with HIV infection (224 CD4 T cells/μm^3) and smear-negative, culture-positive pulmonary tuberculosis after presenting with chronic cough. Chest CT showed left lower lobe interstitial infiltrates. Rapid tuberculosis drug susceptibility testing showed no evidence of drug resistance. The patient was started on isoniazid, rifampin, ethambutol, and pyrazinamide. After 2 weeks, the patient was started on antiretroviral therapy with emtricitabine/tenofovir and dolutegravir. Her cough initially improved but then worsened after about 1 month of tuberculosis treatment. She also developed progressive shortness of breath. A chest x-ray showed new extensive right upper lobe opacities. Sputum smear microscopy was negative.

The patient should now:

A. Switch to an empiric regimen for treatment of multidrug-resistant tuberculosis.
B. Initiate systemic corticosteroids to control symptoms of paradoxical tuberculosis immune reconstitution inflammatory syndrome (IRIS).
C. Enroll in directly observed tuberculosis treatment given the high likelihood of poor adherence to therapy.
D. Begin trimethoprim/sulfamethoxazole for treatment of *Pneumocystis jirovecii* infection.
E. Proceed to open lung biopsy.

18. A 45-year-old man presents to the emergency room with 2 days of severe headache over the left eye and fevers. He reports nearly constant tearing of the left eye and tenderness over the left eye for 24 hours. His medical history is notable for type 1 diabetes mellitus complicated by peripheral neuropathy and chronic kidney disease. His examination is notable for an ill-appearing middle-aged man with chemosis of the left eye and periorbital and palpebral erythema extending over the left side of the nose. Laboratory data are notable for a blood glucose of 527 mg/dL. Urinalysis is remarkable for ketones and glucose. CT of the sinuses reveals opacification of the left frontal, sphenoid, and ethmoid sinuses. Endoscopic evaluation by an otolaryngologist reveals a black eschar over the left middle turbinate.

In addition to treatment with insulin for diabetic ketoacidosis, appropriate management includes:

A. Voriconazole
B. Lipid formulation of amphotericin B
C. Caspofungin
D. Fluconazole
E. Cefepime

19. An obese 57-year-old man with asthma who smokes two packs per day of cigarettes is admitted with 3 days of fever, nonproductive cough, and shortness of breath. Home medications include fluticasone inhaler twice a day and albuterol inhaler as needed for wheezing. Oxygen saturation is 94% on 2 L of oxygen by nasal cannula. Chest x-ray shows dense multifocal consolidations. He is admitted to the medical service and treated with levofloxacin. The following laboratory findings are sent:

Urine legionella antigen: positive
Urine streptococcal antigen: negative
Expectorated sputum Gram stain: no polys, 1+ epithelial cells
Expectorated sputum bacterial culture: 2+ oral flora, 1+ *Candida albicans*

Based on these results the best treatment plan is:

A. Stop levofloxacin and add micafungin.
B. Stop levofloxacin; start azithromycin and micafungin.
C. Continue levofloxacin and add fluconazole.
D. Continue levofloxacin, add fluconazole, and pursue bronchoscopy.
E. Continue levofloxacin and observe.

20. A 25-year-old woman presents to the emergency department with fever and back pain. The patient has been using intravenous heroin for the past few years; she had one prior episode of soft tissue abscess after injection but no other illnesses in the past. She now complains of 2 weeks of fevers, sweats, muscle aches, and some low back pain. On examination she is tachycardic, diaphoretic, febrile (102°F), and ill appearing. Cardiac examination reveals a new systolic murmur. Blood is drawn for basic laboratory findings and blood cultures (two sets). Given her ill appearance, the admitting physician decides to start empiric antibiotics for the most likely pathogens immediately.

The best empiric antibiotic regimen for this patient is:

A. Vancomycin + cefepime
B. Vancomycin + gentamicin + rifampin
C. Vancomycin + caspofungin
D. Ampicillin + gentamicin

21. A 47-year-old male with quadriplegia secondary to a motor vehicle accident as a young adult presents with fever, fatigue, and foul-smelling urine. He has a chronic indwelling Foley catheter due to urinary retention, and he reports multiple hospitalizations for catheter-associated urinary tract infections. On arrival to the emergency department, he is noted to be confused with a temperature of 102.3°F, a respiratory rate of 23 breaths per minute, a heart rate of 116 beats per minute, and a blood pressure of 75/43 mm Hg. Urinalysis finds 3+ leukocyte esterase and positive nitrite with microscopy revealing 100–200 WBC per high-powered field (HPF) with 3+ bacteria. Blood and urine cultures are obtained and laboratory findings are pending.

In addition to administering broad-spectrum antibiotics, the next best step is:

A. Initiation of dopamine as a vasopressor
B. Administration of intravenous hydrocortisone
C. Administration of 30 mL/kg of crystalloid
D. Initiation of norepinephrine as a vasopressor

22. A 23-year-old woman with acute myeloid leukemia (AML) who underwent standard induction chemotherapy with cytarabine and daunorubicin 11 days ago has recurrent fever to 103.1°F associated with malaise and sweats. She also endorses a sore mouth and throat as well as mild diarrhea, which she attributes to her recent chemotherapy. Her laboratory findings are notable for an absolute neutrophil count of 28. She first developed fever and neutropenia 8 days ago and was treated with empiric cefepime. Her fevers resolved within 24 hours, and she remained afebrile until 2 hours ago. When fevers redeveloped, blood cultures were drawn.

Which is the most appropriate antimicrobial agent to add?

A. Fluconazole
B. Vancomycin
C. Caspofungin
D. Meropenem
E. Daptomycin

23. A 22-year-old man presents to his primary care physician's office with fever and sore throat. The patient was feeling well until 1 week ago when he developed fever, malaise, fatigue, and sore throat; he later developed diarrhea. He has lost 5 pounds in the past month. The patient is a student at a local college, he does not smoke, he drinks alcohol a few times per week, and he does not use any recreational drugs. He is sexually active with men and has had two new male partners over the past few months. He is up to date on all of his vaccinations. On examination he is thin, febrile, and mildly tachycardic. His oropharynx is erythematous without exudates; he has palpable small lymphadenopathy in bilateral cervical and groin distribution. He has a maculopapular rash over his chest and back. Laboratory data: WBC 2200/μL, hematocrit 30%, platelets 103,000/μL, blood urea nitrogen (BUN) 20 mg/dL, creatinine 1.0 mg/dL, AST 66/μL, ALT 72/μL, alkaline phosphatase 120/μL, total bilirubin 0.9 mg/dL. Blood cultures are drawn.

Which of the following is the most appropriate panel of tests to order next?

A. Hepatitis A, B, and C serologies
B. Urine gonorrhea and chlamydia probes, syphilis serology
C. Rheumatoid factor (RF), echocardiogram
D. Blood smear, lactate dehydrogenase (LDH), bone marrow biopsy
E. Blood smear, Epstein-Barr virus (EBV) serologies, CMV serologies, HIV 1/2 antigen/antibody, HIV RNA

24. A 48-year-old male presents to the emergency department complaining of shortness of breath worsening over the past 2 days and weakness. Admission chest x-ray reveals pulmonary edema, and laboratory findings are notable for potassium 6.8 mmol/L. On review of his past medical history, you learn that he has severe type 1 diabetes mellitus complicated by nephropathy for which he has been on peritoneal dialysis for the past year. He reports 100% compliance with his peritoneal dialysis regimen at home. Two months ago he was admitted for methicillin-resistant *Staphylococcus aureus* (MRSA) bacteremia related to an infected foot ulcer for which he was treated with a course of intravenous vancomycin. He is admitted for acute management of hyperkalemia and to transition to hemodialysis. On hospital day 4, one day after surgery to create an arteriovenous fistula, he reports an increasingly productive cough and spikes a fever to 101.1°F. A repeat chest x-ray reveals a new consolidative opacity in the right lung.

Based on clinical and radiologic evidence suggesting pneumonia, you recommend:

A. Levofloxacin
B. Ertapenem + vancomycin
C. Piperacillin/tazobactam + amikacin
D. Imipenem + ciprofloxacin
E. Cefepime + levofloxacin + vancomycin

25. A 21-year-old college student with moderate to severe asthma presents to the student health center with a sore mouth for several days. Though it is bothersome, it has not interfered with his eating or drinking. He denies odynophagia. Ten days ago he was hospitalized for 2 days with a severe asthma flare. He was treated with a 2-week prednisone taper for his asthma and with a 5-day course of azithromycin for possible respiratory tract infection. His regular medications include inhaled salmeterol and fluticasone. On examination he is a relatively well-appearing young man with white curd-like plaques adherent to the soft and hard palate.

In addition to education about rinsing the mouth after using a steroid inhaler and considering HIV testing, the next best step is:

A. Clotrimazole troches
B. Chlorhexidine mouthwash
C. Referral to oral medicine for biopsy
D. Oral posaconazole
E. Single-dose intravenous micafungin

26. A 26-year-old female is hospitalized in a burn unit after suffering deep burns over 55% of her body in a house fire. She remains intubated with access via central venous catheter. On hospital day 10, the microbiology lab calls with the result of a blood culture that was sent in the setting of a fever to 102°F. The lab reports that *Acinetobacter baumannii* is growing in the blood, which is testing positive for extended-spectrum beta-lactamases and a carbapenemase.

Based on these results, which antibiotic is most likely to be effective against this pathogen?

A. Meropenem
B. Colistimethate
C. Ciprofloxacin
D. Piperacillin/tazobactam
E. Gentamicin

27. A 37-year-old woman with HIV (CD4 count 523/μL, HIV viral load <20/μL), asthma, and allergic rhinitis presents to her primary care physician office complaining of worsening symptoms of allergic rhinitis. She has had worsening rhinorrhea, itchy and watery eyes, and dry cough over the past few weeks this spring. Her current medications are tenofovir, emtricitabine, darunavir, ritonavir, loratadine, and injectable medroxyprogesterone. She requests an additional medication for control of her allergic rhinitis symptoms.

Which of the following drugs should not be prescribed because of a potentially harmful drug–drug interaction?

A. Oral cetirizine
B. Inhaled albuterol
C. Ophthalmic nedocromil
D. Inhaled fluticasone
E. Oral montelukast

28. A 48-year-old man presents with 4 days of fevers, night sweats, and malaise. He has a history of bicuspid aortic valve with aortic regurgitation. On examination he is febrile (102.4°F) and tachycardic. Blood cultures are drawn. A transthoracic echocardiogram does not show any valvular vegetations or abscess. Based on identification of bacteria grown in blood culture, the suspicion for endocarditis diminishes significantly.

Which of the following bacteria grew in culture?

A. *Haemophilus parainfluenzae*
B. *Eikenella corrodens*
C. *Streptococcus gallolyticus*
D. *Bacteroides fragilis*
E. *Enterococcus faecalis*

29. A 28-year-old woman presents to the emergency department with fever, malaise, abdominal pain, nausea, and vomiting. Initial laboratory findings show WBC 1800/μL, hematocrit 27%, platelets 100,000/μL, AST 170/UL, ALT 195/UL, alkaline phosphatase 422 IU/L, and total bilirubin 2.1 mg/dL. A CT scan of the abdomen and pelvis reveals diffuse lymphadenopathy and hepatosplenomegaly. Further diagnostics reveal that HIV antibody is positive with a CD4 count of 18/μL (4% of total lymphocytes). Biopsy of a lymph node reveals numerous organisms on acid-fast staining. PCR of the sample with numerous organisms is consistent with mycobacterium avium intracellulare (or mycobacterium avium complex [MAC]). The patient is started on treatment with clarithromycin and ethambutol while awaiting the results of resistance testing from mycobacterial isolator blood cultures.

When is the best time to start antiretroviral therapy for this patient?

A. Start three antiretroviral drugs in a staggered fashion, adding one every 2 weeks over the next 6 weeks.
B. A few days after initiation of clarithromycin and ethambutol, but within 2 weeks
C. After 2 weeks on clarithromycin and ethambutol, if no side effects
D. After completion of 6 weeks of clarithromycin and ethambutol, to decrease risk of immune reconstitution inflammatory syndrome (IRIS)
E. After the patient is discharged from the hospital, in the outpatient setting with documented patient capacity for adherence to follow-up and medications

30. A 45-year-old man with a long-standing history of well-controlled HIV presents to his primary care physician for a routine visit. He is feeling well, with no symptomatic complaints. He reports 100% adherence to his antiretroviral regimen: tenofovir, emtricitabine, and rilpivirine. He works in real estate and lives with his husband and their dog. He smokes approximately one pack of cigarettes per day, as he has for the past 20 years. He drinks six alcoholic beverages per week, and he does not use recreational drugs. His family history is notable for coronary artery disease in both parents but no cancer in first-degree relatives. Vital signs: heart rate 82 beats per minute, blood pressure 137/86 mm Hg, BMI 32 kg/m^2, and physical examination is unremarkable. Laboratory findings show CD4 count 470/μL, HIV viral load is <20/μL (undetectable), and complete blood count (CBC) and chem-20 are normal. You plan to continue his current antiretroviral regimen, and you discuss additional health care maintenance efforts with him.

Given his history, which of the following is the most important health care maintenance item to pursue during this visit?

A. Start sulfamethoxazole/trimethoprim for prophylaxis against *Pneumocystis* pneumonia.
B. Counsel patient to decrease alcohol intake, and refer for alcohol dependence treatment.
C. Counsel patient to quit smoking, and discuss medications and supports for smoking cessation.
D. Screen for toxoplasma serostatus to determine risk for toxoplasma reactivation in the future.
E. Refer for early colon cancer screening by colonoscopy.

31. An 84-year-old man with a history of coronary artery disease, diabetes mellitus, and chronic renal insufficiency presents to the emergency room with progressive headache, fevers, and neck pain. The patient was in his usual state of health until 4 days prior when the staff and his friends at his assisted living facility noted he started complaining of feeling ill with headache and nausea. On the morning of presentation he was found in his room confused. In the emergency room he was febrile and confused, and became somnolent during his care there. Head CT showed no acute processes. A lumbar puncture was performed, cerebrospinal fluid (CSF) examination showed glucose 22 mg/dL (serum glucose 112 mg/dL), protein 97 mg/dL, red blood cell (RBC) 7, WBC 489 with 87% neutrophils, 7% monocytes, and 6% lymphocytes. CSF is sent to the microbiology lab for Gram stain and culture.

Which of the following is the most appropriate empiric antibiotic regimen to initiate while awaiting the results of the CSF Gram stain and culture?

A. Vancomycin, ceftriaxone, ampicillin
B. Vancomycin, cefepime, acyclovir
C. Vancomycin, meropenem
D. Ampicillin, gentamicin, acyclovir
E. Ampicillin, trimethoprim-sulfamethoxazole, amphotericin B

32. A 27-year-old woman presents to her primary care physician complaining of fever, cough, sinus pressure, and malaise. She reports onset of symptoms 5 days ago, with fevers for the first 2 days with temperatures as high as 101.1°F. Highest temperature in the past 3 days has been 99.8°F. She reports ongoing symptoms of frequent cough productive of scant white sputum, nasal congestion, mild sinus pressure, and fatigue. The patient has a history of childhood asthma, but she has not used inhalers or other medications for asthma in several years. She is otherwise healthy, and she takes no medications. She has a history of a rash reaction to clarithromycin. On examination, her temperature is 99.0°F, heart rate is 92 beats per minute, blood pressure is 132/85 mm Hg, respiratory rate is 18 breaths per minute, and oxygen saturation is 96% on room air. She appears mildly uncomfortable and is coughing during the examination; she has no lesions in the oropharynx, sclerae are clear, maxillary sinuses are mildly tender on percussion, there is no nasal discharge/drainage, tympanic membranes are clear, and she has a few small (<1.5 cm) palpable cervical lymph nodes. Her lungs are clear except for occasional faint expiratory wheezes.

The most appropriate management is:

A. Oral moxifloxacin, inhaled albuterol, and intranasal oxymetazoline
B. Oral amoxicillin-clavulanate, inhaled fluticasone, and saline nasal irrigation
C. Oral dextromethorphan, inhaled albuterol, and intranasal ipratropium
D. Intramuscular ceftriaxone, oral pseudoephedrine, and inhaled salmeterol
E. Intramuscular influenza vaccine, oral guaifenesin, and inhaled tiotropium

33. A 29-year-old woman who is otherwise healthy presents for a routine prenatal visit at 14 weeks' gestational age. She is feeling well and has no symptomatic complaints, and physical examination is consistent with normal pregnancy, otherwise unremarkable. She has routine prenatal laboratory findings checked, which show the following results: hemoglobin 11.2 g/dL, rubella IgG positive, HIV-1/2 antigen/antibody negative, treponemal IgG (by enzyme immunoassay [EIA]) positive. Follow-up rapid plasma reagin (RPR) is also positive, with a titer of 1:16, and FTA-ABS is also positive. The patient has never had prior syphilis testing. She reports a history of severe allergy to penicillin with a "feeling of throat closing."

The most appropriate management for this patient is:

A. No treatment now due to risk of toxicity; follow clinically and repeat syphilis testing at 20 weeks' gestational age
B. Treat with doxycycline 100 mg orally twice daily for a 21-day course.
C. Treat with ceftriaxone 1 g IM once daily for 10 days.
D. Treat with azithromycin 2 g orally in a single dose.
E. Allergy consultation and admission for desensitization to penicillin in order to facilitate treatment with benzathine penicillin G 2.4 million units IM once weekly for 3 weeks

34. A 24-year-old man with well-controlled HIV presents for routine follow-up primary care visit and notes some dysuria for the past several days. Physical examination is unremarkable. Urinalysis shows 10 WBC, no epithelial cells, 2 RBC, no bacteria per HPF. Urine testing for gonorrhea is positive by nucleic acid amplification test (NAAT) probe, and urine chlamydia NAAT probe is negative. The patient has no known drug allergies.

Which of the following is the recommended treatment regimen?

A. Levofloxacin 500 mg orally once daily for 7 days + doxycycline 100 mg orally twice daily for 7 days
B. Ceftriaxone 250 mg IM single dose
C. Cefixime 400 mg orally single dose + doxycycline 100 mg orally twice daily for 7 days
D. Ceftriaxone 250 mg IM single dose + azithromycin 1 g orally single dose

35. A 32-year-old man presents to his primary care physician complaining of painful perianal lesions. The patient is sexually active with multiple male partners. He has had negative screening for sexually transmitted diseases, including HIV, gonorrhea, and chlamydia, in the past (his last screening tests were 6 months ago). On physical examination he is overall well appearing, but in the perianal area he has multiple shallow ulcerations grouped in the right perianal area. There is no rectal discharge and no palpable lymphadenopathy, but the ulcerations are tender and painful even when not palpated.

The type of diagnostic test that is most likely to confirm the diagnosis of this active condition is:

A. Bacterial culture of a swab of the ulcers
B. Viral culture of a swab of the ulcers
C. Urine NAAT probe
D. Blood serologic test
E. Urinary antigen test

36. A 47-year-old man presents to the emergency department with complaint of hemoptysis. He was born and raised in upstate New York, currently manages a restaurant and bar that he and his siblings own, and is married with two children. His only travel in the last few years was a trip to Montreal. He has been healthy until approximately 6 months prior when he developed sinusitis. He has been treated by his primary care physician with courses of amoxicillin, amoxicillin-clavulanate, and moxifloxacin for episodes of sinusitis over the past few months, but his symptoms persist. He has also had several episodes of epistaxis in the last few months. Over the past 2 weeks he developed a cough, which was initially nonproductive, but during the past 2 days he had a few episodes of hemoptysis. On physical examination he has lost 5 lb since his last examination 1 month prior, he is thin but comfortable, and on sinonasal examination he has septal perforation with no obvious exudates or other abnormalities. Blood tests show white blood cell count of 4200/μL, hemoglobin 9.1 g/dL, and creatinine 2.2 mg/dL. Urinalysis shows too numerous to count red blood cells. Chest x-ray shows some abnormal opacities, so chest CT is obtained, which shows multiple pulmonary nodules.

The test most likely to suggest the diagnosis in this case is:

A. Sputum smear for acid-fast bacilli (AFB)
B. AFB smear of biopsy of a pulmonary nodule
C. Serum test for antineutrophilic cytoplasmic antibodies (ANCA)
D. Serum test for galactomannan
E. Serum interferon-gamma release assay (IGRA)

37. A 62-year-old woman with multiple sclerosis and a neurogenic bladder now has a chronic indwelling urinary catheter, after failing management with intermittent use of urinary straight catheters. She presents for a routine primary care visit and has no current symptomatic complaints. She is interested in discussing strategies to decrease the risk of urinary tract infections in the future. In the past when she has developed urinary tract infections they often precipitated a worsening of her multiple sclerosis, and she often requires hospitalization, so she hopes to prevent the need for hospitalization in the future.

Which of the following strategies would be most successful at achieving her goals?

A. Monitoring for early signs and symptoms of urinary tract infection, with expedited early urinalysis, urine culture, and empiric treatment while awaiting culture results when symptoms develop
B. Routine screening with urinalysis for pyuria at regular intervals with early empiric treatment for urinary tract infection if pyuria is detected, even in the absence of symptoms
C. Addition of gentamicin solution to the catheter drainage bag at regular intervals
D. Chronic prophylaxis with methenamine salts to decrease bacteria
E. Chronic prophylaxis with ciprofloxacin to decrease bacteria and infections

38. A 45-year-old man with a history of prior open reduction and internal fixation (ORIF) of a left femur fracture in the past now presents with his third episode of cellulitis in the left leg. He was well until 1 day prior when he developed sudden onset of malaise, fever, nausea, and erythema and pain in the left leg. He presented to the emergency room overnight and was treated empirically with vancomycin overnight. He improves gradually overnight. In discussion the following day he asks whether there are any strategies to decrease the frequency of his episodes of cellulitis in the future.

Which of the following antibiotics, when taken regularly as prophylaxis, has been shown to decrease the incidence of cellulitis among patients with recurrent cellulitis?

A. Sulfamethoxazole-trimethoprim
B. Doxycycline
C. Clarithromycin
D. Levofloxacin
E. Penicillin

39. A 32-year-old woman presents for routine prenatal care at 12 weeks' gestational age. She is taking prenatal vitamins and is feeling well. She reports that a friend recently gave birth to a daughter who was diagnosed with congenital toxoplasmosis, and she would like to know how to prevent this infection during her pregnancy. She is a kindergarten teacher. She lives with her spouse, who cares for their 10-year-old indoor cat. She likes to garden in her free time.

In addition to washing fruits and vegetables before eating, which of the following lifestyle changes is recommended to reduce risk for acute toxoplasma infection during pregnancy?

A. Cook meat to "well done."
B. Avoid ingestion of pork or any pork products.
C. Give the cat up for adoption.
D. Stop gardening.
E. Take leave from work at the start of the third trimester to avoid transmission from her students.

40. A 74-year-old man with poorly controlled diabetes, coronary artery disease, end-stage renal disease, and peripheral vascular disease presents with pain at a chronic foot ulcer site. The patient has had a nonhealing ulcer on his left great toe for several months but no other symptoms. Over the past few days he developed purulent drainage from the ulcer bed, as well as erythema, pain, and swelling of the toe, which is now tracking up the foot. The margins of the toe ulcer have also started to turn black. He has a fever of 100.7°F at the time of presentation. Laboratory findings reveal a white blood cell count of 13,500 cells/μL. Blood cultures are sent, and debridement—during which cultures of the base will be obtained—is planned for later in the day.

Which of the following antibiotic regimens would be appropriate initial therapy for this patient while awaiting debridement and culture results?

A. Vancomycin
B. Cefazolin and metronidazole
C. Ampicillin-sulbactam
D. Vancomycin and piperacillin-tazobactam
E. Ertapenem

41. A 67-year-old woman presents to the emergency room with right ear pain. She is otherwise healthy at baseline and takes no medications. She lives in New Hampshire and spends time walking her dog in the woods frequently, but she does not remember any specific tick bites. Approximately 10 days earlier she developed upper respiratory infection (URI) symptoms, which improved over a few days and then resolved after 7 days. Over the past 3–4 days she developed right ear pain. On physical examination she is noted to have a right facial droop and some lesions with serous drainage in the right external ear canal. Her mucous membranes are dry.

Which of the following is the most appropriate treatment for this patient?

A. Doxycycline 100 mg orally twice daily for 14 days
B. Valacyclovir 1000 mg orally three times daily for 14 days
C. Ciprofloxacin otic solution to the right ear 4 times per day for 7 days
D. Ciprofloxacin otic solution + amoxicillin-clavulanate 875/125 mg orally twice daily for 10 days
E. Prednisone 60 mg orally once daily for 5 days

42. A 26-year-old man presents with dysuria, which has been persistent for more than 1 week. Urinalysis shows 12 WBC, 1 RBC, and no bacteria per HPF, and the urine culture is negative. Urine NAAT probes for chlamydia and gonorrhea are negative. Serum testing for HIV 1/2 antigen/antibodies is negative.

Which of the following organism is the most likely cause of the patient's symptoms?

A. *Trichomonas vaginalis*
B. Herpes simplex virus (HSV)
C. *Mycoplasma genitalium*
D. *Haemophilus ducreyi*
E. *E. coli*

43. A 71-year-old woman with hypertension develops temporal headaches, fevers, and weight loss. She is diagnosed with giant cell arteritis by temporal artery biopsy and starts treatment with prednisone 50 mg per day. Her symptoms improve markedly, and the prednisone dose is slowly tapered starting 3 weeks later. Ten weeks after starting the prednisone taper she develops fevers in the 100–101°F range despite taking 20 mg of prednisone per day. She also notes a dry cough. She is treated with a course of azithromycin but continues to have a cough and fevers. She also notes dyspnea on exertion. She presents to the emergency department, where she is found to have a temperature of 100.6°F, respiratory rate of 38 breaths per minute, and oxygen saturation of 92% while breathing ambient air. On exam she has no jugular venous distention or peripheral edema. She has faint bilateral crackles in both lungs. A chest x-ray shows bilateral interstitial infiltrates. Serum β-d-glucan is >500 pg/mL.

In addition to treatment with antibiotics for community-acquired pneumonia, which of the following treatments is most appropriate additional empirical therapy?

A. Ivermectin
B. Trimethoprim-sulfamethoxazole
C. High-dose steroids
D. Furosemide
E. Theophylline

44. A 22-year-old man presents to primary care physician for routine follow-up. He is sexually active with men, with three partners in the past year. He had a recent urgent care visit for urethritis, was diagnosed with gonorrhea, and was treated with ceftriaxone and azithromycin. He is now feeling well, with no current symptomatic complaints. The physician focuses this routine visit on sexually transmitted infections (STIs), including risk-reduction counseling, confirming completion of HPV-vaccine series, distribution of condoms, and discussion of preexposure prophylaxis (PrEP) for HIV prevention. The patient is interested in PrEP and inquires about the usual treatment plan and the risks and benefits associated with PrEP.

Which of the following statements about antiretroviral PrEP is true?

A. HIV screening with combination antigen/antibody test should be performed at baseline before initiation of PrEP and annually while on PrEP.
B. Taking tenofovir/emtricitabine once daily with excellent adherence for PrEP can decrease risk of HIV acquisition by about 25%.
C. Patients taking PrEP should have regular screening for other STIs at least every 6 months, including syphilis, gonorrhea, and chlamydia.
D. In the HIV uninfected population there is little risk for tenofovir nephrotoxicity while taking PrEP, so there is no need for monitoring of renal function.
E. In most populations the risks of PrEP outweigh the benefits because patients who are prescribed PrEP have increased sexual risk behaviors and increased incidence of STIs, including HIV when nonadherent to PrEP.

45. A 55-year-old man with a history of hypertension, coronary artery disease, and depression presents with a soft tissue infection on the leg. He has no prior history of soft tissue infections. His current medications are lisinopril, clopidogrel, aspirin, atorvastatin, and duloxetine. He has no known medication allergies. On examination, he has a fever (temperature is 101.2°F) but vital signs are otherwise normal. There is an area of erythema on the lower left leg, originating from a punctate wound where the patient states he sustained a spider bite. The area is warm, swollen, and tender, and there is a central 4-cm area of fluctuance. Incision and drainage of the abscess is performed at the bedside. A culture of drained pus grows methicillin-resistant *Staphylococcus aureus* (MRSA). The patient is treated with vancomycin while an inpatient, and his fevers resolve. He is then discharged with oral linezolid for another 10 days. After 7 days he returns to the emergency room complaining of recurrent fever and malaise. His temperature is 103.7°F, heart rate is 116 beats per minute, blood pressure is 180/92 mm Hg, and oxygen saturation is 98% on room air. On examination he is somewhat agitated and unable to sit still. Lungs are clear to auscultation bilaterally, there are no murmurs on cardiac exam, abdomen is soft and nontender, and the lower left leg prior incision and drainage site is healing.

The most likely cause of this patient's new symptoms is:

A. Drug–drug interaction
B. Recurrent MRSA abscess
C. MRSA bacteremia due to endocarditis
D. Hospital-acquired pneumonia
E. *Clostridium difficile* colitis

46. A 53-year-old man with a prior history of idiopathic thrombocytopenic purpura treated with a course of steroids, rituximab, and ultimately splenectomy 4 months ago now presents with fever and chills. The patient spent a week on Nantucket for a summer vacation and was feeling well until 2 days after he returned from vacation, when he developed fevers as high as 103.2°F, shaking chills, and headache. He presented to a local hospital, where initial complete blood count showed WBC 12,000/μL, hemoglobin 8.2 g/dL, platelets 80,000/μL, normal electrolytes, serum creatinine 2.1 mg/dL, and alkaline phosphatase 206 IU/L. A blood smear showed parasites within the red blood cells; the parasitemia burden was assessed as 12%.

Which of the following is the most appropriate treatment regimen for this patient at this point?

A. Azithromycin and atovaquone/proguanil
B. Quinine and clindamycin and consideration of red cell exchange transfusion
C. Ceftriaxone and doxycycline
D. High-dose corticosteroids, intravenous immunoglobulin, and initiation of plasmapheresis
E. Intravenous artesunate

47. A 36-year-old man with psoriasis, for which he takes methotrexate, traveled to Arizona for 2 weeks for a family reunion and developed a fever 2 days before returning to his home in New York. He was feeling well during the trip and enjoyed the first week of the reunion. He bunked with extended family, including small children and two dogs. He ate food at the hotel and drank primarily bottled water. He went hiking in the desert on three occasions. He swam in the hotel pool but engaged in no fresh water swimming. The weather was dry throughout the trip and very windy at times. Two days before returning home he developed fever, fatigue, malaise, dry cough, and chest pain. He took acetaminophen and rested, then returned home to New York. After 10 days the symptoms had not significantly improved, so he presented to his primary care provider. Physical examination was remarkable only for low-grade fever. Chest x-ray showed subtle left hilar infiltrate and lymphadenopathy. He was treated with a 5-day course of azithromycin with no change in his symptoms.

The best diagnostic test to send at this point would be:

A. Blood serologic test for *Coccidioides*
B. Serum 1,3-β-d-glucan testing
C. Urinary legionella antigen
D. Biopsy of the hilar lymph node for fungal culture
E. Serum galactomannan

48. A 31-year-old man with a prosthetic aortic valve presents with fevers. He had his aortic valve replaced with a mechanical prosthesis at age 24 due to congenital bicuspid aortic valve, and he has been doing well since then. His medications include warfarin and lisinopril. He has no known drug allergies. At the time of admission to the hospital, blood cultures are positive for MRSA. After extensive evaluation, no source for the bacteremia is identified. He is treated for presumed prosthetic valve endocarditis, even in the absence of suggestive findings on transesophageal echocardiogram. His antibiotic regimen is vancomycin, gentamicin, and rifampin. After 3 days the blood cultures clear of bacteria, he clinically improves, and he is eventually discharged to a rehab facility to complete a course of vancomycin, gentamicin, and rifampin. After 3 weeks he returns to the emergency room with an acute stroke, which appears embolic on MRI/MRA of the brain. Laboratory findings show WBC 12,000/μL, hemoglobin 9.8 g/dL, platelets 167,000/μL, creatinine 0.9 mg/dL, liver function tests are normal, partial thromboplastin time 36.0 seconds, and INR 1.2. Blood cultures are negative at 48 hours of incubation.

The most likely cause of the patient's new stroke is:

A. Persistent infectious vegetation on the prosthetic aortic valve
B. Toxicity from gentamicin
C. Aortic valvular dysfunction due to perivalvular abscess
D. Hypercoagulable state due to loss of gut flora while on antibiotics
E. Drug–drug interaction of warfarin with rifampin

49. A 53-year-old woman who is otherwise healthy develops fever, headache, malaise, and then cough, which is persistent and worsens over a couple of days. The patient lives in Missouri, where she works on a dairy farm and also tends sheep for wool as an additional source of income. She spends her spare time hunting deer and rabbits. She is married and is monogamous with her husband. At the time of presentation she was mildly hypoxic and febrile, and her condition rapidly worsened, ultimately requiring mechanical ventilation. Chest imaging showed multifocal infiltrates and progressive pleural effusions, as well as hilar lymphadenopathy. At the time of admission her laboratory findings were normal with the exception of WBC 14,000/μL. However, she developed progressive renal failure and abnormal liver function tests over the first 2 days after admission. Blood, urine, and sputum cultures are all negative repeatedly. She has been treated with vancomycin, cefepime, and metronidazole with no improvement.

The most likely etiologic organism for her current condition is:

A. *Tropheryma whipplei*
B. *Babesia microti*
C. *Borrelia lonestari*
D. *Francisella tularensis*
E. *Anaplasma phagocytophilum*

50. A 22-year-old woman who is healthy at baseline sustains minor blunt trauma to the right thigh after she bumps her leg on the edge of a table. Within hours after the bump she develops fever and severe right leg pain such that she is barely able to walk. She presents to a local emergency room, where she is febrile and hypotensive. Her right thigh appears dusky, and she complains of pain tracking down to the foot and up to the lower abdomen. She is taken immediately to the operating room, where operative exploration reveals necrotizing myositis of the muscles of the thigh without gas formation, with necrotizing soft tissue infection tracking down the leg and up to the groin. Some of the debrided tissue is sent for Gram stain and culture to aid with choice of antibiotics.

The most likely pathogen is:

A. Methicillin-sensitive *Staphylococcus aureus*
B. *E. coli*
C. Group A streptococci
D. Methicillin-resistant *S. aureus*
E. *Aeromonas hydrophila*

Chapter 1 Answers

1. ANSWER: E. Dengue

Leptospirosis can present in many different ways, including headache, muscle aches, and fever, but it is almost always associated with freshwater exposure, such as swimming or white-water rafting. Although all travelers returning with fever should be evaluated for malaria (even in cases where they had reported taking prophylaxis), the normal hematocrit and lack of other laboratory abnormalities in this young woman are reassuring. Typhoid can also present with only headache and fever, and in fact although it is caused by *Salmonella* species. it can often cause little to no gastrointestinal symptoms. The marked thrombocytopenia would be unusual for this diagnosis. Hepatitis A is also a risk for travelers, but the lack of gastrointestinal symptoms and lack of liver enzyme elevation argue against it. Dengue is the second most common cause of systemic febrile illness travelers returning to the United States from foreign travel (12%), after malaria, and dengue was the most frequently identified cause of systemic febrile illness among travelers returning from Southeast Asia. Diagnosis is generally clinical, although acute and convalescent sera can be sent. Treatment is supportive.

Hagmann SH, Han PV, Stauffer WM, et al. Travel-associated disease among US residents visiting US GeoSentinel clinics after return from international travel. *Fam Pract.* 2014;31:678–687.

2. ANSWER: B. Suctioning of subglottic secretions

There are a number of strategies that can help reduce the risk of ventilator-associated pneumonia in an intubated patient. These usually focus around minimizing sedation, preventing aspiration, reducing colonization of the airway and digestive tract, and minimizing contamination of the ventilatory circuit. To prevent aspiration, the head of the bead should be maintained in a semirecumbent position (elevated 30–45 degrees) rather than in a fully recumbent position. One should also use a cuffed endotracheal tube with cuff pressure set at ≥20 cm H_2O with subglottic secretion drainage. To reduce colonization of the airway and digestive tract, orotracheal intubation is preferred to nasotracheal intubation to decrease the risk of sinusitis, acid-reducing medications such a histamine receptor 2 (H_2)–blocking agents and proton pump inhibitors should be avoided except in patients at high risk for ulcers/gastritis, and regular oral care with an antiseptic solution (e.g., chlorhexidine) should be performed. Routine use of oral or intravenous antibiotics for prophylaxis is not recommended. Finally, to minimize contamination of the ventilatory circuit, the tubing should only be changed when visibly soiled or malfunctioning.

Klompas M, Branson R, Eichenwald EC, et al. Strategies to prevent ventilator-associated pneumonia in acute care hospitals: 2014 update. *Infect Control Hosp Epidemiol.* 2014;35:915–936; American Thoracic Society; Infectious Diseases Society of America. Guidelines for the management of adults with hospital-acquired, ventilator-associated, and healthcare-associated pneumonia. *Am J Respir Crit Care Med.* 2005;171:388–416.

3. ANSWER: A. Salmonellosis

Infection risk after solid organ transplantation depends on two key factors: when the transplant occurred and whether the patient has recently been treated for organ rejection. Transplant recipients who underwent transplantation less than a month ago are typically at highest risk for nosocomial infections and infections that result directly from surgery (e.g., wound infection). Those transplanted 1–6 months before or those recently treated for rejection are at risk for opportunistic infections (such as CMV enteritis). Opportunists like CMV are much less likely in those transplanted more than 6 months ago and not treated for rejection recently (as in this case). Patients more than 6 months after transplant who have not been treated for recent rejection are at highest risk for community-acquired pathogens, like *Salmonella* and norovirus. This patient has been in contact with a hamster, which may increase her risk for *Salmonella* infection (hamsters have been associated with *Salmonella* outbreaks). Although she may also be at risk for norovirus infection as a school teacher, *Salmonella* is much more likely in this case based on her history of high fevers and abdominal pain along with diarrhea in the absence of nausea or vomiting. Among medications used for posttransplant immunosuppression, mycophenolate mofetil commonly causes diarrhea; however, the new onset after years of mycophenolate and the associated fevers all make mycophenolate an unlikely cause of this acute illness.

Fishman JA, Rubin, RH. Infection in organ-transplant recipients. *N Engl J Med.* 1998;338:1741–1751; Centers for Disease Control and Prevention. Outbreak of multidrug-resistant *Salmonella typhimurium* associated with rodents purchased at retail pet stores—United States, December 2003-October 2004. *MMWR Morb Mortal Wkly Rep.* 2005;54:429–433.

4. ANSWER: B. Pneumococcal 13-valent conjugate (PCV13) vaccine

This patient is a 24-year-old man with ulcerative colitis for which he takes immunosuppressive medications. Based on his immunocompromised state he should be vaccinated for pneumococcus with both the conjugated and the polysaccharide vaccines. In an immunocompromised patient under 65 years old who has never been vaccinated for pneumococcus, the conjugate vaccine should be given first, followed by the polysaccharide vaccine (Option D) at least 8 weeks later. Although the patient may be due for tetanus vaccination, unless he has a clear history that he previously received the tetanus, diphtheria, acellular pertussis (TDaP) vaccine, the TDaP vaccine should be given now, not the tetanus, diphtheria vaccine (Option A). The Advisory Committee on Immunization Practices (ACIP) recommends that all persons above age 10 should be vaccinated with TDaP once due to outbreaks of pertussis in adolescents and adults related to waning pertussis immunity. This patient has no specific indications for *Haemophilus influenzae* B vaccine at this time (Option C); after standard childhood vaccination this vaccine is typically only indicated in adults in specific circumstances such as stem cell transplantation or splenectomy. The meningococcal B vaccine (Option E, available in two different formulations with different schedules) was first approved in 2014. It is currently recommended for a select population including individuals with asplenia, those with acquired or congenital complement deficiency, or those who were potentially exposed in an outbreak of meningococcus type B infection. Unlike the conjugate meningococcal ACWY vaccine, it is not routinely recommended for young adults between the age of 16 and 23, but it is a consideration.

Kim DK, Bridges CB, Harriman KH, et al. Advisory Committee on Immunization Practices Recommended Immunization Schedule for Adults Aged 19 Years or Older—United States, 2016. *MMWR Morb Mortal Wkly Rep.* 2016;65:88–90; Bennett NM, et al. *MMWR.* 2012;61:816–819; Folaranmi T, Rubin L, Martin SW, et al. Use of serogroup B meningococcal vaccines in persons aged ≥10 years at increased risk for serogroup B meningococcal disease: recommendations of the Advisory Committee on Immunization Practices, 2015. *MMWR Morb Mortal Wkly Rep.* 2015;64:608–612.

5. **ANSWER: C. Chest x-ray to assess for active pulmonary disease**

The patient should undergo chest x-ray to evaluate for active pulmonary tuberculosis. Radiologic disease can be present in the absence of symptoms. Either a tuberculin skin test (PPD) or an interferon gamma release assay alone is acceptable to test for tuberculosis exposure, and a positive test result from either is sufficient to diagnose latent infection. Because interferon gamma release assays are not affected by previous BCG vaccine, this is the preferred screening test for patients who have previously received this vaccine. Sputum evaluation should only be pursued if the patient has concerning symptoms or signs of active disease on chest imaging. The Centers for Disease Control and Prevention (CDC) web site provides updated information about diagnosis and management of latent tuberculosis: http://www.cdc.gov/tb/default.htm.

6. **ANSWER: A. *Campylobacter***

Campylobacter infection can result in Guillain-Barré syndrome (GBS) several weeks after diarrhea. Approximately 1/1000 reported *Campylobacter* illnesses leads to GBS, and up to 40% of GBS in the United States may be triggered by *Campylobacter.* Acute *Campylobacter* gastrointestinal illness can present with diarrhea (possibly bloody), cramping, abdominal pain, and fever, sometimes with nausea and vomiting, and can last from 2 to 10 days. It is not usually spread from one person to another, but most cases are associated with contact with raw or undercooked poultry. As few as 100 organisms can cause illness. Illness can also result from contact with stool of an ill pet dog or cat. Antibiotics are indicated in severe cases.

Hughes RAC, Cornblath DR. Guillain-Barré syndrome. *Lancet.* 2005;366:1653–1666; Vucic S, Kiernan MC, Cornblath DR. Guillain-Barré syndrome: an update. *J Clin Neurosci.* 2009;16:733–741.

7. **ANSWER: C. Nitrofurantoin macrocrystals 100 mg twice daily for 5 days**

In 2010 the Infectious Diseases Society of America (IDSA) updated guidelines for the management of uncomplicated cystitis in premenopausal women. By far the most common cause of uncomplicated cystitis is *E. coli.* Recommended first-line regimens include nitrofurantoin macrocrystals 100 mg orally twice daily × 5 days, trimethoprim-sulfamethoxazole double-strength orally twice daily × 3 days, fosfomycin 3 g single dose, or pivmecillinam 400 mg twice daily × 5 days (not available in the United States). There is no single best agent in this group that is superior to all others for the empiric management of uncomplicated cystitis. The choice between agents should be individualized and based on the patient's history, including allergies, local resistance patterns, drug availability, and cost. Trimethoprim-sulfamethoxazole is effective and inexpensive, but allergic reactions are more common, and in some US geographic areas, resistance rate among community-acquired *E. coli* isolates exceeds 20% and therefore it is not recommended in this type of setting. Nitrofurantoin is more expensive but effective. Fosfomycin is not as effective and is also expensive. However, they both exert little "collateral damage." This term refers to the indirect adverse effects of antibiotic agents, including their propensity to select drug-resistant organisms and promote colonization and infection with multidrug-resistant bacteria. A 3-day regimen of fluoroquinolones such as ciprofloxacin is highly efficacious in the management of uncomplicated cystitis. However, fluoroquinolones are no longer recommended as first-line empiric agents due to their potential to impact gastrointestinal flora and also for potential side effects. Beta-lactam antibiotics, including amoxicillin and cephalexin, tend to have inferior efficacy and more adverse effects compared to the recommended agents. They are therefore considered second-line agents for uncomplicated cystitis and are recommended when other agents cannot be used.

Gupta K, Hooton TM, Naber KG, et al. International clinical practice guidelines for the treatment of acute uncomplicated cystitis and pyelonephritis in women: A 2010 update by the Infectious Diseases Society of America and the European Society for Microbiology and Infectious Diseases. *Clin Infect Dis.* 2011;52:e103–e120; Food and Drug Administration Safety Announcement; July 26, 2016; http://www.fda.gov/Drugs/DrugSafety/ucm511530.htm.

8. **ANSWER: E. Reactivation of hepatitis B infection**

Rituximab, a monoclonal antibody to CD-20 (a B-lymphocyte marker), is a well-described cause of hepatitis B reactivation characterized by redevelopment of high levels of circulating hepatitis B virus, transaminitis, and in some cases a symptomatic hepatitis flare. Inactive carriers of hepatitis B (surface antigen positive, but with normal liver function tests [LFTs] and low amounts of circulating virus) and also patients with serologic evidence of previous hepatitis B infection (hepatitis B core IgG positive, surface antigen negative) are both at risk for reactivation after therapy with rituximab. Reactivation tends to occur early (weeks to months) after rituximab therapy in "inactive carriers," whereas it is more often a late complication of rituximab therapy in patients with serologic evidence of previous infection, occurring up to a year after rituximab therapy ends.

There is very low risk of developing hepatitis C infection as a consequence of blood transfusion in the United States (<1 in 2 million transfusions), and hepatitis C infection does not frequently cause an acute illness as described here (Option A). Transaminitis would be an unusual manifestation of relapse of lymphoma (Option B). Hepatitis A can cause an acute symptomatic hepatitis similar to this case presentation, but this patient was immune to hepatitis A based on prechemotherapy serologies so it is unlikely here (Option C). Isoniazid can cause idiosyncratic drug-induced liver injury characterized by significantly elevated transaminases, but this would be an unlikely cause of new elevation in LFTs many months after the treatment course ended (Option D).

Perrillo RP, Gish R, Falck-Ytter YT. American Gastroenterological Association Institute technical review on prevention and treatment of hepatitis B virus reactivation during immunosuppressive drug therapy. *Gastroenterology.* 2015;148:221–244.

9. ANSWER: C. Start empiric azithromycin for a 5-day course.

The clinical incubation of *Bordetella pertussis* is 5–21 days, and patients are considered infectious until 3 weeks after symptom onset. *B. pertussis* is a highly communicable disease, and patients with suspected infection should be treated pending test results. All nonpregnant patients who present with 3 weeks or less of symptoms (6 weeks or less if pregnant) are potentially contagious and so should be treated. The treatment of choice for adults is azithromycin, clarithromycin, or erythromycin. The CDC recommends trimethoprim-sulfamethoxazole as the second-line agent to treat those with macrolide antibiotic allergies or intolerance. Fluoroquinolones have not been shown to be effective as therapy. Neither vaccination nor administration of immunoglobulin would adequately treat *B. pertussis* infection.

Tiwari T, Murphy TV, Moran J, et al. Recommended antimicrobial agents for the treatment and postexposure prophylaxis of pertussis: 2005 CDC Guidelines. *MMWR Recomm Rep.* 2005;54(RR14):1–16.

10. ANSWER: E. Doxycycline 200 mg by mouth × 1

In the mid-Atlantic and Northeast, including Delaware, the deer tick *Ixodes scapularis* is the vector for *Borrelia burgdorferi*, which causes Lyme disease. Individuals bitten by ticks in an endemic area where there is clear evidence that the bite was due to a deer tick and the tick was attached for long enough to transmit the infection (at least 36 hours) are at substantial risk for developing Lyme disease. The IDSA recommends either of two potential management strategies in this case: a single oral dose of doxycycline 200 mg × 1 within 72 hours of tick removal or close observation for rash or other symptoms of early Lyme disease. A full treatment course for Lyme disease (Options B and D) or a single dose of antibiotics that might be active against Lyme other than the doxycycline regimen above (Option A) are not recommended. Serologies are unlikely to be helpful in a case of recent exposure as seroconversion within 1–2 days or exposure is unlikely (Option C).

Wormser GP, Dattwyler RJ, Shapiro ED, et al. The clinical assessment, treatment, and prevention of Lyme disease, human granulocytic anaplasmosis, and babesiosis: clinical practice guidelines by the Infectious Diseases Society of America. *Clin Infect Dis.* 2006;43:1089–1134.

11. ANSWER: C. Trimethoprim-sulfamethoxazole

This patient has a purulent skin and soft tissue infection that was appropriately drained and cultured, which is the mainstay of treatment. Uncomplicated **purulent** skin and soft tissue infections are most often caused by *Staphylococcus aureus.* Although in the absence of systemic illness this type of infection can be managed with drainage alone, a recent study comparing drainage and trimethoprim-sulfamethoxazole to drainage and placebo found high clinical cure rates in those treated with trimethoprim-sulfamethoxazole. Antibiotics active against *S. aureus*, MRSA in particular, are recommended while cultures of purulent material are pending. Appropriate antibiotics include trimethoprim-sulfamethoxazole or doxycycline, both of which are usually active against methicillin-sensitive and resistant strains of *S. aureus.* Some of the other antibiotic options in this question have limited activity against *S. aureus* (levofloxacin, clarithromycin), but none of the other options are recommended for the treatment of **purulent** skin and soft tissue infection. Penicillin may be active against susceptible *S. aureus* infection, but this susceptibility pattern is rare; penicillin is more appropriate to treat uncomplicated **nonpurulent** cellulitis, which is more often due to streptococci. Notably, rifampin is an oral antibiotic with good oral bioavailability and activity against *S. aureus.* However, rifampin should not be used as monotherapy in the treatment of these infections due to a low barrier to resistance.

Talan DA, Mower WR, Krishnadasan A, et al. Trimethoprim-sulfamethoxazole versus placebo for uncomplicated skin abscess. *N Engl J Med.* 2016;374:823–832; Stevens DL, Bisno AL, Chambers HF, et al. Practice guidelines for the diagnosis and management of skin and soft tissue infections: 2014 update by the Infectious Diseases Society of America. *Clin Infect Dis.* 2014;59:147–159.

12. ANSWER: E. Oral amoxicillin-clavulanate

Splenectomy results in increased vulnerability to overwhelming infection and sepsis due to certain organisms, including *Streptococcus pneumoniae, Haemophilus influenzae, Neisseria meningitidis*, and *Capnocytophaga canimorsus. C. canimorsus* is an anaerobic gram-negative rod that is part of canine and feline oral flora. When inoculated into humans, *C. canimorsus* can cause severe infection in certain hosts, including those without a spleen. Given this risk, typically asplenic patients who sustain a dog or cat bite in which the skin is broken are treated with a short course of preventative oral antibiotics. First-generation cephalosporins (such as cephalexin) and trimethoprim-sulfamethoxazole are not typically active; beta-lactam/beta-lactamase inhibitors and third-generation cephalosporins are usually active. In this case the patient is well clinically so has no indication for intravenous antibiotics (ceftriaxone); thus amoxicillin-clavulanate is the most appropriate choice. Rabies is unlikely in this case because the puppy is a domestic pet.

Butler T. *Capnocytophaga canimorsus:* an emerging cause of sepsis, meningitis, and post-splenectomy infection after dog bites. *Eur J Clin Microbiol Infect Dis.* 2015;34:1271–1280.

13. ANSWER: C. Use of a chlorine-containing cleaning agent to address environmental contamination

Standard environmental cleaning detergents are not sporicidal. To adequately clean the room of a patient with *Clostridium difficile* infection, it is necessary to use a chlorine-containing cleaning agent (1000–5000 ppm available chlorine) or other sporicidal agent. Even in outbreak settings, routine identification of asymptomatic carriers is not recommended and treatment is not effective in reducing horizontal transmission. Strict adherence to contact precautions, including gowning and gloving on entry to a patient's room and hand hygiene with soap and water, are key measures in reducing horizontal transmission of *C. difficile.* The spore form of *C. difficile* is resistant to killing by alcohol. Contact precautions should continue at least for the duration of the diarrhea, with many hospitals continuing contact precautions for the duration of the inpatient admission. There is no evidence at this time to support the use of prophylactic antibiotics to prevent horizontal transmission.

Cohen SH, Gerding DN, Johnson S, et al. Clinical practice guidelines for *Clostridium difficile* infection in adults: 2010 update by the Society for Healthcare Epidemiology of America (SHEA) and the Infectious Diseases Society of America (IDSA). *Infect Control Hosp Epidemiol.* 2010;31:431–455.

14. ANSWER: D. Start intravenous caspofungin.

The most likely cause of yeast in blood cultures in this patient with recent antibiotic exposure and an indwelling hemodialysis catheter is *Candida* species. Based on IDSA guidelines for the management of *Candida* infections, an echinocandin antifungal (caspofungin, micafungin, anidulafungin) is the first-line agent for treating candidemia in an ill patient such as this. Fluconazole may also be a reasonable agent to use initially in select patients (such as the elderly or diabetic patients) who are hemodynamically stable, have not previously been treated with an antifungal in the azole class, and are not at risk for resistant fungi. In addition, fluconazole is renally cleared and therefore the dose offered in Option A would not be appropriate for a patient on hemodialysis. Isavuconazonium (Option C) and liposomal amphotericin (Option E) also likely have activity against *Candida*, but neither are recommended as first-line agents for this indication. In most cases, central venous catheters need to be removed in the setting of candidemia (Option B), but candidemia needs to be treated as quickly as possible—fast treatment can portend better outcomes, so Option B is incorrect.

Pappas PG, Kauffman CA, Andes DR, et al. Clinical practice guideline for the management of candidiasis: 2016 update by the Infectious Diseases Society of America. *Clin Infect Dis.* 2016;62:e1–50.

15. ANSWER: A. *Bartonella henselae*

All of the pathogens listed including *Bartonella henselae, Toxocara cati, Toxoplasmosis gondii*, and *Yersinia pestis* can be transmitted to humans by cats. The most likely cause of this patient's symptoms is *B. henselae.* Systemic bartonellosis can sometimes present with a primary lesion that develops 3–10 days following inoculation from a bite or scratch from an infected cat (usually kitten). Tender lymphadenopathy may develop proximally after 1–10 weeks with overlying erythema that can suppurate and may last weeks. Rare complications include neuroretinitis (stellate macular exudates; "macular star"), encephalopathy/transverse myelitis, or endocarditis. In immune-suppressed individuals, disseminated illness can present as bacillary angiomatosis. *T. cati* is a helminthic infection that can be passed from cats to humans via fecal oral transmission; it is typically asymptomatic but can cause cutaneous larva migrans. Toxoplasmosis is a protozoan infection that similarly can be spread from cats to humans via fecal oral transmission. This infection is also often asymptomatic in normal hosts but can cause a mono-like illness with cervical adenopathy and occasionally can cause retinal disease in normal hosts. *Y. pestis*, the cause of plague, is transmitted uncommonly by feline fleas and is generally a rare illness in the United States.

Goldstein EJC, Abrahamian FM. Diseases transmitted by cats. *Microbiol Spectr.* 2015;3:IOL5-0013-2015.

16. ANSWER: D. Country of birth

The US Preventive Services Task Force updated recommendations for hepatitis B screening in 2014 based on extensive review of available data. Individuals who should be screened for hepatitis B infection include those born in countries where the prevalence of HBV infection is higher than 2%, those born in the United States to parents born in countries or regions where the prevalence of hepatitis B infection is higher than 8% and were not vaccinated in infancy, those who are HIV-infected, injection drug users, men who have sex with men, and household contacts or sexual partners of individuals with chronic hepatitis B infection. Based on these recommendations, the reason that this patient needs to be screened for hepatitis B infection is her country of birth. The estimated prevalence of hepatitis B infection in Vietnam and Asia in general is above 2%. Other regions of high hepatitis B infection prevalence include Africa and parts of the Middle East and Central and South America. In addition to the above screening recommendations, the CDC also recommends hepatitis B screening for all individuals in whom immunosuppressive therapy (including chemotherapy) is planned, individuals on hemodialysis, blood and body fluid donors, all pregnant women, and infants of HBV-infected mothers.

LeFevre ML. Screening for hepatitis B virus infection in nonpregnant adolescents and adults: U.S. Preventive Services Task Force recommendation statement. *Ann Intern Med.* 2014;161:58–66; Weinbaum CM, Williams I, Mast EE, et al. Recommendations for identification and public health management of persons with chronic hepatitis B virus infection. *MMWR Recomm Rep.* 2008;57:RR-8.

17. ANSWER: B. Initiate systemic corticosteroids to control symptoms of paradoxical tuberculosis immune reconstitution inflammatory syndrome (IRIS).

The clinical syndrome is classic for paradoxical tuberculosis IRIS, which is characterized by new or worsening findings of tuberculosis disease within 2–3 months of initiation of antiretroviral therapy. Manifestations can be seen within lung parenchyma, the central nervous system, and at serosal surfaces (pleural effusions, ascites, or pericardial effusions). Mild symptoms can be controlled with nonsteroidal antiinflammatory medications, but moderate to severe symptoms often require systemic corticosteroids. Multidrug-resistant tuberculosis is unlikely given the negative drug susceptibility test. The rapid onset of symptoms is not consistent with loss of control of tuberculosis infection due to poor adherence. *Pneumocystis jirovecii* is in the differential diagnosis but less likely given the CD4 T cell count above 200 cells/μL^3.

Panel on Antiretroviral Guidelines for Adults and Adolescents. Guidelines for the use of antiretroviral agents in HIV-1-infected adults and adolescents. Department of Health and Human Services. <http://aidsinfo.nih.gov/contentfiles/lvguidelines/AdultandAdolescentGL.pdf/>; accessed 08.05.16.

18. ANSWER: B. Lipid formulation of amphotericin B

The case patient's presentation is consistent with a severe sinus infection with an angioinvasive mold resulting in a rapidly progressive infection with an intranasal eschar. The most common infection syndromes in this clinical context include mucormycosis and aspergillosis. Appropriate empiric antifungal therapy in suspected cases of fungal sinusitis includes an antifungal agent active against Mucorales and *Aspergillus* species such as amphotericin B or a lipid formulation of amphotericin (which may be less nephrotoxic in this individual with chronic kidney disease). Voriconazole and caspofungin are active against *Aspergillus* species but do not have activity against Mucorales when given alone. Fluconazole has no activity in *Aspergillus* species or Mucorales. Two azole antifungal drugs, posaconazole and isavuconazole, have in vitro activity against Mucorales, though typically a lipid formulation of amphotericin in combination with surgical debridement is the treatment of choice for initial management of these types of infections.

Chitasombat MN, Kontoyiannis DP. Treatment of mucormycosis in transplant patients: role of surgery and of old and new antifungal agents. *Curr Opin Infect Dis.* 2016;29:340–345.

19. ANSWER: E. Continue levofloxacin and observe.

This patient has *Legionella* pneumonia based on a clinical syndrome consistent with community-acquired pneumonia and a positive urinary *Legionella* antigen, which has high specificity for the diagnosis of *Legionella* serotype 1. Therefore treatment of *Legionella* with either levofloxacin or azithromycin, which are considered first-line therapy for *Legionella* pneumonia, is indicated. Gram stain and culture of the expectorated sputum in this case suggest that the specimen was orally contaminated and does not represent the lower respiratory tract.

The growth of *Candida* species from sputum typically indicates colonization and does not require antifungal treatment as described in the IDSA guidelines for the management of *Candida* infections (thus Options A–D are incorrect). This patient may have been orally colonized with *Candida* due to the use of inhaled fluticasone (particularly if he is not rinsing his mouth after use).

Phin N, Parry-Ford F, Harrison T, et al. Epidemiology and clinical management of Legionnaires' disease. *Lancet Infect Dis.* 2014;14:1011–1021; Pappas PG, Kauffman CA, Andes DR, et al. Clinical practice guideline for the management of candidiasis: 2016 update by the Infectious Diseases Society of America. *Clin Infect Dis.* 2016;62:e1–50.

20. ANSWER: A. Vancomycin + cefepime

This patient most likely has bacterial endocarditis. Because this patient is febrile and ill appearing, it is appropriate to start empiric antibiotics as soon as blood cultures have been drawn in order to prevent further complications of infection. The most common pathogens in this type of presentation in an intravenous drug user include *Staphylococcus aureus,* coagulase-negative staphylococci, viridans streptococci (β-hemolytic streptococci, oral flora), and occasionally aerobic gram-negative bacilli or fungi. Empiric therapy should target these bacteria. Enterococci are a less frequent cause of endocarditis, though still important to consider—empiric treatment for staphylococci and streptococci will also include empiric treatment for enterococci. *Candida* endocarditis occurs in injection drug users but is less common than the bacterial pathogens.

The best empiric therapy among the choices given is vancomycin and cefepime, which would treat *S. aureus* (including MRSA), enterococci, streptococci, and aerobic gram-negative organisms (including *Pseudomonas*). Another reasonable regimen would include vancomycin and ceftriaxone. Although Option B, which includes vancomycin, gentamicin, and rifampin, would have activity against the organisms of concern, this is the regimen recommended for treatment of prosthetic valve MRSA endocarditis. Rifampin has a low barrier of resistance to bacteria so is not typically used during active bacteremia and is typically only indicated to treat staphylococcal prosthetic valve endocarditis or specific rare causes of endocarditis such as *Brucella*. The remaining antibiotic treatment options do not adequately target the most common pathogens as listed above.

Baddour LM, Wilson WR, Bayer AS, et al. Infective endocarditis in adults: diagnosis, antimicrobial therapy, and management of complications: a scientific statement for healthcare professionals from the American Heart Association. *Circulation.* 2015;132:1435–1486.

21. ANSWER: C. Administration of 30 mL/kg of crystalloid

This patient is at risk for sepsis based on the clinical criteria of altered mental status, increased respiratory rate (>22 breaths per minute), and low systolic blood pressure (<100 mm Hg), which make up the quick Sequential Organ Failure Assessment (qSOFA). The qSOFA and the more detailed SOFA score, which is based on Pao_2, platelet count, bilirubin, mean arterial pressure, Glasgow coma scale, serum creatinine, and urine output, allow clinicians to identify patients with sepsis who are at increased risk for mortality to allow for appropriate early intervention.

The Surviving Sepsis Campaign recommends that the following be completed within 3 hours: measurement of lactate, obtaining blood cultures before administration of antibiotics, administration of broad-spectrum antibiotics, and administration of 30 mL/kg of crystalloid for hypotension or lactate ≥4 mmol/L. There is good evidence that early antibiotics (within 1 hour of recognizing sepsis) improves patient outcomes. Norepinephrine is the first-choice vasopressor to maintain a mean arterial pressure ≥65; however, vasopressors should be reserved for hypotension that is nonresponsive to fluid resuscitation. Dopamine is not recommended except in highly select circumstances. Likewise, intravenous hydrocortisone is not recommended if hemodynamic stability is restored with fluid resuscitation and vasopressors.

Singer M, Deutschman CS, Seymour CW, et al. The Third International Consensus Definitions for Sepsis and Septic Shock (Sepsis-3). *JAMA.* 2016;315:801–810; Dellinger RP, Levy MM, Rhodes A, et al. Surviving sepsis campaign: international guidelines for management of severe sepsis and septic shock: 2012. *Crit Care Med.* 2013;41:580–637.

22. ANSWER: C. Caspofungin

Neutropenic patients with fever that persists or recurs after 4–7 days of empiric antibiotics are at high risk for fungal infection, particularly due to *Candida* and *Aspergillus* species. Neutropenic patients with this fever pattern should be treated with empiric antifungal therapy. Based on IDSA guidelines, appropriate antifungal therapy at this juncture would include an echinocandin (such as caspofungin or micafungin), voriconazole, or a preparation of amphotericin.

Freifeld AG, Bow EJ, Sepkowitz KA, et al. Clinical practice guideline for the use of antimicrobial agents in neutropenic patients with cancer: 2010 update by the Infectious Diseases Society of America. *Clin Infect Dis.* 2011;52:e56–e93.

23. ANSWER: E. Blood smear, EBV serologies, CMV serologies, HIV 1/2 antigen/antibody, HIV RNA

This patient has a "mono-like illness," characterized by fever, sore throat, malaise, fatigue, rash, and lymphadenopathy. Mild hepatitis and pancytopenia may also be a part of the syndrome. The most common causes of this syndrome in young adults are viral pathogens, including EBV and CMV for those who were not already infected during childhood. Serologies for both EBV and CMV are helpful diagnostics here. Acute retroviral syndrome, or acute HIV, may also present as a mono-like illness, often with concurrent diarrhea and weight loss just as this patient had. The incidence of new HIV infections in the United States is highest among men who have sex with men at present, so this patient has a documented risk factor as well. Acute HIV is the most likely diagnosis for this patient. In acute HIV, the HIV antibody is often still negative, before seroconversion, but the HIV p24 antigen is positive. Fourth-generation HIV tests check serum for HIV antibodies and p24 antigen. The CDC recommends the following testing algorithm for patients with suspected established or acute HIV infection: initial HIV 1/2 antigen/antibody testing; if the test is reactive, then the sample is reflexively tested specifically for HIV1 and HIV2 antibodies. This antibody differentiation test would be positive for either HIV1 or HIV2 antibodies in established infection, whereas it may be negative in acute infection. Thus patients with discordant results on the HIV 1/2 antigen/antibody and antibody differentiation test (positive/negative) should have further testing with an HIV RNA (or viral load), which should be positive and is usually very high in acute HIV. In cases where suspicion is high for acute HIV, like this case, it is also reasonable to check HIV RNA upfront because it becomes positive in acute infection a few days before the HIV antigen/antibody test.

Although hepatitis serologies may be helpful at some point if the liver function tests continue to be abnormal, viral hepatitis would not explain the full constellation of this patient's symptoms or lab abnormalities, and the transaminases are not high enough to be consistent with acute viral hepatitis, so these would not be the appropriate next tests to order. It is appropriate to consider the possibility of new sexually transmitted infections (STIs) given his new sexual partners, and secondary syphilis can also present with fever and rash and lymphadenopathy but would be unlikely to present with diarrhea, weight loss, and pancytopenia. An echocardiogram might be an appropriate test if the blood cultures are positive, but there are no other clues specific to endocarditis here aside from the fever. A blood smear and LDH may be appropriate tests at this point given the patient's pancytopenia of uncertain etiology, but a bone marrow biopsy should not be pursued until further noninvasive diagnostics have been performed.

Centers for Disease Control and Prevention and Association of Public Health Laboratories. Laboratory testing for the diagnosis of HIV infection: updated recommendations. Available at <http://stacks.cdc.gov/view/cdc/23447/>. Published June 27, 2014. Accessed 08.05.16.

24. ANSWER: E. Cefepime + levofloxacin + vancomycin

This patient has hospital-acquired pneumonia (HAP), which is defined as "pneumonia not incubating at the time of hospital admission and occurring 48 hours or more after admission" by the IDSA. The appropriate antibiotic choice in this setting depends on three patient factors:

1. Risk for infection with MRSA
   - Risk for MRSA is increased if the patient has received IV antibiotic therapy in the last 90 days or is hospitalized in a unit where more than 20% of *S. aureus* isolates are methicillin-resistant or if this statistic is not known.
2. Risk for mortality
   - Risk for mortality is increased if the patient requires ventilatory support for or has septic shock due to HAP.
3. Risk for infections due to multidrug-resistant organisms including *Pseudomonas* species.
   - Risk for resistant organisms is increased if the patient has received IV antibiotic therapy in the last 90 days.

Based on the patient's previous course of IV antibiotics for bacteremia within the last 3 months, he is at increased risk for both multidrug-resistant pathogens and MRSA. For patients in this setting or in those at high risk for mortality, two drugs that treat *Pseudomonas,* including beta-lactams, quinolones, or aminoglycosides (but preferably not to include two agents in the same class), and a single agent to treat for *S. aureus,* including MRSA (either vancomycin or linezolid), are recommended. Therefore among the choices given, cefepime, levofloxacin, and vancomycin would be the best choice. Current guidelines emphasize the importance of referring to local antibiograms data to choose the best antibiotic combination for patients at each center. Antibiotics can be adjusted based on clinical improvement and culture results at 48 to 72 hours.

Kalil AC, Metersky ML, Klompas M, et al. Management of adults with hospital-acquired and ventilator-associated pneumonia: 2016 clinical practice guidelines by the Infectious Diseases Society of America and the American Thoracic Society. *Clin Infect Dis.* 2016;63:e61–e111.

25. ANSWER: A. Clotrimazole troches

The patient in this case has clinical evidence of oral candidiasis (thrush). He recently received treatment with systemic steroids and antibiotics and is also on a chronic inhaled steroid, all of which raise his potential risk for thrush. In order to minimize the possibility that the thrush resulted from the use of an inhaled steroid, reviewing proper oral hygiene after use could be helpful. Despite these risk factors, it is also reasonable to consider HIV testing; the CDC currently recommends testing for all patients in the health care setting. Appropriate treatment for mild thrush includes clotrimazole troches or miconazole buccal tablets; oral nystatin solution or pastilles is also an alternative. Systemic oral fluconazole is typically reserved for moderate or severe oral thrush. Posaconazole and micafungin are broader spectrum systemic antifungal agents than fluconazole and are not indicated for the treatment of mild oral thrush in a normal host, though posaconazole is sometimes used for fluconazole-refractory thrush in a compromised host. Chlorhexidine mouthwash is approved for treatment of gingivitis but does not have antifungal activity and will not treat oral thrush.

Pappas PG, Kauffman CA, Andes DR, et al. Clinical practice guideline for the management of candidiasis: 2016 update by the Infectious Diseases Society of America. *Clin Infect Dis.* 2016;62:e1–50.

26. ANSWER: B. Colistimethate

Acinetobacter baumannii is an aerobic gram-negative coccobacillus that can cause hospital outbreaks with high rates of mortality. Outbreaks are typically associated with colonized respiratory support equipment, irrigation solutions, and intravenous solutions. The most common infections include ventilator-associated pneumonia, infection of surgical wounds and burns, and bacteremia. Over 50% of *A. baumannii* isolates in US hospitals are multidrug resistant. Colistimethate (colistin) is virtually always active in vitro. The presence of a beta-lactamase means that both cefepime and piperacillin/tazobactam, the two most active beta-lactam antibiotics against *A. baumannii*, are likely to be ineffective. The presence of a carbapenemase means that imipenem/cilastatin, meropenem, and doripenem are all unlikely to be effective. Finally, most multidrug-resistant *A. baumannii* isolates are resistant to fluoroquinolones. Even if the isolate tests susceptible to a fluoroquinolone, resistance often develops during use.

Fishbain J, Peleg AY. Treatment of *Acinetobacter* infections. *Clin Infect Dis.* 2010;51:79–84.

27. ANSWER: D. Inhaled fluticasone

There are many possible problematic drug–drug interactions with antiretroviral medications and commonly prescribed drugs. Physicians should review medication lists for any possible drug–drug interactions before prescribing new medications to patients who are currently taking antiretroviral medications. Computer software applications that predict drug interactions from a physician-entered medication list are particularly helpful in this setting. The most problematic antiretroviral agent in terms of risk of drug interactions is ritonavir. Ritonavir is the most potent cytochrome P450 3A4 inhibitor of all currently available medications. The other protease inhibitors, such as atazanavir and darunavir, and the pharmacologic booster agent cobicistat (available in several coformulations and alone), also inhibit CYP 3A4. These medications interact with many commonly prescribed drugs, including warfarin, the statins, combination estrogen/progesterone oral contraceptives, clarithromycin, rifampin, amiodarone, benzodiazepines, carbamazepine, phenytoin, sildenafil, tadalafil, meperidine, methadone, and peripherally administered corticosteroids. Peripherally administered corticosteroids (inhaled fluticasone, in this case) may reach systemic levels in patients who are taking ritonavir, which can lead to corticosteroid excess (features of Cushing syndrome) and then later lead to corticosteroid insufficiency when the medication is withdrawn. The systemic effects of peripherally administered corticosteroids with ritonavir are unpredictable and thus are difficult to monitor and treat. Peripherally administered corticosteroids, including inhaled, intranasal, injected (joint injections for treatment of pain), and even ophthalmic, should be avoided in patients taking ritonavir. If these medications are necessary, then an HIV specialist should be consulted. In addition to the aforementioned list of drug–drug interactions, there are other common drug–drug interactions with antiretroviral medications. Both atazanavir and rilpivirine require stomach acid for absorption to therapeutic levels, so coadministration of acid blockers (H_2 blockers and especially proton pump inhibitors) can lead to decreased blood levels, and therefore decreased efficacy, of these agents. Efavirenz is both a substrate and inducer of isoforms of the cytochrome P450 system, but interactions with efavirenz are generally less common and less severe, though the interaction with methadone is unpredictable and can be problematic. Inhaled albuterol, ophthalmic antihistamines, oral cetirizine, and oral montelukast would not be expected to cause a problematic drug interaction for this patient.

Panel on Antiretroviral Guidelines for Adults and Adolescents. Guidelines for the use of antiretroviral agents in HIV-1-infected adults and adolescents. Department of Health and Human Services. Available at http://www.aidsinfo.nih.gov/ContentFiles/AdultandAdolescentGL.pdf. Accessed 08.08.16.

28. ANSWER: D. *Bacteroides fragilis*

Bacteroides fragilis is an anaerobic gram-negative bacteria that colonizes the intestines and is cultured from the blood in the setting of bowel perforation. It is not a common cause of endocarditis. Common pathogens that cause endocarditis include *Staphylococcus aureus*, the viridans streptococci, *Streptococcus gallolyticus* (previously known as *Streptococcus bovis*), the HACEK organisms (*Haemophilus parainfluenzae, Haemophilus aphrophilus, Haemophilus paraphrophilus, Actinobacillus, Cardiobacterium hominis, Eikenella corrodens, Kingella kingae*), and enterococci (community acquired, without another obvious source). Positive blood cultures from at least two separate cultures with any of those organisms are considered major criteria for the diagnosis of endocarditis by the modified Duke criteria, or highly positive antibody titer to *Coxiella burnetii* (because this organism is exceedingly difficult to culture). The other major criterion for diagnosis of endocarditis is an echocardiogram with findings consistent with infective endocarditis (mobile intracardiac mass, abscess, new dehiscence of prosthetic valve, or new valvular regurgitation). A diagnosis of endocarditis by Duke criteria requires fulfillment of either two major criteria (as listed previously), or one major and three minor criteria, or five minor criteria. This patient meets two minor criteria for the diagnosis of endocarditis at the time of presentation: fever and predisposing cardiac lesion (the bicuspid valve with regurgitation). Other minor criteria are as follows: other predisposing risk (injection drug use), evidence of emboli (arterial emboli, pulmonary infarcts, Janeway lesions, conjunctival hemorrhage), immunologic complications (glomerulonephritis, Osler nodes), or positive blood cultures that do not meet the major criteria or serologic evidence of an infection with an organism consistent with infective endocarditis not satisfying a major criterion (e.g., *Bartonella henselae*). The diagnosis of infective endocarditis is "possible" if only one major and one minor criteria are fulfilled, or if three minor criteria are fulfilled.

Baddour LM, Wilson WR, Bayer AS, et al. Infective endocarditis in adults: diagnosis, antimicrobial therapy, and management of complications: a scientific statement for healthcare professionals from the American Heart Association. *Circulation.* 2015;132:1435–1486.

29. ANSWER: B. A few days after initiation of clarithromycin and ethambutol, but within 2 weeks

Antiretroviral therapy (ART) should be started within 2 weeks of diagnosis of most opportunistic infections, with the exception of cryptococcal meningitis and tuberculosis meningitis. There is a risk of immune reconstitution inflammatory syndrome (IRIS) in patients who start ART with low CD4 count, high viral load, and active opportunistic infection. IRIS may be less pronounced if the opportunistic infection is treated first. However, IRIS may be treated with corticosteroids if needed. Patients have increased mortality from AIDS-related causes if ART is not started early enough. It may be appropriate to start treatment for opportunistic infections first to ensure tolerance of those medications for a couple of days prior to ART and start control of those infections, but then ART should be started soon afterwards, within 2 weeks of the diagnosis of opportunistic infection. There is no reason to wait until hospital discharge to start ART. ART may be started during hospitalization and transitioned to the outpatient setting in the same way that other new medications (e.g., statins, beta-blockers, and clopidogrel after new cardiac event) are started during hospitalization and transitioned to the outpatient setting. ART should not be started in a staggered fashion, one at a time over weeks.

Zolopa A, Andersen J, Powderly W, et al. Early antiretroviral therapy reduces AIDS progression/death in individuals with acute opportunistic infections: a multicenter randomized strategy trial. *PLOS One.* 2009;4:e5575; Panel on Antiretroviral Guidelines for Adults and Adolescents. Guidelines for the use of antiretroviral agents in HIV-1-infected adults and adolescents. Department of Health and Human Services. Available at http://www.aidsinfo.nih.gov/ContentFiles/AdultandAdolescentGL.pdf. Accessed 08.08.16.

30. ANSWER: C. Counsel patient to quit smoking, and discuss medications and supports for smoking cessation.

This patient has well-controlled HIV with a CD4 count well above the range that would be concerning for opportunistic infections. If he continues to take his antiretrovirals regularly, then he should continue to have a robust immune system and low risk of opportunistic infections. In fact, patients with HIV who are diagnosed early (before diagnosis of AIDS), started on antiretroviral therapy quickly, and maintained on antiretroviral therapy without interruptions are estimated to have a life expectancy that approaches that of the general population. Although this patient is unlikely to develop AIDS-related complications, such as opportunistic infections and AIDS-related malignancies (e.g., Kaposi sarcoma), there are other risks with prolonged HIV infection. Prolonged HIV infection is associated with increased risk of cardiovascular disease and non–AIDS-related malignancies, such as lung cancer. Health care maintenance, including addressing modifiable risk factors and pursuing age-appropriate cancer screening, is extremely important in these patients. For this patient the most important modifiable risk factor for cardiovascular disease and malignancy is his smoking. Among all of the health care maintenance items that could be addressed with the patient during this visit, smoking cessation (if this can be achieved) is the most likely to lead to a reduction in morbidity and mortality. It is important to address smoking cessation with him through counseling (use of motivational interviewing is especially helpful here) and discussion of nicotine replacement therapy (nicotine patches, etc.) and other medications to aid in smoking cessation (varenicline, bupropion). This patient does not meet criteria to start prophylaxis for *Pneumocystis* pneumonia because his CD4 count is well above 200, and he is not at risk for reactivation of latent toxoplasmosis because his CD4 count is greater than 100. A discussion about alcohol use to screen for warning signs of abuse or dependence may be appropriate at this visit, but his current reported number of alcoholic beverages per week is below the threshold of concern for men, so this is less important to address than smoking cessation. The patient should be referred for colonoscopy screening at age 50, but in the absence of symptoms or a personal or family history of polyps or colon cancer, there is no indication to refer for early colonoscopy screening.

31. ANSWER: A. Vancomycin, ceftriaxone, ampicillin

This patient is an elderly man who is living in a close community at his assisted living facility, now presenting with probable bacterial meningitis. The most common pathogens in this case are *Streptococcus pneumoniae, Neisseria meningitidis*, and *Listeria monocytogenes.* The combination of vancomycin and high-dose ceftriaxone is used empirically when *S. pneumoniae* meningitis is a possibility because of the small but significant prevalence of penicillin-resistant and even cefotaxime-resistant *S. pneumoniae.* Ampicillin is used for treatment of *Listeria* meningitis. The other antibiotic options that are listed are not appropriate for this patient. This patient has no history of neurosurgical procedures, so he does not need empiric treatment with an antipseudomonal cephalosporin, such as cefepime or ceftazidime, or a carbapenem, such as imipenem or meropenem.

The CSF examination of this patient shows definite predominance of neutrophils with minimal lymphocytes and low glucose, which is more suggestive of bacterial meningitis rather than viral meningitis, so acyclovir is not required for initial treatment. The combination of ampicillin and gentamicin may be useful for such pathogens as ampicillin-sensitive enterococci or *Streptococcus agalactiae* (group B *Streptococcus*), but it does not include appropriate empiric treatment for *S. pneumoniae* or *N. meningitidis.* Fungal meningitis is rare, seen primarily in patients who are immunocompromised or those who have been instrumented or undergone epidural injections with contaminated material such as in the 2012 outbreak involving steroid injections contaminated with *Exserohilum rostratum.* This patient does not have a history of immunocompromise, instrumentation, or epidural injections of medications, so fungal meningitis is extremely unlikely, and empiric therapy with amphotericin B is not appropriate.

Kainer MA, Reagan DR, Nguyen DB, et al. Fungal infections associated with contaminated methylprednisolone in Tennessee. *N Engl J Med.* 2012;367:2194–2203; Tunkel AR, Hartman BJ, Kaplan SL, et al. Practice guidelines for the management of bacterial meningitis. *Clin Infect Dis.* 2004;39:1267–1284.

32. ANSWER: C. Oral dextromethorphan, inhaled albuterol, and intranasal ipratropium

This patient has rhinosinusitis that is improving without antibiotic treatment already, based on cessation of fevers 3 days ago and only mild residual symptoms. Acute rhinosinusitis ("sinusitis") is an extremely common condition, especially among adults age 45–74 years, and the cause is viral in more than 90% of cases, with bacterial infection accounting for less than 10% of cases. Symptoms of upper respiratory tract infections or sinusitis may include nasal congestion, headache, ear pain, cough, fever, and purulent nasal discharge. The indications for antibiotic treatment of sinusitis are when symptoms suggest bacterial infection with any one or combination of three patterns: (1) persistent or not improving symptoms (≥10 days); (2) severe symptoms for ≥3–4 days (including temperature >39°C or 102°C, or 3–4 consecutive days of sinus pain at the beginning of the illness); or (3) worsening or "double-sickening" (onset of new/worsening symptoms as viral upper respiratory infection is starting to resolve after 5–6 days, indicating bacterial superinfection). This patient meets none of these criteria; therefore antibiotic treatment including moxifloxacin (Option A), amoxicillin-clavulanate (Option B), and ceftriaxone (Option D) are not indicated. Furthermore, for patients who do meet criteria for therapy and are not penicillin-allergic, quinolones and third-generation cephalosporins are no longer considered first-line therapy; amoxicillin-clavulanate remains the treatment of choice for patients who do need treatment. Influenza vaccine, although not contraindicated in this situation because the patient is now afebrile, is never indicated as a part of treatment of an acute illness, so Option E is incorrect. This patient should be treated with supportive care, including symptom management—all of the medications in Option C may be used for symptom management, so this is the correct answer.

Chow AW, Benninger MS, Brook I, et al. IDSA clinical practice guideline for acute bacterial rhinosinusitis in children and adults. *Clin Infect Dis.* 2012;54:e73–e112.

33. ANSWER: E. Allergy consultation and admission for desensitization to penicillin in order to facilitate treatment with penicillin G 2.4 million units IM once weekly for 3 weeks

Syphilis infection during pregnancy can have serious consequences for both the mother and fetus if left untreated. Therefore it is important to treat immediately with the most aggressive, data-supported effective treatment for syphilis, which is penicillin. Pregnant women who are diagnosed with syphilis should always be treated with penicillin, even if this requires hospitalization for desensitization to penicillin, in the case of penicillin allergy. All other treatments for syphilis are potentially less effective, and doxycycline is contraindicated during pregnancy. This patient may be presumed to have late latent syphilis, as she is asymptomatic with infection of unknown duration, so treatment with weekly IM penicillin for 3 weeks would be appropriate. Follow-up RPR titers should be monitored to ensure that they decrease appropriately.

Workowski KA, Bolan GA. Sexually transmitted diseases treatment guidelines, 2015. *MMWR Recomm Rep.* 2015;64:1–137.

34. ANSWER: D. Ceftriaxone 250 mg IM single dose + azithromycin 1 g orally single dose

This patients has uncomplicated gonococcal urethritis. Fluoroquinolone-resistant strains of *Neisseria gonorrhoeae* are now disseminated throughout the United States. So, fluoroquinolones have *not* been recommended for treatment of gonorrhea in the United States since 2007 (Option A). In addition, Asian and European countries have reported cefixime-resistant strains and treatment-failures. In the United States, gonorrhea surveillance in the last decade has also suggested that the efficacy of cefixime may be reduced, and strains not susceptible to cefixime are also typically not susceptible to tetracyclines like doxycycline. In 2015 the CDC changed their recommendations for the treatment of uncomplicated cervical, urethral, and rectal gonorrhea infection to a single preferred regimen of intramuscular ceftriaxone and single-dose oral azithromycin. Ceftriaxone, also a third-generation cephalosporin like cefixime, remains part of the regimen of choice because the intramuscular delivery leads to long-lasting high levels of antibiotic relative to a single oral dose of cefixime.

Cefixime remains an alternative option for treatment of uncomplicated gonorrhea when given with a single dose of azithromycin, but not in combination with doxycycline (Option C). Concurrent treatment with azithromycin in either case is important because most gonococci are also susceptible to azithromycin even with diminished susceptibility to cephalosporins. Concurrent treatment may also decrease the rates of development of antibiotic-resistant gonorrhea and also treats for the possibility of concomitant *Chlamydia* coinfection in cases where this infection is present.

Workowski KA, Bolan GA. Sexually transmitted diseases treatment guidelines, 2015. *MMWR Recomm Rep.* 2015;64:1–137.

35. ANSWER: B. Viral culture of a swab of the ulcers

The most likely diagnosis in this case is anogenital herpes simplex virus (HSV) infection. The features that are consistent with this diagnosis are the grouped ulcerations, which are painful, with absence of significant lymphadenopathy or rectal discharge, which would be expected with some other conditions such as gonorrhea or lymphogranuloma venereum (LGV). Diagnostics for active HSV infection are somewhat limited, and the diagnosis is often made clinically followed by somewhat empiric treatment. Viral culture of a swab of the lesion has a high specificity, but the sensitivity is limited and operator dependent. In certain institutions the direct fluorescent antibody testing (DFA) of a scraping of the base of the lesion may be highly sensitive and specific, but it is also operator dependent and therefore not consistent across institutions. PCR for HSV is both sensitive and specific from CSF during episodes of HSV meningitis and can also be checked from a swab of an ulcer. Serologic testing for HSV type-specific antibodies will demonstrate infection that was acquired at some point in the past if the patient is having a recurrent outbreak and will develop within the first several weeks of infection for new exposures, but serologies are not helpful in diagnosing an active outbreak. Urine NAAT probes are helpful for diagnosis of gonorrhea or chlamydia but not helpful for diagnosis of HSV. Bacterial studies would not be expected to be positive during active HSV infection, which is a viral infection.

Workowski KA, Bolan GA. Sexually transmitted diseases treatment guidelines, 2015. *MMWR Recomm Rep.* 2015;64:1–137.

36. ANSWER: C. Serum test for antineutrophilic cytoplasmic antibodies (ANCA)

This question stem describes a patient with an "infection mimicker," which can be diagnostically challenging. Many of the features of this patient's illness may be consistent with an infectious etiology—chronic sinusitis, especially in immunocompromised patients, may be due to fungal infection. Pulmonary nodules and hemoptysis may be due to fungal infection or tuberculosis, or nontuberculous mycobacterial infection. However, when the entirety of the patient's history is reviewed, the salient points are as follows: no obvious risk factors for tuberculosis or immunosuppression at baseline, chronic sinusitis that was unresponsive to repeated treatments with antibiotics, new pulmonary nodules and hemoptysis, and blood tests showing anemia and hematuria. Taken together, this syndrome is most consistent with granulomatosis with polyangiitis (previously known as Wegner granulomatosis). The American College of Rheumatology–endorsed diagnostic criteria for granulomatosis with polyangiitis stipulate that patients should meet at least 2 of 4 criteria that include "nasal or oral inflammation," abnormal chest imaging, abnormal urinary sediment, and granulomatous inflammation of biopsy. Most patients with active granulomatosis will have positive serum ANCA testing (up to 80%), especially if the disease is severe, but biopsy would be definitive. AFB smears from sputum or from biopsy samples would be positive if the patient had tuberculosis or nontuberculous mycobacterial infection. Serum galactomannan would be positive if the patient had invasive aspergillosis. Serum IGRA may be positive in patients with tuberculosis.

Leavitt RY, Fauci AS, Bloch DA, et al. The American College of Rheumatology 1990 criteria for the classification of Wegener's granulomatosis. *Arthritis Rheum.* 1990;33:1101–1107.

37. ANSWER: A. Monitoring for early signs and symptoms of urinary tract infection, with expedited early urinalysis, urine culture, and empiric treatment while awaiting culture results when symptoms develop

Patients with chronic indwelling urinary catheters often have pyuria and bacteria even in the absence of other signs or symptoms of active urinary tract infection. Routine screening with urinalysis and urine culture is not recommended in these patients because this will lead to overtreatment of asymptomatic patients, and it increases the risk for antibiotic-resistant infections in the future. Early diagnosis and treatment, based on prior available culture results while waiting for pending acute cultures, is the safest approach to management to decrease the risk of overtreatment. Antibiotic treatments into the urinary drainage bag are not recommended, and chronic prophylaxis with methenamine salts or empiric broad antibiotics (such as ciprofloxacin) without any review of culture data or prior infections are not recommended.

Hooton TM, Bradley SF, Cardenas DD, et al. Diagnosis, prevention, and treatment of catheter-associated urinary tract infection in adults: 2009 International Clinical Practice Guidelines from the Infectious Diseases Society of America. *Clin Infect Dis.* 2010;50:625–663.

38. ANSWER: E. Penicillin

Recurrent cellulitis with episodes as described for this patient (sudden onset of fever, systemic symptoms, and pain and erythema of the leg) is commonly attributed to recurrent streptococcal infection, though the microbiologic diagnosis is not confirmed in most cases. Risk factors for recurrent cellulitis may include prior surgery or prior infections in the affected limb, lower-extremity edema, poor hygiene status, skin ulcerations, and onychomycosis. A randomized, placebo-controlled trial of chronic suppressive/prophylactic oral penicillin showed that this was an effective strategy to decrease recurrences of cellulitis; incidence of cellulitis was 37% among placebo recipients and 22% among penicillin recipients during the follow-up period. Many of the antibiotic options listed have good efficacy at treating staphylococcal infections, and some have good efficacy at treating streptococcal infections (e.g., levofloxacin), but only penicillin has been proven to reduce risk of recurrence of cellulitis in a placebo-controlled clinical trial.

Thomas KS, Crook AM, Nunn AJ, et al. Penicillin to prevent recurrent leg cellulitis. *N Engl J Med.* 2013;368:1695–1703; Stevens DL, Bisno AL, Chambers HF, et al. Practice guidelines for the diagnosis and management of skin and soft tissue infections: 2014 update by the Infectious Diseases Society of America. *Clin Infect Dis.* 2014;59:147–159.

39. ANSWER: A. Cook meat to "well done."

Toxoplasma gondii is a parasite found in soil and contaminated or undercooked foods. Cats are the definitive host and shed oocytes that eventually become infectious to humans or other animals if consumed (typically through poorly washed produce, undercooked meat, or inadequate hand washing after soil exposure). Acute infection may be associated with malaise, fever, and lymphadenopathy, but it is often asymptomatic. Acute infection during pregnancy may result in congenital infection of the newborn, which can cause long-term complications such as blindness. Early diagnosis and treatment during pregnancy is essential to preventing complications. However, prevention of infection is ideal. The CDC and the American College of Obstetrics and Gynecology recommend that pregnant women be advised about several lifestyle changes to reduce the risk of exposure. This includes careful washing of fruits and vegetables before consumption because they may be contaminated with cysts from the soil. All meats should be cooked to "well done" because uncooked meats may also carry infection. Although pork products may also carry infection, they do not need to be universally avoided as long as they are cooked properly. Lastly, pregnant women should wear gloves and carefully wash hands afterwards when they anticipate soil exposure, such as with gardening (but it need not be given up as long as gloves are worn). Toxoplasmosis is not typically spread directly from human to human in a teacher-student relationship, and pregnant women can keep a pet cat as long as contact with feces is minimized (e.g., another person cleans the litter box) and hands are washed carefully after any potential exposure.

Montoya JG, Remington JS. Management of *Toxoplasma gondii* infection during pregnancy. *Clin Infect Dis.* 2008;47(4):554–566; American College of Obstetricians and Gynecologists. Practice bulletin no. 151: cytomegalovirus, parvovirus B19, varicella zoster, and toxoplasmosis in pregnancy. *Obstet Gynecol.* 2015;125:1510–1525; Lopez A, Dietz VJ, Wilson M, et al. Preventing congenital toxoplasmosis. *MMWR Recomm Rep.* 2000;49:59–68.

40. ANSWER: D. Vancomycin and piperacillin-tazobactam

This patient has poorly controlled diabetes with a new progressive soft tissue infection arising from a nonhealing toe ulcer. The black areas of the toe are concerning for necrotic tissue, which in this case would raise the concern for "wet gangrene," or infected gangrenous tissue. This patient requires surgical debridement and may require amputation of the toe, depending on the extent of the infection. Based on the presence of his local symptoms (purulent drainage, tenderness, pain), the size of the ulcer (>2 cm), and his systemic signs and symptoms of infection (fever >100.4°F and white blood cell count >12,000 cells/μL), this patient has a severe infection based on IDSA classifications. Antibiotics should be started immediately while awaiting results of cultures and operative management. Cultures should be obtained from deep tissue typically by biopsy or debridement after the wound has been cleaned, as cultures obtained from superficial swabs of the wound may be less accurate. For severe infections, empirical therapy for *Staphylococcus aureus*, including MRSA, as well as gram-negative bacilli, including *Pseudomonas aeruginosa* when risk factors such as a high prevalence of *Pseudomonas* infection are present, is indicated. Of the listed antibiotic regimens, only piperacillin-tazobactam and vancomycin treat for these possibilities.

Lipsky BA, Berendt AR, Cornia PB, et al. 2012 Infectious Diseases Society of America clinical practice guideline for the diagnosis and treatment of diabetic foot infections. *Clin Infect Dis.* 2012;54:132–173.

41. ANSWER: B. Valacyclovir 1000 mg orally three times daily for 14 days

This patient has Ramsay Hunt syndrome type II, otherwise known as herpes zoster oticus. This is a rare syndrome that is caused by reactivation of herpes zoster virus in the geniculate ganglion, which leads to a triad of symptoms including (1) ear pain, tinnitus, and vertigo, (2) ipsilateral peripheral facial nerve paralysis, and (3) vesicles in the external auditory canal, ear, mouth, or anterior two-thirds of the tongue. Patients may also experience altered sensation in the ear canal and loss of moisturization of the eyes and mouth. The concurrence of facial droop with ear canal symptoms, changes in mucous membranes moisture, and skin lesions make this syndrome unique. This zoster reactivation is treated with acyclovir or valacyclovir. The addition of corticosteroids, such as prednisone to antiviral therapy, is controversial but has not been shown to be of benefit in a randomized study. The facial droop alone can be a symptom of Lyme disease (especially with the epidemiologic risk factors listed for this patient) and would be appropriately treated with doxycycline but would not explain the patient's other symptoms. Otitis externa may be treated with otic ciprofloxacin drops, and if concurrent otitis media was suspected, then additional treatment with amoxicillin-clavulanate would be appropriate.

Worme M, Chada R, Lavallee L. An unexpected case of Ramsay Hunt syndrome: case report and literature review. *BMC Res Notes.* 2013;6:337; Kansu L, Yilmaz I. Herpes zoster oticus (Ramsay Hunt syndrome) in children: case report and literature review. *Int J Pediatr Otorhinolaryngol.* 2012;76:772–776.

42. ANSWER: C. *Mycoplasma genitalium*

This patient has nongonococcal urethritis (NGU) based on the clinical diagnosis of urethritis and the negative testing for gonorrhea. The most common cause of NGU is *Chlamydia* infection, which causes an estimated 15%–40% of all NGU, but this patient also had negative testing for *Chlamydia.* Other organisms that cause NGU include *Mycoplasma genitalium, Trichomonas vaginalis,* HSV, and occasionally adenovirus. After *Chlamydia, M. genitalium* is likely the next most common cause of NGU at about 15%–25% and is treated with azithromycin. Notably, this organism is less responsive to doxycycline, and, furthermore, azithromycin resistance with this infection is thought to be increasing in the United States. In patients with NGU who do not respond to azithromycin, *M. genitalium* is the most common cause and retreatment with moxifloxacin is indicated. *Trichomonas* is a less common cause of urethritis but is a consideration in men who have sex with women and do not respond to empiric therapy for NGU with azithromycin or doxycycline, particularly in areas where *Trichomonas* infection is prevalent. *Haemophilus ducreyi* is the causative organism in chancroid, which is an ulcerative STI and does not typically cause urethritis.

Workowski KA, Bolan GA. Sexually transmitted diseases treatment guidelines, 2015. *MMWR Recomm Rep.* 2015;64:1–137.

43. ANSWER: B. Trimethoprim-sulfamethoxazole

This patient has *Pneumocystis jirovecii* pneumonia, also still commonly known as PCP. Besides HIV infection or AIDS, PCP is most commonly seen in immunocompromised patients treated with corticosteroids. Risk for PCP in patients treated with corticosteroids depends on the dose and duration of the steroids. In a study of 116 patients with PCP who did not have HIV, 91% had been on corticosteroids when PCP was diagnosed, and the mortality rate was 49%. The median steroid dose and duration in this study was 30 mg of prednisone per day for 12 weeks, but it was seen in patients on doses as low as 16 mg per day and for durations as short as 8 weeks.

The features of the presentation that are consistent with *Pneumocystis* pneumonia include prolonged corticosteroid exposure (especially in the context of recent tapering), cough and shortness of breath, which are progressive despite antibiotics; significant hypoxia on presentation; and bilateral infiltrates on chest imaging. The serum β-d-glucan assay may be positive in the setting of *Pneumocystis* pneumonia, especially in immunocompromised patients, and also in some other fungal infections. Treatment is with trimethoprim-sulfamethoxazole, and corticosteroids should be added when there is severe disease as evidenced by a large A–a gradient.

Ivermectin would be used to treat *Strongyloides stercoralis* hyperinfection, which can cause respiratory failure in patients who are latently infected and then receive corticosteroids, but it is less common in the United States and is typically manifested with other symptoms and problems also including diarrhea, abdominal pain, gram-negative sepsis, or meningitis related to increased worm burden and transit. Though fevers could suggest flaring of her giant cell arteritis such that increased steroids are necessary, her pulmonary symptoms and lack of recurrent headaches make this less likely. Pulmonary edema is also a consideration, but on exam she has no evidence of congestive heart failure and this would not explain the fevers.

Yale SH, Limper AH. *Pneumocystis carinii* pneumonia in patients without acquired immunodeficiency syndrome: associated illness and prior corticosteroid therapy. *Mayo Clin Proc.* 1996;71:5–13; Kermani TA, Ytterberg SR, Warrington KJ. *Pneumocystis jiroveci* pneumonia in giant cell arteritis: a case series. *Arthritis Care Res.* 2011;63:761–765.

44. ANSWER: C. Patients taking PrEP should have regular screening for other STIs at least every 6 months, including syphilis, gonorrhea, and chlamydia.

The CDC recommends tenofovir/emtricitabine once daily for PrEP for HIV prevention for patients with high risk of HIV acquisition, including men who have sex with men as well as heterosexual men and women with increased sexual risk, and injection drug users. The CDC has extensive online resources on PrEP for both patients and providers at http://www.cdc.gov/hiv/risk/prep/. Providers should follow these online guidelines when prescribing PrEP, including baseline and regular HIV testing every 3 months (not 12), regular STI screening, and monitoring renal function because there is risk for nephrotoxicity with tenofovir. Taking tenofovir/emtricitabine for PrEP with excellent adherence can reduce the risk of HIV acquisition by as much as 92% in this patient population. Since the advent of PrEP, many providers have raised concerns that patients taking PrEP would compensate with increased sexual risk behaviors, resulting in increased incidence of STIs. However, the PROUD study of PrEP in a real-world setting demonstrated no increased incidence of STIs in the PrEP arm, and no evidence of increased risky behaviors in the PrEP arm.

US Public Health Service. Preexposure prophylaxis for the prevention of HIV infection in the United States—2014. Available at: http://www.cdc.gov/hiv/pdf/prepguidelines2014.pdf. Accessed 29.09.16; McCormack S, Dunn DT, Desai M, et al. Pre-exposure prophylaxis to prevent the acquisition of HIV-1 infection (PROUD): effectiveness results from the pilot phase of a pragmatic open-label randomised trial. *Lancet.* 2016;387:53–60.

45. ANSWER: A. Drug–drug interaction

This patient has serotonin syndrome due to interaction of linezolid with duloxetine. Linezolid is a mild monoamine oxidase inhibitor, and when combined with certain medications including selective serotonin reuptake inhibitors, drug-induced serotonin excess can result. The syndrome is characterized by autonomic instability, cognitive/behavioral changes, and neuromuscular excitability; thus the signs and symptoms of serotonin syndrome can include tachycardia, hyperthermia, hypertension, agitation, restlessness, and confusion. This condition can be fatal if not addressed quickly, which is why there is a black-box warning on linezolid to avoid concurrent administration with selective serotonin reuptake inhibitors, serotonin-norepinephrine reuptake inhibitors, and some other serotonin-active medications. Based on the history given, there is no evidence of recurrent soft tissue infection on physical exam and no reason to suspect MRSA bacteremia without another source, without murmurs on cardiac exam, and without evidence of sepsis (blood pressure is high, rather than low). The abdominal examination is normal, and there are no reported abdominal symptoms, so *C. difficile* infection is also unlikely.

Lawrence KR, Adra M, Gillman PK. Serotonin toxicity associated with the use of linezolid: a review of postmarketing data. *Clin Infect Dis.* 2006; 42:1578–1583.

46. ANSWER: B. Quinine and clindamycin and consideration of red cell exchange transfusion

This patient has severe babesiosis. Intraerythrocytic parasites (protozoa) are diagnostic of either malaria (caused by multiple different *Plasmodium* species) or babesiosis (in the United States most often caused by *Babesia microti*). This patient has traveled to Nantucket, where babesiosis is a relatively common tick-borne illness (*Ixodes scapularis*), and has no reported travel history to a malaria-endemic area, so it is presumed that the infection in this case is babesiosis rather than malaria. Severe babesiosis, as in this case, is defined as infection resulting in renal, hepatic, or pulmonary end-organ dysfunction, high grade parasitemia (>10%), or significant hemolysis. Mild babesiosis may be treated with azithromycin and atovaquone (but not with proguanil, so Option A is wrong). Severe babesiosis is generally treated with quinine (oral quinine or intravenous quinidine when necessary) and clindamycin. The major risk factors for severe babesiosis in this patient are his history of splenectomy and rituximab therapy within the last 6–12 months. His age (i.e., >50 years old) is also a risk factor for severe disease. Patients with severe babesiosis should be evaluated for red cell exchange transfusion, especially if the patient also has a history of splenectomy and/or recent rituximab therapy. This patient meets many criteria for red cell exchange transfusion, and it should be pursued immediately to prevent further complications from this disease. Plasmapheresis, steroids, and IVIG (Option D) are not used to treat babesiosis. Ceftriaxone and doxycycline (Option C) may be used to treat other tick-borne infections (Lyme disease and anaplasmosis) but would not be effective treatment for babesiosis. Notably, babesiosis, Lyme disease, and anaplasmosis are transmitted by the same species of tick, *I. scapularis*, and so coinfection should be considered in ill patients. Intravenous artesunate is appropriate therapy for severe malaria but not for babesiosis.

Wormser GP, Dattwyler RJ, Shapiro ED, et al. The clinical assessment, treatment, and prevention of Lyme disease, human granulocytic anaplasmosis, and babesiosis: clinical practice guidelines by the Infectious Diseases Society of America. *Clin Infect Dis.* 2006;43:1089–1134; Krause PJ, Gewurz BE, Hill D, et al. Persistent and relapsing babesiosis in immunocompromised patients. *Clin Infect Dis.* 2008;46:370–376.

47. ANSWER: A. Blood serologic test for *Coccidioides*

This patient most likely has primary pulmonary coccidioidomycosis, or "valley fever." The features of his presentation that are consistent with this diagnosis are as follows: exposure in an endemic area (hiking in dry windy climate in the American Southwest), somewhat immunosuppressed (due to his psoriasis and methotrexate treatment), and acute-onset illness with fever, fatigue, chest pain, and cough, which all persisted despite antibiotic therapy. The chest x-ray may show an infiltrate, or it may be normal. Laboratory findings often also show new eosinophilia, but this may also be normal. This patient has ongoing symptoms, but they are not worsening, so his disease is relatively mild and uncomplicated, despite his underlying treatment with methotrexate. Serologic testing for *Coccidioides* (IgM and IgG) is often diagnostic in these cases—if the serology is positive, then the patient most likely has active *Coccidioides* infection, because serologic reactivity tends to wane within months of an infection. However, it sometimes takes months for antibody tests to be positive, so sputum culture may be the only way to diagnose early infection. Many patients with this infection will have self-limited disease, often even subclinical. Directed treatment, with antifungals such as itraconazole or liposomal amphotericin, is generally only required in severe, disseminated, or prolonged infection.

Although the fungal antigen 1,3-β-d-glucan (Option B) can be positive in active coccidioidomycosis, it is not a specific test because it can also be positive in the setting of other invasive fungal infections such as disseminated candidiasis and histoplasmosis. CT imaging would similarly be abnormal but not specific for coccidioidomycosis. Hilar lymph node biopsy (Option D) may also reveal the diagnosis but would not be an initial diagnostic test of choice. Serum galactomannan (Option E) is only helpful for making the diagnosis of aspergillosis typically in an immunocompromised host.

Galgiani JN, Ampel NM, Blair JE, et al. 2016 Infectious Diseases Society of America (IDSA) clinical practice guideline for the treatment of coccidioidomycosis. *Clin Infect Dis.* 2016;63:e112–e146.

48. ANSWER: E. Drug–drug interaction of warfarin with rifampin

Rifampin is not a commonly prescribed antibiotic, but it is used in several specific situations and has numerous drug–drug interactions because it is a potent inducer of cytochrome P450 3A. Patient medication lists should be reviewed carefully for potential interactions whenever rifampin is started, and a plan for monitoring or adjustment in treatment should be made whenever possible. In this case, rifampin induces the metabolism of warfarin so that the patient has approximately half the previously available warfarin dose after rifampin is started. If the INR is not monitored carefully in order to facilitate warfarin dose adjustments, then patients will quickly become subtherapeutic in this setting. Even with proper monitoring and dose adjustments, some patients are unable to achieve therapeutic warfarin levels while on rifampin and may require concurrent treatment with enoxaparin or other medications. This patient had a recent transesophageal echocardiogram, which did not show any valvular vegetations or perivalvular abscess, and the blood cultures on this presentation are negative, so there is no evidence to suggest treatment failure at this point. Gentamicin has many associated potential toxicities, but it does not cause stroke. Loss of gut flora while on antibiotic therapy often leads to decreased vitamin K production and therefore hypocoagulable state, rather than hypercoagulable state.

Lee CA, Thrasher KA. Difficulties in anticoagulation management during coadministration of warfarin and rifampin. *Pharmacotherapy.* 2001;21:1240–1246.

49. ANSWER: D. *Francisella tularensis*

Tularemia is the infection caused by *Francisella tularensis*, which is a gram-negative bacterium. People may develop tularemia infection after contact with infected animals or via insect vectors such as ticks. Most of the cases in the United States are reported in Arkansas, Missouri, Kansas, South Dakota, Oklahoma, and California. After exposure, patients may be asymptomatic, or they may develop any one of the six major clinical forms of tularemia: ulceroglandular tularemia, glandular tularemia, oculoglandular tularemia, pharyngeal (oropharyngeal) tularemia, typhoidal tularemia, or pneumonic tularemia. Ulceroglandular and pneumonic tularemia are the two most commonly diagnosed forms of the disease. This patient has pneumonic tularemia. Primary pneumonic disease occurs after inhalation of the organism from a source, such as an infected animal—this is most common among farmers, sheep workers, landscapers, and hunters. Pneumonic tularemia may present similarly to pneumonic plague (caused by *Yersinia pestis*), except that pulmonary disease often consists of peribronchial infiltrates or lobar consolidations in pneumonic tularemia, whereas it is often rounded and cavitated pulmonary infiltrates or nodules in setting of pneumonic plague. Patients may have some laboratory abnormalities, including elevated or depressed WBC and abnormal liver function tests, but laboratory findings may also be normal. Patients may develop respiratory failure and empyema with pneumonic tularemia, and infection may even spread beyond the lungs, with complications such as meningitis and endocarditis. Diagnosis is primarily by serologies and clinical suspicion, but the organism may be cultured (with difficulty) if cultures are specifically requested on cysteine-containing supportive media. When tularemia is suspected, the laboratory must be notified in order to take special precautions because it is highly transmissible in the laboratory setting. Treatment is with doxycycline or ciprofloxacin for mild disease, and with streptomycin or gentamicin for severe disease.

Tropheryma whipplei is the etiologic agent in Whipple disease, which commonly presents with abdominal pain, diarrhea, weight loss, and joint pains. *Babesia microti* is a parasite that is transmitted by ticks primarily in New England and to some extent in the upper Midwest; babesiosis is characterized by fever, anemia, thrombocytopenia, and often respiratory distress, but this patient had no anemia or parasites visualized on initial laboratory findings. *Borrelia lonestari* is thought to be the causative agent in Southern tick–associated rash illness (STARI), which is a Lyme disease–like infection described in patients in the southeastern and south-central United States. *Anaplasma phagocytophilum* causes anaplasmosis, formerly known as human granulocytic ehrlichiosis, which is another tick-borne illness that often presents with fever, headache, and lab abnormalities but rarely causes pulmonary disease.

Centers for Disease Control and Prevention. Tularemia—United States, 2001-2010. *MMWR Morb Mortal Wkly Rep.* 2013;62:963–966.

50. ANSWER: C. Group A streptococci

This patient has a necrotizing soft tissue infection with myonecrosis after blunt trauma. This is most often caused by group A beta-hemolytic streptococci. Treatment is emergent surgical debridement and aggressive antibiotics, preferably with high-dose IV penicillin and clindamycin to reduce toxin formation once the pathogen is identified. If antibiotics are started in the absence of Gram stain results, then a more broad-spectrum regimen would be appropriate until culture data are available, including vancomycin and piperacillin-tazobactam or a carbapenem. Staphylococci, including methicillin-resistant or methicillin-sensitive, can cause necrotizing soft tissue infections, which is more often polymicrobial and purulent as compared with this presentation of "streptococcal gangrene." Necrotizing soft tissue infections can also be caused by polymicrobial flora, which can include *E. coli*, other gram-negative pathogens, and anaerobes; this type of necrotizing skin and soft tissue infection most commonly occurs in the groin and genital area ("Fournier gangrene"). *Clostridium* species including *C. perfringens* and *C. septicum* also cause necrotizing skin and soft tissue infection with gas formation (which was not present in this nonclostridial case) and myonecrosis. *Aeromonas hydrophila* is a rare cause of necrotizing skin and soft tissue infection associated with trauma in or exposed to fresh water. The history for this patient was not consistent with this pathogen.

Stevens DL, Bisno AL, Chambers HF, et al. Practice guidelines for the diagnosis and management of skin and soft tissue infections: 2014 update by the Infectious Diseases Society of America. *Clin Infect Dis.* 2014;59:147–159.

Acknowledgment

The authors and editors gratefully acknowledge the contributions of the previous authors—Michael Calderwood, Rebeca Plank, Dylan Tierney, and Sigal Yawetz.

2 Hematology and Oncology

AMY BESSNOW AND ANN S. LACASCE

1. An 80-year-old man presents with several months of epigastric pain, weight loss, fatigue, and dyspnea. The patient was diagnosed with pernicious anemia 5 years ago and has been receiving regular vitamin B_{12} injections. At that time, he had a colonoscopy, which was notable for extensive sigmoid diverticulosis. His complete blood count (CBC) today reveals a hematocrit of 24% and a mean cell volume (MCV) of 75 fL.

   What malignancy is most likely responsible for his symptoms?
   A. Myelodysplastic syndrome
   B. Gastric cancer
   C. Colon cancer
   D. Mucosa-associated lymphoid tissue (MALT) lymphoma
   E. Pancreatic cancer

2. A 45-year-old man presents with back pain, jaundice, and weight loss of 20 pounds. A CT scan of the abdomen reveals a large mass in the pancreatic head. His cancer antigen (CA) 19-9 is elevated at 496 U/mL. The patient's family history is notable for the following. His father was diagnosed with colon cancer at age 72. His mother is an only child and was diagnosed with breast cancer at age 51. His maternal grandfather died of pancreatic cancer at age 55. His sister was diagnosed with ovarian cancer at 52 and is currently in remission.

   The patient is most likely to have which of the following hereditary cancer syndromes?
   A. Lynch syndrome
   B. *BRCA2* mutation
   C. *CDKN2A* mutation
   D. Li-Fraumeni syndrome
   E. *CDH1* mutation

3. A 60-year-old healthy woman undergoes a CT scan of the abdomen for signs and symptoms of nephrolithiasis. The scan confirms a small right kidney stone but also reveals a 2-cm cystic lesion involving the main pancreatic duct. After spontaneously passing the kidney stone, the patient follows up in your clinic stating that she feels entirely well. She denies jaundice, abdominal or back pain, weight loss, or any other symptoms. Her CA 19-9 is drawn and found to be normal. You refer the patient for magnetic resonance cholangiopancreatography (MRCP), which confirms a 1.9-cm mucinous lesion involving the main pancreatic duct, with classic features of an intraductal papillary mucinous neoplasm of the pancreas (IPMN).

   What is the proper next step in management?
   A. Follow-up CT scan in 6 months
   B. Follow-up MRCP in 6 months
   C. Referral to a pancreatic surgeon for resection
   D. See the patient in 6–12 months to assess symptoms, but obtain no further imaging studies.
   E. This is a benign finding; no specific follow-up is required.

4. A 35-year-old woman originally from the Dominican Republic comes to the clinic for her first visit. She has no significant medical problems and has had two children. After the birth of her second child 3 years ago, she was told to take iron tablets twice daily. Aside from an oral contraceptive, this is her only medication. Results of her laboratory studies are shown in Table 2.1.

   What is the most appropriate management?
   A. Phlebotomy for hemochromatosis
   B. Continue current iron therapy and initiate workup for chronic inflammatory process.
   C. Switch therapy from oral iron sulfate to iron dextran.
   D. Discontinue iron therapy; send for ferritin and hemoglobin electrophoresis.

5. A 74-year-old man with diabetes mellitus controlled with an oral agent presents for routine follow-up. His other medical problems include hypertension, for which he takes an angiotensin-converting enzyme (ACE) inhibitor, and benign prostatic hypertrophy. On review of his records, you note that his hematocrit has been gradually declining over the past 3 years. Results of his laboratory studies are shown in Table 2.2.

   What is the most likely etiology of his anemia?
   A. Combined iron and vitamin B_{12} deficiency
   B. Medication effect from the ACE inhibitor

TABLE 2.1 Laboratory Results for Question 4

White blood cell count	4600/mm³	(4000–10,000)
Hematocrit	35%	(36–48)
Mean cell volume	66 fL	(80–95)
Red blood cell count	6.0	(4.2–5.6)
Platelets	256,000/mm³	(150,000–450,000)
Iron	150 μg/dL	(40–159)
Total iron-binding capacity	275 μg/dL	(250–400)

TABLE 2.2 Laboratory Results for Question 5

White blood cell count	7000/mm³	(4000–10,000)
Hematocrit	28%	(36–48)
Mean cell volume	84 fL	(80–95)
Red blood cell distribution width	15	(10–14.5)
Platelets	340,000/mm³	(150,000–450,000)
Blood urea nitrogen	35 mg/dL	(9–25)
Creatinine	1.9 mg/dL	(0.7–1.3)
Lactate dehydrogenase	230 U/L	(107–231)

C. Erythropoietin deficiency
D. Anemia due to marrow replacement by metastatic prostate cancer

6. A 50-year-old man presents complaining of dyspnea on exertion. He was in a car accident 5 years ago with multiple abdominal injuries, resulting in a splenectomy and a resection of several feet of his terminal ileum. After a prolonged recovery, he returned to work and his normal activities. For the last 4–6 months, he has had trouble climbing the stairs to his bedroom without stopping to catch his breath. He is on no medications, has not lost weight, and has a well-balanced diet (see Table 2.3 for CBC). Peripheral smear showed macrocytic erythrocytes, hypersegmented neutrophils, and decreased platelets.

What is the most likely diagnosis?
A. Myelodysplastic syndrome
B. Vitamin B_{12} deficiency
C. Sideroblastic anemia
D. Hemolytic anemia

7. An 18-year-old woman is referred for the evaluation of mild jaundice. She thinks she has had it intermittently for years. She thinks that she has always tired more easily than her friends, and she has been told several times that she is anemic. She has been treated on several occasions with iron pills, but not in the past 2 years. Her physical examination reveals that she has scleral icterus and a spleen tip palpable below the left costal margin (Table 2.4).

The patient is most likely to respond to which of the following?
A. Corticosteroids
B. Intravenous iron
C. Splenectomy
D. Eculizumab

TABLE 2.3 Complete Blood Count Results for Question 6

Hemoglobin	5.6 g/dL
Hematocrit	17%
Mean cell volume	123 fL
White blood cell count	3500/mm³
Platelets	70,000/μL
Bilirubin	2.3 mg/dL

TABLE 2.4 Laboratory Results for Question 7

Hemoglobin	11.6 g/dL
Hematocrit	31%
Mean cell volume	83 fL
Reticulocytes	7.0%
Platelets	220,000/mm³
White blood cell count	6500/mm³
Blood smear	Spherocytes, increased reticulocytes
Coombs test	Negative

8. A 39-year-old man with sickle cell anemia is admitted for management of pneumonia. He presented with a 2-day history of a dry, nonproductive cough and fever to 101°F, and he was found to have a right lower lobe infiltrate. On admission, his oxygen saturation was 94% on room air, and he was not short of breath. He is placed on cefuroxime and given intravenous hydration (Table 2.5). One day later, he complains of increasing shortness of breath and is found to have an oxygen saturation of 86% on room air. Chest radiography reveals bilateral lower lobe opacities.

What are the best next steps?
A. Continue current antibiotic coverage and administer supplemental O_2.
B. Continue current antibiotic coverage, administer supplemental O_2, and obtain a V/Q scan.

TABLE 2.5 Laboratory Results for Question 8

CBC on Admission		
White blood cell count	18,000/mm^3	(4000–10,000)
Hematocrit	21%	(36–48)
Platelets	247,000/mm^3	(150,000–450,000)

TABLE 2.6 Laboratory Studies in the Emergency Room for Question 9

White blood cell count	14,000/mm^3	(4000–10,000)
Hematocrit	20%	(36–48)
Platelets	317,000/mm^3	(150,000–450,000)
Reticulocyte count	0.3%	(0.6–2.8)
Total bilirubin	1.8 mg/dL	(0.2–1.2)
Direct bilirubin	0.3 mg/dL	(0.0–0.3)
Lactate dehydrogenase	240 U/L	(135–225)

C. Continue current antibiotic coverage, administer supplemental O_2, and transfuse packed red blood cells (PRBCs).
D. Add coverage for atypical organisms and administer supplemental O_2.
E. Add coverage for atypical organisms, administer supplemental O_2, and exchange transfuse.

9. A 54-year-old African American man with sickle cell anemia presents to the emergency room with a 2-day history of fatigue and pain in his back and lower extremities. He scores his pain at 5 out of 10. He has had episodes of pain in the past and is well known to the emergency department staff. His temperature is 99°F, heart rate is 108 beats per minute, blood pressure is 120/70 mm Hg, and oxygen saturation on room air is 96% (see Table 2.6). He is started on intravenous (IV) normal saline and morphine.

What is the best next step?
A. Admit to the hospital and start broad-spectrum antibiotics.
B. Admit to the hospital and transfuse packed red blood cells (PRBCs).
C. Admit to the hospital and arrange for emergent RBC exchange transfusion.
D. Manage pain aggressively and discharge home with close hematology follow-up.
E. Manage pain aggressively and discharge home on oral antibiotics.

10. In which of the following patients should yearly screening with low-dose computed tomography for lung cancer *not* be considered?
A. A 47-year-old woman with a 2-pack-per-day active tobacco use habit and a history of lung cancer in both her mother and father
B. A 57-year-old woman with a history of a 1-pack-per-day tobacco use habit from ages 15 to 50
C. A 70-year-old man with a history of asbestos exposure and 50-pack-year history of cigarette smoking who quit smoking 12 years ago
D. A 75-year-old woman who has smoked a half-pack of cigarettes per day since age 30
E. A 60-year-old man with a 50-pack-year history of cigarette smoking whose last cigarette was after a heart attack at age 50

11. A 47-year-old woman required emergency craniotomy and repair of an aneurysm. On postoperative day 2, she develops left calf pain and is found to have thrombus in the popliteal vessel. Intravenous (IV) unfractionated heparin is started given her recent neurosurgery. Two days later, warfarin is started. On postoperative day 7, she is found to have right leg swelling and dyspnea. Evaluation reveals pulmonary emboli and thrombus in the right common femoral vein. Her platelet count is noted to be 87,000/μL, down from 320,000/μL at the time of surgery.

Next steps in her management include:
A. Immediately stop all heparin exposure, including IV line flush.
B. Start IV direct thrombin inhibitor such as argatroban or bivalirudin.
C. Give 10 mg IV vitamin K to reverse warfarin.
D. Test for heparin-platelet factor 4 antibodies.
E. All of the above

12. A 32-year-old woman 8 weeks postpartum is seen by her obstetrician for fevers, fatigue, and bruising. In addition to elevated temperature as well as some bruises and petechiae on examination, she is found to have a hematocrit of 21%, platelet count of 23,000/μL, and creatinine of 2.4 mg/dL. Values at time of delivery were normal. While waiting to get more laboratory serum tests, she develops right arm weakness and confusion. She is sent directly to the emergency room and admitted to the intensive care unit.

What should your immediate next step be?
A. Request neurology consult for electroencephalogram (EEG).
B. Transfuse with platelets.
C. Give IV fluids for dehydration.
D. Check peripheral smear and find schistocytes; initiate plasmapheresis.
E. Send for ADAMTS13 level and wait for results before treating.

13. A 39-year-old man is seen by a new primary care physician. "von Willebrand disease (vWD)" is listed in his past medical history, but the patient does not know many details of this. He had an episode of gastrointestinal (GI) bleeding in college requiring hospitalization and RBC transfusion when taking nonsteroidal antiinflammatory drugs (NSAIDs). He was told he has vWD and to avoid aspirin and NSAIDs. Review of systems is negative for recent episodes of bleeding, bruising, or epistaxis. His father has had some bleeding episodes in the past.
   What tests do you send to evaluate for vWD?
   A. Factor VIII activity
   B. vWF antigen level
   C. Ristocetin cofactor
   D. vWF multimer gel electrophoretic analysis
   E. All of the above

14. A 43-year-old woman undergoes elective cholecystectomy for gallstones. Her past medical history is unremarkable, and she is on no medications. On postoperative day 4, she develops left lower-extremity calf pain and is found to have popliteal vein thrombus by compression ultrasound (US). She has no past history of thrombosis. She weighs 68 kg and has normal renal function.
   Which is the best treatment option?
   A. Compression stockings
   B. Aspirin 325 mg once daily
   C. Low-molecular-weight heparin overlapping with warfarin targeting international normalized ratio 1.5–2.0
   D. Rivaroxaban 15 mg twice daily × 3 weeks, then 20 mg once daily
   E. Intravenous unfractionated heparin (IV UFH)

15. The patient in Question 14 has no past history of thrombosis, despite two pregnancies. Her father had a deep vein thrombosis (DVT) at age 43, and his father had a pulmonary embolism in his 60s. She has two daughters, ages 12 and 15.
   She should be tested for thrombophilia:
   A. True
   B. False

16. A 32-year-old woman undergoes laparoscopic resection of a benign complex ovarian cyst by her gynecologist. One week later she presents complaining of increasing lower back and abdominal pain. On examination, she has a 7-cm × 4-cm subfascial hematoma from the umbilicus to the right lower quadrant and a 6-cm × 3-cm suprapubic ecchymosis. Her prothrombin time (PT) is 12.3 seconds (normal 11.2–13.4 seconds), and her activated partial thromboplastin time (aPTT) is 72.4 seconds (normal 23.8–36.6 seconds). Repeat testing reveals PT 12.8 seconds and aPTT 81.5 seconds.
   What is the next test to evaluate an isolated elevated aPTT?
   A. Factor XIII level
   B. Fibrinogen
   C. Mixing study
   D. Platelet aggregation studies
   E. D-Dimer

17. A 63-year-old man with type 2 diabetes mellitus and hypertension presents with recurrent painless hematuria. He undergoes a CT scan of the abdomen and pelvis, which shows an enhancing 6.3-cm left kidney mass highly suspicious for a renal cell carcinoma. There were multiple retroperitoneal enlarged lymph nodes, and the lung bases showed four or five pulmonary nodules, with the largest measuring 1.1 cm. The patient has a good performance status. His CBC and comprehensive metabolic panel (CMP) results were within normal limits, except for a hemoglobin of 11.5 g/dL.
   The next steps would include all *except:*
   A. Biopsy of the kidney mass
   B. Biopsy of the lung lesions
   C. Chest CT, brain magnetic resonance imaging (MRI), bone scan
   D. Initiating sunitinib or pazopanib
   E. Proceed with cytoreductive nephrectomy.

18. A 72-year-old man who is an active smoker presents with dysuria and vague abdominal/pelvic pain. His urinalysis reveals 10–20 RBCs/high-power field. He undergoes an abdominal ultrasound that is unremarkable except for potential thickening of the bladder wall on the left side. Cystoscopy shows a 5-cm bladder mass. The patient undergoes transurethral resection of bladder tumor (TURBT), which reveals high-grade urothelial cancer with focal invasion into the lamina propria. No muscle is available in the specimen.
   The next step would be:
   A. Radical cystectomy
   B. Partial cystectomy (left bladder wall)
   C. Proceed with bacille Calmette-Guérin (BCG) immunotherapy.
   D. Repeat TURBT
   E. Chemoradiation to the bladder mass

19. A 51-year-old woman presents with recurrent urinary tract infections (UTIs) for the past 6 months and pelvic pain for 6 weeks. A CT scan of her pelvis shows a large bladder mass. Cystoscopy followed by TURBT shows a poorly differentiated urothelial carcinoma. Tumor is invading into the muscularis propria. Chest and abdominal CT do not show distant metastases or enlarged lymph nodes. Her serum creatinine is 0.75 mg/dL. Her bone scan is normal. The patient has an excellent performance status.
   Which is the correct statement?
   A. Neoadjuvant cisplatin-based chemotherapy is indicated based on a 15% absolute reduction in death.
   B. Adjuvant cisplatin-based chemotherapy is indicated based on a 15% absolute reduction in death.

C. Neoadjuvant cisplatin-based chemotherapy is indicated based on a 5% absolute reduction in death.
D. Adjuvant cisplatin-based chemotherapy is indicated based on a 5% absolute reduction in death.
E. Proceed with radical cystectomy.

20. A 59-year-old man, previously healthy and taking only one 81-mg aspirin per day, was referred for prostate biopsy after a screening showed a serum prostate-specific antigen (PSA) of 4.8 ng/mL and unremarkable digital rectal examination (DRE). A 12-core needle biopsy was performed, revealing two cores on the left with Gleason 3 + 3 adenocarcinoma involving up to 20% of each core. All other cores showed no evidence of disease. The patient asks you about imaging to complete his diagnostic workup.
What would you advise?
A. Endorectal coil MRI only
B. CT scan of the abdomen/pelvis only
C. Bone scan only
D. CT scan of the abdomen/pelvis and bone scan
E. No further workup necessary

21. A 61-year-old man presents with a history of hypertension and hyperlipidemia, and he is taking aspirin, hydrochlorothiazide, and simvastatin daily. He has been undergoing PSA screening. His digital rectal examination has been normal, but a recent PSA of 5.4 ng/mL prompted a prostate biopsy. Biopsy demonstrated 1 of 12 cores positive for Gleason 4 + 3 prostate cancer involving 15% of the core. His urologist ordered an endorectal coil MRI that showed a 1.6-cm left-sided lesion suspicious for tumor. There was no evidence of extracapsular extension, seminal vesicle involvement, or enlarged lymph nodes. A bone scan was also ordered, but it showed no evidence of metastases. The patient is anxious about the side effects associated with prostate cancer treatment and asks for your guidance.
Which of the following is *not* a recommended option for primary management of this patient's prostate cancer?
A. Active surveillance
B. Radical prostatectomy
C. External beam radiation therapy
D. Interstitial brachytherapy
E. All of the options above are acceptable.

22. A 66-year-old man presented with hip pain and was ultimately diagnosed with prostate cancer that had metastasized to the ribs and pelvic bones. His PSA at the time of diagnosis was 180 ng/mL. He was started on androgen deprivation therapy with leuprolide, a gonadotropin-releasing hormone (GnRH) agonist. After 6 months on treatment, his pain resolved and his PSA has decreased to 0.8 ng/mL. He presents to the clinic to discuss side effects of his therapy.
Which of the following is *not* a risk associated with androgen deprivation therapy?
A. Osteoporosis and bone fracture
B. Prolactinoma
C. Hot flashes
D. Anemia
E. Increase in subcutaneous adipose tissue

23. Immune therapy with programmed death receptor 1 (PD-1) inhibition can be effective and is often well tolerated in patients with a variety of advanced malignancies. In which of the following patients should immune therapy with PD-1 inhibition *not* be considered?
A. A patient with metastatic squamous cell carcinoma of the epiglottis that recurs after platinum-based therapy and unknown tumor programmed death receptor ligand 1 (PD-L1) expression
B. A patient with newly diagnosed metastatic nonsmall cell lung cancer, poor performance status, and 10% tumor PD-L1 expression
C. A patient with metastatic nonsmall cell lung cancer refractory to platinum-based chemotherapy and 0% tumor PD-L1 expression
D. A 30-year-old patient with recurrent classic Hodgkin lymphoma after autologous transplant and brentuximab vedotin
E. An elderly patient with metastatic melanoma and heart disease

24. A 76-year-old woman with stage IV nonsmall cell lung cancer has been receiving nivolumab for the past 3 months after her disease recurred following chemotherapy with carboplatin and pemetrexed. She was feeling quite well, but a few days after her last infusion she calls to report rapidly progressive shortness of breath and dry cough over the past 24 hours. On evaluation, she has no fever, she is tachycardic to the 110s, her blood pressure is mildly elevated at 155/90 mm Hg, and she her respiratory rate is 22 breaths per minute. Her lungs are clear to auscultation bilaterally, and she is able to speak in full sentences easily, although she becomes dyspneic walking briskly across the room. She is referred to the ER, where her chest radiograph is unremarkable and electrocardiogram shows only tachycardia. Pulmonary embolism (PE)-protocol CT is without visualized clot but is notable for diffuse ground-glass opacities and areas of mildly increased interstitial markings.
Which of the following interventions is indicated?
A. A course of antibiotics for suspected pneumonia
B. Enoxaparin for suspected small-vessel PE
C. Prednisone at least 1 mg/kg or equivalent
D. A and C
E. A course of antibiotics and inhaled corticosteroids

25. A 40-year-old woman with a strong family history of breast cancer is considering taking tamoxifen for chemoprevention. She calls to discuss potential side effects of the medication. She reports she does not want to experience premature menopause, weight gain, or depression.

What do you advise her?

A. Tamoxifen causes none of these side effects.
B. She should take raloxifene instead.
C. She should take exemestane instead.
D. Tamoxifen may cause weight gain and depression, but not premature menopause.
E. She should wait until after menopause to start tamoxifen.

26. A 68-year-old man with a 40-pack-year smoking history and chronic obstructive pulmonary disease (COPD) presented to his local emergency room after falling on his bathroom rug and hitting his head and right ribs. A noncontrast head CT scan did not show evidence of bleeding. A chest radiograph did not show any broken ribs, but it did incidentally show a spiculated right upper lobe lung mass measuring 3.6 × 2.4 cm. A subsequent biopsy confirms nonsmall cell lung cancer.

Which of the following radiographic studies is *not* recommended as part of a subsequent staging evaluation?

A. Brain MRI with gadolinium
B. Chest CT with IV contrast
C. Positron emission tomography (PET)-CT
D. Skeletal survey with plain films

27. A 63-year-old woman who had smoked two packs of cigarettes daily for 30 years presents with several weeks of increasing cough and dyspnea with exertion, followed over the last few days with lethargy and swelling of her face and arms. Initial evaluation in the emergency room reveals a serum sodium of 120 mEq/L, blood urea nitrogen (BUN) 17 mg/dL, and creatinine 0.8 mg/dL. Chest CT with IV contrast is negative for pulmonary embolus but demonstrates a 5.5-cm right hilar mass with associated mediastinal adenopathy and compression of the superior vena cava; furthermore, there appear to be multiple osseous and hepatic metastases.

What is the most likely diagnosis?

A. Breast cancer
B. Bronchial carcinoid tumor
C. Non-Hodgkin lymphoma
D. Small cell lung cancer
E. Thymoma

28. A 70-year-old man with a history of kidney stones and a 20-pack-year smoking history underwent CT of the abdomen as part of an evaluation for flank pain. CT demonstrated recurrence of nephrolithiasis but also demonstrated an incidental, peripheral, 5-mm left lower lobe (LLL) lung nodule. Chest CT was performed and again showed the small LLL nodule but did not demonstrate other nodules or mediastinal or hilar adenopathy.

What is the most appropriate next step for follow-up of the lung nodule?

A. Repeat chest CT in 3 months
B. Repeat chest CT in 6 months
C. Repeat chest CT in 2 years
D. PET/CT now
E. Referral for CT-guided biopsy

29. A 58-year-old woman with minimal prior medical history and with good performance status is found to have a new 2.2-cm peripheral right lower lobe mass. Complete staging evaluation demonstrates only the solitary lung mass, with no other sites of disease in the mediastinum or distantly. CT-guided biopsy confirms a diagnosis of nonsmall cell lung cancer, adenocarcinoma histology.

What is the most appropriate next step in management?

A. Chemotherapy
B. Cryoablation
C. Repeat CT scan in 6 months
D. Stereotactic radiation
E. Surgical resection

30. A 25-year-old woman presents with a dry cough, intermittent drenching night sweats, and diffuse pruritus without identifiable rash. On physical examination, she appears tired. Her vital signs are notable for a temperature of 99.9°F, heart rate of 110 beats per minute, blood pressure of 100/80 mm Hg, respiratory rate of 18 breaths per minute, and oxygen saturation of 98% on room air. Her physical examination is notable for the absence of peripheral lymphadenopathy. Her chest is clear to auscultation bilaterally. Cardiac examination reveals tachycardia with a soft systolic ejection murmur. She had no splenomegaly. Her lower extremities are notable for linear excoriations. Laboratory studies reveal a white blood cell count of 14,300/μL with 80% neutrophils and 5% lymphocytes, 10% eosinophils, and 5% monocytes. Her basic metabolic panel is normal.

What is the next most appropriate step in her management?

A. Obtain a lactate dehydrogenase (LDH) level.
B. Order a PET/CT scan.
C. Refer to dermatology for evaluation.
D. Obtain a chest x-ray.
E. Send for Epstein-Barr virus (EBV) serologies.

31. A 70-year-old man presents to the emergency department for evaluation of upper respiratory symptoms with low-grade fevers. He appears clinically well. His physical examination is notable for a 1-cm palpable lymph nodes in the bilateral neck and axilla. His spleen tip is palpable just below the left costal margin.

Laboratory studies reveal a white blood cell count of 18,000/μL with 75% lymphocytes, with smudge cells, 15% neutrophils, and 5% monocytes. His chemistries are normal, including LDH.

What is the next most appropriate step?

A. Obtain peripheral blood flow cytometry.
B. Refer for excisional lymph node biopsy.
C. Order a PET/CT to evaluate the best node for biopsy.
D. Perform a bone marrow aspiration and biopsy.
E. Treat with antibiotics and recheck CBC in 1 month.

32. A 65-year-old woman presents complaining of a mass in the left neck without fevers, night sweats, weight loss, or localizing symptoms. On examination, she has normal vital signs and is found to have a 2.5-cm left anterior cervical node, a 2-cm left axillary node, and a 3-cm right inguinal node. Her examination is otherwise normal. Laboratory studies, including a CBC with differential, basic metabolic panel, and LDH, are normal.

What is the next most appropriate step in her management?

A. Refer to interventional radiology for a needle biopsy of the most easily accessible lymph node.
B. Refer to otolaryngology for fine-needle aspiration of the neck mass.
C. Refer to a surgeon for an excisional lymph node biopsy.
D. Obtain a PET/CT scan.
E. Send for peripheral blood flow cytometry.

33. A 66-year-old postmenopausal woman with hypertension and hypothyroid is diagnosed with stage IA ER/PR-positive, HER2/neu-negative invasive ductal carcinoma. She undergoes lumpectomy followed by radiation, and chemotherapy is deferred based on a low risk of recurrence and low likelihood of benefit. She is started on an aromatase inhibitor (AI).

For which of the following is she now at significantly increased risk due to her aromatase inhibitor?

A. DVT/PE
B. Hypothyroid
C. Osteoporosis
D. Endometrial cancer
E. Glucose intolerance

34. A 35-year-old woman with a history of regular menses presents with complaints of bilateral galactorrhea. She notes that her menses have been more irregular over the last year and that her last menstrual period was approximately 6 weeks ago. She reports occasional headaches but otherwise feels well. She does not take any medication or herbal supplements. Laboratory testing reveals a negative pregnancy test, thyroid-stimulating hormone (TSH) of 2.2 mIU/L, and prolactin of 360 ng/mL. You suspect a prolactinoma and order a pituitary MRI, which reveals a 10-mm × 12-mm pituitary lesion. There is no cavernous sinus invasion or compression of the optic nerves by the pituitary tumor.

You advise the patient that the initial treatment of choice is:

A. Medical therapy with a somatostatin analogue
B. Observation only
C. Transsphenoidal pituitary tumor resection
D. Medical therapy with a dopamine agonist
E. Radiation therapy to the pituitary

35. Which of the following antidepressants is preferred in women taking tamoxifen for hormone receptor–positive breast cancer?

A. Paroxetine
B. Fluoxetine
C. Venlafaxine
D. Bupropion
E. Duloxetine

36. Which of the following patients would be a good candidate for novel oral anticoagulant (NOAC) therapy?

A. A 65-year-old woman with rheumatic heart disease and a metal prosthetic mitral valve
B. A 35-year-old woman with a newly diagnosed PE, history of multiple second-trimester pregnancy losses, and positive antiphospholipid antibodies
C. A 60-year-old man with new-onset nonvalvular atrial fibrillation and a history of a diverticular bleed 5 years ago
D. A 60-year-old man with a newly diagnosed PE and metastatic nonsmall cell lung cancer
E. A 60-year-old man with newly diagnosed DVT and renal insufficiency

37. A 64-year-old woman presents with abdominal bloating, early satiety, and constipation. On bimanual exam, an enlarged right ovary is noted. Ultrasound demonstrates a complex 10-cm × 8-cm mass highly concerning for malignancy as well as a moderate amount of free fluid in the pelvis.

Which of the following is *not* potentially indicated?

A. Abdominal/pelvic CT
B. Laboratory testing for cancer antigen 125 (CA-125)
C. Colonoscopy
D. Referral to gynecologic oncology for consideration of surgery
E. Referral to interventional radiology for needle-guided biopsy of the adnexal mass

38. A 22-year-old man presents with headache and peripheral vision loss. Brain imaging reveals a large sellar mass with both solid and cystic components that is compressing the optic chiasm. Humphrey visual field testing demonstrates bitemporal hemianopsia. He has no previous medical history, his body mass index (BMI) is 20 kg/m^2, and he is taking no medications. His initial pituitary functional evaluation revealed central hypogonadism and central hypothyroidism. His adrenal function was normal. MRI characteristics suggested the mass was a craniopharyngioma. He was taken to surgery to remove the pituitary mass in attempts to decompress the optic chiasm and restore his vision. He did well in the immediate postoperative period, but within 24 hours, he began to develop polyuria. His urine output increased to 400 mL/h and was very dilute with a urine specific gravity of less than 1.001. He complained of extreme thirst. His serum sodium increased to 148 mEq/L, and his fasting glucose was elevated at 106 mg/dL.

What diagnosis are you suspecting in this patient?

A. Syndrome of inappropriate antidiuretic hormone secretion (SIADH)
B. Diabetes mellitus, type 2
C. Central diabetes insipidus
D. Nephrogenic diabetes insipidus
E. None of the above

39. A 55-year-old woman was involved in a motor vehicle accident as an unrestrained driver. Although she did not lose consciousness, she sustained a significant head trauma and was brought by ambulance to the emergency department. She was evaluated and found to have a normal neurologic examination, but due to the mechanism of her accident, brain imaging by noncontrast CT scan was performed. She was incidentally found to have a large sellar lesion, estimated at approximately 2 cm in greatest diameter. No acute intracranial hemorrhage was identified. She had a laceration on her forehead that was repaired, and because she was otherwise clinically stable, she was discharged with a plan to follow up with her primary care provider for further evaluation of this pituitary mass.

In evaluating a patient with a newly discovered pituitary mass, what are the important initial clinical considerations?

A. Evaluation for mass effects (headaches, visual loss, cranial nerve abnormalities)
B. Evaluation for pituitary hormonal hypersecretion
C. Evaluation for pituitary hormonal hypofunction
D. All of the above
E. None of the above

40. A 22-year-old college student notes increasing fatigue over the past few weeks that she attributes to staying up late studying for final examinations. Over the past 2–3 days she has noted several new bruises on her upper and lower extremities. She does not recall antecedent trauma leading to the bruising. This morning she developed a bloody nose lasting 20 minutes. She presents to Student Health for evaluation. Her physical examination is notable for scattered, quarter-sized bruises on her upper arms and thighs. Laboratory studies are notable for a white blood cell count of 500/μL, hemoglobin of 7 g/dL, and platelets of 50,000/μL. A peripheral smear is notable for 80% large atypical cells with folded, bilobed, kidney-shaped nucleoli and elongated, bluish-red rods within the cytoplasm.

What translocation is the defining feature of this disease?

A. t(11;14)
B. t(15;17)
C. t(9;22)
D. t(8;14)
E. t(14;18)

41. A 65-year-old man with past medical history of hypertension presents to his primary care physician (PCP) with several weeks of fatigue and dyspnea on exertion (DOE). He notes feeling more winded during his 3-mile walks. His vital signs are stable. His blood pressure is 120/60 mm Hg, and his O_2 saturation is 97% on room air. He had no hepatosplenomegaly. His complete blood count is notable for white blood cell count of 4000/μL with 60% neutrophils, hemoglobin of 9 g/dL, and platelets of 110,000/μL. The laboratory findings are notable for a vitamin B_{12} of 700 pg/mol, folate of 20 ng/mL, TSH of 1.2 mIU/mL, testosterone of 400 ng/dL, and erythropoietin of 90 U/L. A bone marrow biopsy is done and is remarkable for dysplastic erythroid precursors and megakaryocytes with 1% blasts. Cytogenetics are normal. He has 2 points—1 for Hgb of 9 g/dL and 1 for normal cytogenetics—based on his Revised International Prognostic Scoring System (IPSS-R) score.

What would be the most appropriate recommendation for therapy for his myelodysplastic syndrome?

A. Allogeneic stem cell transplant
B. Induction chemotherapy with an anthracycline + cytarabine
C. Lenalidomide
D. Erythropoiesis-stimulating agent (ESA)
E. No treatment necessary

42. A 35-year-old woman presents to her PCP for her annual visit. She has been feeling well. She denies fevers, night sweats, and weight loss. She denies GI symptoms, including nausea, vomiting, abdominal pain, and early satiety. She denies easy bleeding, bruising, or history of clots. On examination, her spleen is palpable two fingerbreadths below the costal margin. A complete blood count is notable for a white blood cell count of 60,000/μL, hemoglobin of 10 g/dL, and platelets of 600,000/μL. Review of the peripheral smear is notable for a large percentage of basophils and eosinophils, along with myelocytes and metamyelocytes. JAK2 V617F mutation is negative.

What is the most appropriate next step in management?

A. Start hydroxyurea.
B. Check blood cultures and start empiric antibiotics for possible infection.
C. Start high-dose aspirin (325 mg twice daily).
D. Send peripheral blood for cytogenetics to evaluate for the t(9;22) chromosome translocation.
E. Determine a leukocyte alkaline phosphatase (LAP) score.

43. A 60-year-old woman with past medical history of hypertension and COPD is brought to the emergency room by her daughter. She is lethargic and is having difficulty walking. She has noted increasing difficulty breathing over the past few hours. Her physical examination is notable for temperature of 100.7°F, blood pressure of 150/70 mm Hg, respiratory rate of 24 breaths per minute, and O_2 saturation of 88% on room air. She has difficulty with finger-to-nose and rapid alternating movements. She has fine crackles bilaterally. A complete blood count is notable for a white blood cell count of 110×10^6, hemoglobin of 8, and platelets of 75,000/μL. A chest x-ray shows bilateral infiltrates.

What would be the appropriate next step in management of this patient?

A. Give a unit of PRBCs.
B. Start antibiotics for possible pneumonia and follow for symptom improvement before initiating more invasive procedures.
C. Start steroids and antibiotics for COPD flare.
D. Start leukapheresis while establishing diagnosis.
E. Establish diagnosis and start appropriate therapy.

44. A 32-year-old woman presents in active labor on a Friday evening. She tells the admitting obstetrician who is covering for a group practice that she has a history of heavy periods and mucosal bleeding and was told she has von Willebrand disease. She uses a nasal inhaler at the start of her periods, and it reduces bleeding. Her mother and sister have similar bleeding histories. You find laboratory values done prior to her pregnancy showing vWF antigen of 42%, vWF activity of 38%, and factor VIII of 49%. All of these are below the lower limits of normal. There is a note stating that the values are compatible with type I von Willebrand disease.

Which of the following statements is/are true?

A. von Willebrand factor levels go down during pregnancy.
B. Placement of an epidural catheter is contraindicated in a patient with von Willebrand disease.
C. The correct treatment would be infusion of recombinant coagulation factor VIIa (NovoSeven).
D. von Willebrand factor levels become normal during pregnancy in patients with type I disease.
E. Despite normal vWF levels, pregnant women with vWD have increased risk of bleeding during delivery and should be treated prophylactically with Humate-P.

45. A 68-year-old lifelong-nonsmoking woman in excellent general health is brought to the ER after seizure-like activity was observed by her family during dinner. She is somnolent on arrival but within 30 minutes is alert and oriented and without focal neurologic findings. Noncontrast head CT shows no bleed, and brain MRI with and without contrast demonstrates three foci of enhancement measuring up to 2 cm and located in the right parietal, occipital, and left frontal lobes. There is surrounding vasogenic edema, particularly of the largest lesion in the left frontal cortex. However, there is no mass effect or shift. CT of the chest, abdomen, and pelvis demonstrate a spiculated left upper lobe lung mass and multiple bony lesions. Biopsy of the left upper lobe mass demonstrates poorly differentiated adenocarcinoma consistent with lung primary.

Which step would *not* be included in the management of this patient?

A. Radiation oncology consultation for consideration of urgent whole-brain radiotherapy (WBRT)
B. Intravenous dexamethasone
C. Initiation of levetiracetam
D. Radiation oncology consultation for consideration of stereotactic radiosurgery (SRS)
E. Molecular testing of tumor specimen for targetable mutations

46. In which of the following patients would you be most concerned about initiating therapy with ibrutinib for symptomatic chronic lymphocytic leukemia (CLL)?

A. A patient with bulky nodal disease and anemia
B. A patient with a p53 mutation and rapid disease recurrence after fludarabine, cyclophosphamide, and rituximab
C. A patient with a history of pneumocystis pneumonia and recurrent varicella zoster virus infections
D. A patient with poorly controlled atrial fibrillation and platelets of 20,000/μL
E. A patient with a history of immune colitis

47. Your patient is a 56-year-old schoolteacher who presented with about 2 months' history of intermittent blood in the toilet bowl with bowel movements. A colonoscopy is performed that demonstrates a mass in the midsigmoid, and biopsy confirms adenocarcinoma. He undergoes laparoscopic hemicolectomy, and final pathology reveals a 3-cm, moderately differentiated adenocarcinoma invading through the muscle layer into the serosa with two of nine lymph nodes positive.

What would be the next step?

A. Reoperate for more complete lymph node dissection.
B. Referral to medical oncologist for consideration of chemotherapy

C. Follow-up colonoscopy in 1 year
D. Referral to radiation oncologist for postoperative radiation

48. A 42-year-old man newly diagnosed with Burkitt lymphoma presents to the emergency room 3 days after beginning chemotherapy. He complains of decreased urine output. Laboratory data show serum potassium of 6.5 mg/dL, BUN of 48 mg/dL, serum creatinine of 2.4 mg/dL, uric acid of 10.9 mg/dL, and phosphorus of 6.4 mg/dL, with uric acid crystals on his urinalysis. He is already on allopurinol.
What treatment is *least* likely to be effective at this point?
A. Hydration and furosemide, monitoring urine output and weight to maintain euvolemia
B. Acute management of hyperkalemia with calcium gluconate and insulin and dextrose
C. Initiation of hemodialysis if diuresis does not occur
D. A recombinant uricase, such as rasburicase
E. Increase in dose of allopurinol

49. A 69-year-old man with prostate cancer and widespread bone metastases complains of worsening lumbosacral back pain for 2 weeks. His physical examination is normal except for localized tenderness over L4, with no neurologic deficits.
What is the best next step?
A. Increase his scheduled pain medications and see him for follow-up in 1 month.
B. Arrange for an urgent MRI of the spine to evaluate for possible cord compression.
C. Arrange for radiation therapy within 24 hours for probable cord compression.
D. Emergency neurosurgical evaluation for suspected spinal cord compression

50. Which one of the following statements is true regarding superior vena cava (SVC) syndrome?
A. Establishing a tissue diagnosis is the most important step in management of most patients with SVC syndrome.
B. SVC syndrome should be treated with IV thrombolytics and stenting of the vena cava.
C. Diagnosis is usually established by chest x-ray, then venography if needed.
D. Breast cancer and germ cell tumors are the most common malignant causes of SVC syndrome.

Chapter 2 Answers

1. **ANSWER: B. Gastric cancer**
Pernicious anemia is an autoimmune disorder that is characterized by autoantibodies against intrinsic factor, destruction of gastric parietal cells, vitamin B_{12} deficiency, and gastric achlorhydria. Over time, the condition progresses to chronic atrophic gastritis, intestinal metaplasia, dysplasia, and ultimately gastric adenocarcinoma. The patient described here has developed occult upper gastrointestinal (GI) bleeding from gastric cancer, stemming from long-standing pernicious anemia and atrophic gastritis. Myelodysplastic syndrome has not been associated with pernicious anemia, nor is it associated with iron deficiency. Although the patient likely has iron-deficiency anemia, pernicious anemia is also not associated with colon cancer. Additionally, an advanced colon cancer would be unlikely, given the patient's colonoscopy findings 5 years previously. MALT lymphoma is highly linked to *Helicobacter pylori* infection, not pernicious anemia. Although some reports indicate an increased risk of pancreatic cancer associated with pernicious anemia, pancreatic cancer would not cause iron-deficiency anemia.

2. **ANSWER: B. *BRCA2* mutation**
This patient presents with a likely diagnosis of pancreatic adenocarcinoma. In addition to his young age, his family history raises concern for a possible hereditary cancer syndrome. The patient's maternal family history, including early breast cancer, ovarian cancer, and pancreatic cancer, is highly suggestive of *BRCA* mutation. Both *BRCA1* and *BRCA2* mutations are associated with increased risk of pancreatic cancer, but *BRCA2* is much more strongly associated. *BRCA2* mutation is thought to be responsible for approximately 15% of familial pancreatic cancer. Although Lynch syndrome (hereditary nonpolyposis colorectal cancer [HNPCC]) is associated with a modestly increased risk of pancreatic cancer, his father's diagnosis of colon cancer at age 72 is not highly suggestive of Lynch syndrome. Li-Fraumeni syndrome results from a mutation in the *p53* tumor suppressor gene, and it is most notably associated with early diagnosis of sarcoma, brain tumors, breast cancer, and leukemia, but not pancreatic cancer. Mutations in *CDKN2A* result in the familial atypical multiple-mole melanoma syndrome, which is associated with markedly increased risk of melanoma and pancreatic cancer. Germline mutations in CDH1 (E-cadherin) are associated with a very high risk of diffuse gastric cancer and breast cancer, but not pancreatic cancer.

3. **ANSWER: C. Referral to a pancreatic surgeon for resection**
The patient was incidentally found on an imaging study to have a main duct IPMN. IPMNs are premalignant lesions of the pancreatic ductal epithelium, which have the potential to progress to pancreatic adenocarcinoma. IPMNs involving the side branches of the pancreatic ductal system (so-called branch duct

IPMNs) carry an approximate 10%–20% risk of progressing to pancreatic cancer. For patients with branch duct IPMNs who do not wish to have surgery, active surveillance with serial MRI or pancreas protocol CT is considered an acceptable option. This patient has an IPMN of the main pancreatic duct, which carries approximately a 70% risk of progression to pancreatic adenocarcinoma. For this reason, all patients diagnosed with a main duct IPMN, without significant contraindications to surgery, should be referred to an experienced pancreatic surgeon for consideration of resection.

Tanaka M, Fernández-del Castillo C, Adsay V, et al. International consensus guidelines 2012 for the management of IPMN and MCN of the pancreas. *Pancreatology.* 2012;12(3):183–197.

4. **ANSWER: D. Discontinue iron therapy; send for ferritin and hemoglobin electrophoresis.**

This young woman has a microcytic anemia despite 3 years of oral iron therapy. Because patients are frequently noncompliant with oral iron, one must always consider that the patient has not taken the medication. Although the best measure of iron stores would be to check serum ferritin, her iron and total iron-binding capacity (TIBC) show an iron saturation of over 50%, so it seems unlikely that she remains iron deficient. A ferritin level will allow you to determine if she is iron replete or iron overloaded. The profound microcytosis in the face of a near-normal hematocrit, mildly elevated RBC count, and presumed adequate iron stores should lead one to consider a diagnosis of thalassemia minor. Indeed, an MCV this low is extremely rare in iron deficiency and would never occur in the absence of profound anemia. Beta-thalassemia minor can be diagnosed by hemoglobin electrophoresis, and it is established by the demonstration of an elevated hemoglobin A_2 (>4%). Given the minimal anemia, it is even more likely that this represents alpha-thalassemia, which can be diagnosed only by DNA studies, because it does not result in an abnormal hemoglobin electrophoresis.

Peters M, Heijboer H, Smiers F, Giordano PC. Diagnosis and management of thalassaemia. *BMJ.* 2012;344:e228.

5. **ANSWER: C. Erythropoietin deficiency**

The patient has a normochromic, normocytic anemia. The most likely reason for the gradual decrement in his hematocrit is that he has had a gradual decline in his erythropoietin level coincident with his moderate renal insufficiency. This can be readily assessed by checking an erythropoietin level, which should be several hundred with a hemoglobin/hematocrit in this range.

Although this could be a result of combined iron and vitamin B_{12} deficiency, one would expect the red blood cell distribution width (RDW) to be abnormally high. Furthermore, vitamin B_{12} deficiency (which can be a complication of metformin) should also depress the white blood cell count and the platelet count. ACE inhibitors are not typically associated with anemia. In a patient with benign prostatic hypertrophy, the sudden development of prostate cancer leading to marrow infiltration and anemia with a normal white count and platelet count and a normal lactate dehydrogenase (LDH) would seem highly unlikely.

6. **ANSWER: B. Vitamin B_{12} deficiency**

This patient has megaloblastic anemia secondary to malabsorption of vitamin B_{12}, which is absorbed in the terminal ileum. Because people with a good diet usually have substantial body stores of vitamin B_{12}, patients typically do not develop vitamin B_{12} deficiency until several years following failure of vitamin B_{12} absorption. Megaloblastic anemia causes pancytopenia because the failure of DNA synthesis affects all rapidly dividing cells. Patients may also have mouth ulcers, symptoms of malabsorption, smooth tongue, and neurologic abnormalities.

Sideroblastic anemia typically presents with a microcytic anemia. Hemolytic anemia should not cause leukopenia or thrombocytopenia. Although myelodysplasia can be associated with macrocytosis, it rarely causes an MCV over 100–110 fL. Furthermore, although you may see pseudo Pelger-Huët anomaly (bilobed neutrophils) in the neutrophils in patients with myelodysplastic syndrome, hypersegmented polys are seen only in megaloblastic anemia.

Stabler SP. Vitamin B_{12} deficiency. *N Engl J Med.* 2013; 368(21):149–160.

7. **ANSWER: C. Splenectomy**

The patient has anemia with increased reticulocytes, and spherocytes are seen on the peripheral smear. The diagnostic distinction to be made is between a congenital hemolytic anemia and an immune hemolytic anemia. The patient's long history of jaundice and the relatively well-compensated hemolysis is most suggestive of hereditary spherocytosis. Hereditary spherocytosis, if severe enough to require therapy, responds very well to splenectomy.

The negative Coombs test makes autoimmune hemolytic anemia (AIHA) unlikely, although about 10% of patients with AIHA may have a negative Coombs test. Steroids are the preferred first-line therapy for AIHA. The reticulocytosis makes iron deficiency extremely unlikely. Although hemolysis is the hallmark of paroxysmal nocturnal hemoglobinuria (PNH), patients with PNH have intravascular hemolysis secondary to surface activation of complement and therefore do not present with spherocytes in the peripheral blood.

8. ANSWER: E. Add coverage for atypical organisms and administer supplemental O_2, and exchange transfusion.

The patient presented with a clearly defined right lower lobar pneumonia that progressed to acute chest syndrome (ACS). ACS is an acute illness characterized by a constellation of fever, chest pain, shortness of breath, hypoxia, and a new infiltrate(s) on chest radiograph. ACS is a life-threatening complication of sickle cell disease often caused by atypical organisms such as *Mycoplasma pneumoniae.* It is not uncommon for adults with sickle cell disease to present with a pain crisis or pneumonia and deteriorate in the hospital to ACS. The treatment for ACS is antibiotic coverage for typical and atypical organisms, red blood cell exchange transfusion to a goal hemoglobin S (sickle) <30% and other supportive care. While simple transfusion can be very helpful to increase the oxygen-carrying capacity of blood and blood volume itself, it does not rapidly decrease the percentage of circulating sickle cells. Thus in situations such as ACS where sickling of RBCs is the chief problem, exchange transfusion is the preferred treatment. A pulmonary embolus would not explain this patient's new pulmonary infiltrates.

Vichinsky EP, Neumayr LD, Earles AN, et al. Causes and outcomes of the acute chest syndrome in sickle cell disease. *N Engl J Med.* 2000;342(25):1855–1865.

9. ANSWER: B. Admit to the hospital and transfuse packed red blood cells.

Vasoocclusive pain crises are the hallmark of sickle cell disease, and patients may be admitted to the hospital very frequently for pain control. However, not all presentations of individuals with sickle cell disease are for a pain crisis. A significant finding in this presentation is anemia accompanied by reticulocytopenia. This patient has transient red cell aplasia (TRCA) due to parvovirus B19. His anemia is likely to worsen because of the shortened lifespan of sickled red blood cells (about 20 days) and the inability of his bone marrow to produce reticulocytes. Reticulocytopenia begins about 5 days postexposure and continues for 7 to 10 days. Recovery is spontaneous, but support with RBC transfusions is necessary. The two indications for RBC exchange transfusion are stroke/TIA and acute chest syndrome. This patient has no indication for broad-spectrum antibiotics.

Serjeant BE, Hambleton IR, Kerr S, et al. Haematological response to parvovirus B19 infection in homozygous sickle-cell disease. *Lancet.* 2001;358(9295):1779–1780.

10. ANSWER: A. A 47-year-old woman with a 2-pack-per-day active tobacco use habit and a history of lung cancer in both her mother and father

Low-dose CT screening in high-risk patient populations has been associated with the potential for a significant reduction in lung cancer mortality. The National Lung Screening Trial (NLST) compared annual low-dose chest CT to chest x-ray for 3 years in high-risk populations, which demonstrated a statistically significant decrease in lung cancer deaths in the CT-screened group (lung cancer mortality reduction of 20% [CI 3.8–26.7], all-cause mortality reduction of 6.7% [CI 1.2–13.6]). Several other screening studies are underway or under analysis. Additionally, there are multiple guidelines as to appropriate populations in which to consider screening. The broadest guidelines include individuals with all the following characteristics:

- Aged 55–79
- At least a 30-pack-year smoking history
- Active tobacco use within the past 15 years

The duration of screening is unclear, but all guidelines recommend yearly screening for a minimum of 3 years and a maximum recommendation of yearly screening until patients no longer meet high-risk criteria. There are no data at this time to suggest a mortality benefit in screening patients under age 50.

National Lung Screening Trial Research Team. Reduced lung-cancer mortality with low-dose computed tomographic screening. *N Engl J Med.* 2011;365(5):395–409.

11. ANSWER: E. All of the above

This patient has a clinical diagnosis of heparin-induced thrombocytopenia (HIT) with development of new clots while on heparin for 5 days, and with a platelet count decrease greater than 50% of initial count. Despite recent neurosurgery, lifesaving treatment requires doing A, B, and C immediately. Although testing should be sent to confirm diagnosis, waiting for results before starting treatment is contraindicated and can lead to poor outcome, including death.

Greinacher A. Heparin-induced thrombocytopenia. *N Engl J Med.* 2015; 373(3):252–261.

12. ANSWER: D. Check peripheral smear and find schistocytes; initiate plasmapheresis.

This patient has the classic pentad of findings associated with thrombotic thrombocytopenic purpura (TTP). Although disseminated intravascular coagulation (DIC) from retained products of conception could result in microangiopathic changes and thrombocytopenia, DIC is not usually associated with renal failure or focal neurologic findings. Risk factors for TTP include pregnancy, HIV infection, autoimmune disorders, and others. Rapid initiation of plasmapheresis is critical, even if confirmatory laboratory test results are not available.

George JN, Nester CM. Syndromes of thrombotic microangiopathy. *N Engl J Med* 2014;371(7):654–666.

13. ANSWER: E. All of the above

This patient gives a good history for vWD, with mucosal bleeding in the setting of impaired platelet function due to NSAIDs that was severe enough to require red cell transfusion. All of the tests listed above are required to make a diagnosis of vWD and determine the type (I, II, or extremely unlikely III). vWF antigen level measures the actual vWF protein level, but vWF also functions to carry FVIII and prolong its plasma half-life as well as bind to platelets—hence the need to measure factor VIII activity and ristocetin cofactor activity, a functional surrogate assay for patient vWF platelet binding. vWF multimer gel electrophoresis determines vWF multimer size, which is needed in order to classify vWD type II subtypes.

Leebeek FWG, Eikenboom JCJ. Von Willebrand's disease. *N Engl J Med.* 2016;375(21):2067–2080.

14. ANSWER: D. Rivaroxaban

This patient is an ideal candidate for treatment of acute deep vein thrombosis (DVT) with rivaroxaban—she is young, has no significant health problems or medications, and has limited duration of therapy for provoked venous thromboembolism (VTE). This dose (15 mg twice daily for 3 weeks followed by 20 mg once daily) is the treatment dose for acute DVT or pulmonary embolism.

Aspirin or compression stockings are inadequate treatment for acute VTE. A target INR of 1.5–2.0 is too low for acute VTE treatment. Although IV UFH could be considered, at 96 hours postoperatively, she should have adequate hemostasis to allow oral anticoagulant therapy with a short-acting new oral anticoagulant.

15. ANSWER: A. True

Although she has had a provoked DVT, her father had a DVT at a young age and she has two daughters who might consider oral contraceptive pill (OCP) use. Finding an inherited thrombophilia in this patient would not change current management or duration of anticoagulation treatment for provoked DVT (3 months), but if present, it would prompt testing of her daughters prior to OCP use. Additionally, results could affect management of potential future pregnancies of her daughters.

16. ANSWER: C. Mixing study

A mixing study should be done next to determine if the aPTT is prolonged due to the absence of a coagulation factor in the intrinsic coagulation pathway or to the presence of a circulating inhibitor. A mixing study is performed by mixing patient plasma with normal pooled plasma in a 1:1 ratio. The normal plasma supplies enough of the coagulation factors to correct a congenital deficiency and normalize the aPTT. If an inhibitor is present, such as an acquired FVIII inhibitor, lupus anticoagulant, or even drugs such as unfractionated heparin or bivalirudin, the addition of plasma will not correct the aPTT, because the factors in the normal plasma will be affected. If the mixing study corrects the aPTT, then individual factor levels can be performed to determine which is deficient (XII, XI, IX, VIII). If the aPTT does not correct, tests for inhibitors need to be performed.

Factor XIII activity is not measured by the aPTT. Because the PT is normal, fibrinogen levels should be normal. Platelets have no impact on the aPTT. D-Dimer results would not be of help in determining the etiology of prolonged aPTT in this postoperative patient with normal PT.

17. ANSWER: D. Initiating sunitinib or pazopanib

It is mandatory to have tissue diagnosis prior to initiating systemic therapies. Although renal cell carcinoma (RCC) is statistically by far the most likely diagnosis, transitional cell cancer (TCC) of the renal pelvis is a consideration. In that case, removal of the primary would not be indicated, and the patient would proceed with a different systemic therapy.

18. ANSWER: D. Repeat TURBT

It is very important to have muscle present on the biopsy report to document whether muscle invasion is present for appropriate staging and to guide therapy.

Superficial disease: BCG for high-risk superficial disease.

Muscle-invasive disease: neoadjuvant chemotherapy + cystectomy.

19. ANSWER: C. Neoadjuvant cisplatin-based chemotherapy is indicated based on a 5% absolute reduction in death.

In patients with good performance status and good kidney function, neoadjuvant cisplatin-based chemotherapy is standard. It is associated with a 5% absolute reduction in death and 15% relative reduction in death. Data for adjuvant therapy are limited, although in practice it is frequently considered in patients who did not receive neoadjuvant therapy. The preferred approach in this healthy patient with normal renal function is neoadjuvant cisplatin-based chemotherapy followed by radical cystectomy.

Bellmunt J, Orsola A, Leow JJ, et al. Bladder cancer: ESMO Practice Guidelines for diagnosis, treatment and follow-up. *Ann Oncol.* 2014;25(suppl 3):iii40–iii48.

20. ANSWER: E. No further workup necessary

The most common sites of prostate cancer metastases are bone and lymph nodes. For patients with low-risk disease (T1c [normal DRE] or T2a [tumor involving one-half or less of one lobe] *and* PSA <10 ng/mL *and* Gleason score <7), the likelihood of spread of disease visible by imaging is exceedingly low. Further workup is not recommended for these patients. CT of the abdomen/pelvis and bone scan are recommended for men with serum PSA >20 ng/mL, or serum PSA >10 ng/mL with a positive DRE, or a Gleason ≥8 tumor, or evidence of tumor extension through the prostate capsule. Several institutions use endorectal coil MRI as part of the initial workup, but the clinical utility of this modality is not yet clear.

Mohler JL, Armstrong AJ, Bahnson RR, et al. Prostate cancer, version 1.2016. *J Natl Compr Canc Netw.* 2016;14(1):19–30.

21. ANSWER: A. Active surveillance

Given the long natural history of prostate cancer, the frequency of indolent disease in a high percentage of patients, and significant morbidity associated with local treatment, active surveillance is increasingly recommended by urologists and medical oncologists. Prospective series clearly demonstrate that active surveillance (serial PSAs and physical examinations every 3–4 months along with repeat biopsies every 1–2 years) can safely be used to manage certain patients, avoiding (or at the very least forestalling) life-altering therapies. However, not all patients are good candidates for active surveillance. For patients <70 years old, criteria for entry into most active surveillance series include early-stage disease, Gleason score ≤6, and serum PSA ≤10 ng/mL. There are data suggesting that low-volume Gleason 3 + 4 disease can be managed successfully by active surveillance, particularly for patients older than age 70. However, a diagnosis of localized Gleason 4 + 3 disease in a patient with life expectancy >10 years, as in the case above, warrants definitive treatment.

Mohler JL, Armstrong AJ, Bahnson RR, et al. Prostate cancer, version 1.2016. *J Natl Compr Canc Netw.* 2016;14(1):19–30.

22. ANSWER: B. Prolactinoma

Androgen deprivation therapy (ADT) is the first-line treatment for advanced prostate cancer and is used as neoadjuvant treatment along with radiation therapy for intermediate- and high-risk localized disease. After about 1 week on ADT, GnRH receptors in the pituitary are downregulated, and LH and FSH production are diminished. This results in a profound reduction in testosterone production by the testicles and induces tumor responses in 80%–90% of patients. Castrate testosterone levels are associated with several common side effects: loss of libido, osteopenia/osteoporosis, hot flashes, decrease in lean body mass, increase in subcutaneous adipose tissue, thinning of body hair, decrease in penile and testicular size, gynecomastia, anemia, and mild fatigue. More rarely, treatment may be associated with cognitive decline or depression. Some studies have observed an increased incidence of cardiovascular events in those receiving ADT; others have found no convincing association. Associations between ADT and development of colorectal cancer have also been reported, but a true causal relationship has not been firmly established. There is no known association with other cancers.

23. ANSWER: B. A patient with newly diagnosed metastatic lung cancer and 10% tumor programmed death receptor ligand 1 (PD-L1) expression

Immune therapy with PD-1 inhibition is currently approved in several malignancy types and settings, with many more indications under study. PD-1 is a checkpoint protein expressed on T cells, and activation of PD-1 leads to downregulation of the immune response. PD-L1 is expressed on some tumor cells and can bind to PD-1 on T cells, one strategy for tumor evasion of the immune response. Blockade of PD-1 with pharmaceutical inhibitors (currently approved agents: nivolumab, pembrolizumab) can result in increased immune recognition and killing of tumor cells. PD-1 inhibition is currently approved in all of the settings in this question with the exception of up-front therapy for stage IV lung cancer where tumor PD-L1 expression is less than 50%. In most instances, quantification of tumor PD-L1 expression is not required for initiation of therapy, although response rates appear to be higher in many cases in tumors with increased PD-L1 expression. The exception is frontline therapy for metastatic lung cancer, where >50% PD-L1 expression is required. Studies of frontline platinum doublet chemotherapy versus PD-1 inhibition failed to demonstrate improved outcomes for immune therapy in patients with tumors with lower or no PD-L1 expression and thus are not recommended in this setting.

Giroux Leprieur E, Dumenil C, Julie C, et al. Immunotherapy revolutionises non-small-cell lung cancer therapy: results, perspectives and new challenges. *Eur J Cancer.* 2017 Apr 10;78:16–23.

24. ANSWER: D. A and C

PD-1 and PD-L1 inhibition, though often well tolerated, are associated with a wide variety of autoimmune toxicities. Among the most common are endocrine dysfunction (hyper- or hypothyroid, pituitary dysfunction), colitis, pneumonitis, and rash. Less common toxicities include pancreatitis, nephritis, hepatitis, diabetes, and myocarditis. Pneumonitis and colitis are the most frequently cited causes of life-threatening or even fatal toxicities. The mainstay of therapy for severe reactions is permanent cessation of drug and immediate initiation of immune suppression with corticosteroids. Milder toxicities can often be managed with temporary cessation of drug plus or minus courses of oral corticosteroids. The optimal dose and corticosteroid type for severe reactions is unknown, but the equivalent of at least 1 mg/kg of prednisone is a widely accepted minimum. In this patient with cough, dyspnea, absence of fever, and the listed CT findings, nivolumab-induced pneumonitis is highly likely. Pneumonitis is a diagnosis of exclusion, however, and other etiologies must be considered and evaluated. Because atypical pneumonia could have a similar presentation, it is prudent to treat this patient for both infection and pneumonitis.

Maughan BL, Bailey E, Gill DM, Agarwal N. Incidence of immune-related adverse events with program death receptor-1- and program death receptor-1 ligand-directed therapies in genitourinary cancers. *Front Oncol.* 2017;7:56.

25. ANSWER: A. Tamoxifen causes none of these side effects.

In placebo-controlled, randomized trials of tamoxifen for breast cancer prevention among patients without a personal history of breast cancer, there was no increased risk of premature menopause, weight gain, or depression. Both raloxifene and exemestane have data only for postmenopausal women.

26. ANSWER: D. Skeletal survey with plain films

In the case of lung cancer, the most common sites of involvement are the mediastinum and contralateral lung, liver, bone, brain, and adrenal glands. The appropriate radiographic staging workup of lung cancer should include imaging of all of those sites.

Brain imaging is required for all patients with small cell lung cancer, patients with nonsmall cell lung cancer of stage IB or greater, or any patient with lung cancer with any neurologic symptom. In this case, the unexplained fall in the setting of new lung cancer warrants dedicated brain imaging. MRI is preferred over CT for brain imaging, though CT with contrast is a reasonable alternative. Regardless of modality, IV contrast (gadolinium for MRI, iodinated contrast for CT) is required for sufficient detection of brain metastases. The prior noncontrast head CT is insufficient.

A chest CT with IV contrast that is performed specifically for lung cancer staging should be expanded to include the liver and adrenal glands. The administration of IV contrast enhances the ability to detect hepatic metastases. Furthermore, by delineating the mediastinal vasculature with IV contrast, the clinician can better assess the size and extent of mediastinal lymph nodes.

PET/CT or bone scan is the best modality to look for bone metastases in lung cancer. PET/CT is the preferred modality. A plain film skeletal survey is not sensitive enough to detect occult bone metastases in lung cancer.

Ettinger DS, Wood DE, Aisner DL, et al. *Non-small cell lung cancer*, version 5.2017, NCCN Clinical Practice Guidelines in Oncology. *J Natl Compr Canc Netw.* 2017;15(4):504–535.

27. ANSWER: D. Small cell lung cancer

The findings of a large hilar mass with superior vena cava (SVC) syndrome, hepatic and bony metastases, and hyponatremia in a 63-year-old woman with a significant smoking history are most consistent with a small cell lung cancer (SCLC). SCLC is the tumor type most closely associated with smoking: About 95% of patients with SCLC have a smoking history. SCLC tends to occur in the central chest, so SVC syndrome or tracheal compression can be presenting symptoms. In fact, SCLC is the most common cause of SVC syndrome. SCLC tends to be aggressive in its course, with metastatic disease found at the time of initial diagnosis in 60%–70% of patients with SCLC. SCLC can also be associated with a number of paraneoplastic syndromes. The most common of these is hyponatremia due to the syndrome of inappropriate antidiuretic hormone secretion (SIADH).

28. ANSWER: B. Repeat chest CT in 6 months

The Fleischner Society has published guidelines for the follow-up and management of nodules <8 mm detected incidentally at nonscreening CT. These guidelines make a distinction between low- and high-risk patients, and nodule sizes ≤4 mm, >4–6 mm, >6–8 mm, and >8 mm. High-risk patients are defined as those with a history of smoking or other known risk factors. In this case, a 5-mm nodule in a patient with a 20-pack-year smoking history merits a follow-up CT in 6–12 months. For a nodule that small, it would be difficult to reliably perform a CT-guided biopsy, and it may be below the size threshold for fluorodeoxyglucose avidity on PET/CT (Table 2.7).

29. ANSWER: E. Surgical resection

The gold standard therapy for newly diagnosed early-stage lung cancer is anatomic resection. In patients with good performance status and adequate

TABLE 2.7 Guidelines for Management of Small Pulmonary Nodules Detected on CT Scans: A Statement From the Fleischner Society

Nodule Size (mm)[a]	Low-Risk Patient	High-Risk Patient
≤4	No follow-up needed	Follow-up CT at 12 months; if unchanged, no further follow-up
>4–6	Follow-up CT at 12 months; if unchanged, no further follow-up	Initial follow-up CT at 6–12 months, then at 18–24 months if no change
>6–8	Initial follow-up CT at 6–12 months, then at 18–24 months if no change	Initial follow-up CT at 3–6 months, then at 9–12 and 24 months if no change
>8	Follow-up CT at around 3, 9, and 24 months; dynamic contrast-enhanced CT; PET; and/or biopsy	Same as for low-risk patient

NOTE: Newly detected indeterminate nodule in persons 35 years of age or older.
Nonsolid (ground-glass) or partly solid nodules may require longer follow-up to exclude indolent adenocarcinoma.
[a]Average of length and width.

From MacMahon H, Austin JH, Gamsu G, et al. Guidelines for management of small pulmonary nodules detected on CT scans: a statement from the Fleischner Society. *Radiology.* 2005;237(2):395–400.

lung function, the goal is anatomic resection (i.e., resection of the mass and its associated lymphatic drainage). This is classically achieved via lobectomy, though segmentectomy (resection of an anatomic segment of a lung lobe) may be adequate for some tumors that are small enough and in the right location.

For patients who are poor operative candidates, stereotactic body radiation therapy (SBRT) can be considered. The potential use of stereotactic radiation for early-stage lung cancer may be limited by tumor size and location. In general, tumors >4 cm are not generally amenable to definitive control with stereotactic radiation. Furthermore, there have been concerns about stereotactic radiation to central tumors because early trials of this modality raised concerns about collapse of adjacent airways.

Chemotherapy is not considered a curative modality in lung cancer, and it has not been shown to be an appropriate up-front therapy for potentially resectable early-stage nonsmall cell lung cancer.

Modalities such as cryoablation and radiofrequency ablation continue to be investigated in lung cancers but are not currently considered a standard curative treatment option in early-stage lung cancer.

More recent data suggest that this may be achieved by segmentectomy, depending on a tumor's size and location. For patients who are poor operative candidates, consider stereotactic radiation.

Ettinger DS, Wood DE, Aisner DL, et al. *Non-small cell lung cancer*, version 5.2017, NCCN Clinical Practice Guidelines in Oncology. *J Natl Compr Canc Netw.* 2017;15(4):504–535.

30. ANSWER: D. Obtain a chest x-ray.

This young woman presents with signs and symptoms worrisome for lymphoma, particularly Hodgkin lymphoma (HL). Although pruritus is a frequent symptom in patients with HL, intense pruritus without a rash is quite rare. On the other hand, B symptoms (fevers, drenching night sweats, and unexplained weight loss) are common in this disease. In addition, she is a young adult at the median age of presentation of HL. Finally, the leukocytosis with lymphopenia and elevated eosinophils may be seen with HL. Given that she does not have peripheral lymphadenopathy, the next most logical step in her management is to obtain a chest x-ray to look for a mediastinal mass. LDH is rarely elevated in HL. A PET/CT scan is done as part of staging once a diagnosis has been established. She does not have symptoms typical for EBV infection.

31. ANSWER: A. Obtain peripheral blood flow cytometry.

This patient presents with the classic findings of a patient with CLL with diffuse lymphadenopathy and splenomegaly with a lymphocytosis and smudge cells on a peripheral smear. The diagnosis of CLL may be established using peripheral blood flow cytometry. Excisional lymph node biopsy and bone marrow biopsy are not necessary, given that the diagnosis may be established using flow cytometry. PET/CT is not necessary in the evaluation of CLL. CT scans may be obtained in patients with adverse cytogenetics, such as 11q and 17p deletion, but they are not necessary at this time. The patient's symptoms are suggestive of a viral infection, and antibiotics are not indicated.

32. ANSWER: C. Refer to a surgeon for an excisional lymph node biopsy.

The patient presents with diffuse, asymptomatic lymphadenopathy suggestive of involvement by an indolent lymphoma. To establish the diagnosis, an adequate tissue biopsy is critical. Given that she has palpable peripheral lymphadenopathy, referral to a surgeon for an excisional lymph node biopsy is the most appropriate way to obtain adequate diagnostic tissue. Needle biopsies lack adequate tissue to evaluate for architecture. Peripheral blood flow cytometry is unlikely to yield a diagnosis in the setting of a normal white blood cell count and differential. PET/CT scan is indicated for staging in aggressive lymphomas and Hodgkin lymphoma after a diagnosis has been established.

33. ANSWER: C. Osteoporosis

Aromatase inhibitors are associated with estrogen deficiency–induced bone loss. Patients starting an AI should undergo baseline bone density testing, and testing should continue periodically for the duration of the course of therapy. Although formal guidelines do not exist, many experts recommend testing every 2 years while a patient is on AI therapy. If identified, osteopenia and osteoporosis should be managed aggressively and according to expert guidelines. Additionally, all women should be counseled regarding lifestyle optimization for bone health, including physical activity, smoking cessation, and adequate calcium and vitamin D intake.

Increased risk for DVT/PE and endometrial cancer (Answers A and D) are associated with tamoxifen. Hypothyroid and glucose intolerance are not known adverse effects of hormonal therapy for breast cancer.

Patel S. Disruption of aromatase homeostasis as the cause of a multiplicity of ailments: a comprehensive review. *J Steroid Biochem Mol Biol.* 2017;168:19–25.

34. ANSWER: D. Medical therapy with a dopamine agonist

Medical therapy with a dopamine agonist is considered the first-line initial therapy for symptomatic prolactinomas. Dopamine agonists have both antiproliferative and antisecretory effects on prolactin-producing pituitary cells and typically result in both decreased prolactin secretion and tumor shrinkage. Cabergoline is preferred over bromocriptine for most patients due to its increased efficacy and tolerability. Somatostatin analogues are used in the treatment of acromegaly.

Transsphenoidal surgery is reserved for patients who do not tolerate or are not responsive to the dopamine agonists. Radiation would be considered only in very rare cases of advanced or progressive prolactinomas that have failed medical or surgical interventions. Observation alone would not be the preferred approach in a patient with a macroadenoma (size >10 mm), because control of tumor growth would be desired.

35. ANSWER: C. Venlafaxine

There are multiple drug interactions between tamoxifen and antidepressants based on the potential for CYP2D6 inhibition by many antidepressants. CYP2D6 converts tamoxifen to endoxifen, its active form. Venlafaxine has the least effect on CYP2D6 of the commonly used antidepressants. Paroxetine, fluoxetine, and bupropion are strong inhibitors and should be avoided if possible. Duloxetine and sertraline are moderate inhibitors. Citalopram and escitalopram are mild inhibitors. Desvenlafaxine and mirtazapine likely have minimal effect on tamoxifen/endoxifen, but direct studies are lacking.

36. ANSWER: C. A 60-year-old man with new-onset nonvalvular atrial fibrillation and a history of a diverticular bleed 5 years ago

NOACs (rivaroxaban, edoxaban, apixaban, dabigatran) are approved in nonvalvular atrial fibrillation and DVT/PE. Current contraindications include patients with active malignancies (studies underway), metallic heart valves, the antiphospholipid antibody syndrome (studies underway), and renal insufficiency (glomerular filtration rate [GFR] <15 mL/min for edoxaban and apixaban, and GFR <30 mL/min for rivaroxaban and dabigatran). Data are insufficient regarding safety in pregnant or lactating women. Prior GI bleeding is not an absolute contraindication to NOAC use.

Steinberg BA. How I use anticoagulation in atrial fibrillation. *Blood.* 2016;128(25):2891–2898.

37. ANSWER: E. Referral to IR for needle-guided biopsy of the adnexal mass

If clinical suspicion of ovarian malignancy is high, any of the above evaluations is reasonable (although only referral to gynecologic oncology is required), with the exception of needle biopsy due to the potential risk for malignant seeding of the needle tract. Colonoscopy should be considered in women who are found to have mucinous histology at surgical resection, or for women in whom colorectal cancer is clinically suspected at presentation.

38. ANSWER: C. Central diabetes insipidus

The symptoms and presentation in this case are most concerning for the development of postoperative central diabetes insipidus. Diabetes insipidus is a syndrome of hypotonic polyuria and is due to either a deficiency of arginine vasopressin, also known as antidiuretic hormone (ADH), or an inadequate renal response to ADH. Patients with diabetes insipidus often complain of extreme thirst and will excrete large amounts of very dilute urine. Without this hormone, individuals cannot adequately concentrate their urine and, if not allowed access to liquids, may develop severe, life-threatening hypernatremia. Central diabetes insipidus is due to deficiency, either partial or complete, of ADH. Central diabetes insipidus can occur after any pituitary surgery. It can be transient or permanent and is seen more frequently in patients with larger tumors or tumors that tend to invade the pituitary stalk, such as craniopharyngiomas. The diagnosis is not likely SIADH, because this condition is typically associated with hyponatremia. Type 2 diabetes mellitus would also not be a likely cause of this patient's acute severe polyuria and polydipsia, because his BMI is normal and his fasting glucose is only mildly elevated. Given the clinical presentation of a pituitary lesion, his diabetes insipidus would be much more likely be central than nephrogenic.

Lobatto DJ, de Vries F, Zamanipoor Najafabadi AH, et al. Preoperative risk factors for postoperative complications in endoscopic pituitary surgery: a systematic review. *Pituitary.* 2017 Sep 15. [Epub ahead of print]

Prete A, Corsello SM, Salvatori R. Current best practice in the management of patients after pituitary surgery. *Ther Adv Endocrinol Metab.* 2017;8(3):33–48.

39. ANSWER: D. All of the above

This patient was found to have an incidental pituitary lesion. All three of the answer choices are important for the initial evaluation of the patient. A thorough history must be obtained to elicit symptoms of mass effects and pituitary dysfunction (both hypersecretion and hypofunction). Having a complete understanding of pituitary physiology will help guide the questions related to determining the function of each hormonal axis. The clinician should look for both signs and symptoms to suggest hormonal hypersecretion (i.e., hyperprolactinemia, growth hormone excess, or hypercortisolism) or hormonal hypofunction (i.e., central adrenal insufficiency, central hypothyroidism, central hypogonadism, GH deficiency, diabetes insipidus). Laboratory evaluation should be performed to assess pituitary hormonal function. MRI should be performed to better characterize the structure of the mass. Taken together, both laboratory and imaging studies will help guide further evaluation and treatment of the patient presenting with a pituitary mass.

40. ANSWER: B. t(15;17)

The age distribution of patients with acute promyelocytic leukemia (APL) differs from other forms of acute myeloid leukemia (AML). APL is uncommon in the first decade of life; its incidence increases during the second decade, reaches a plateau during early adulthood, and then remains constant until it decreases after age 60 years. The median age is 40 years old, thus considerably lower than for other myeloid leukemias.

APL is a medical emergency defined by the presence of a reciprocal translocation between the long arms of chromosomes 15 and 17, with the creation of a fusion gene, PML-RARA, which links the retinoic acid receptor alpha (RARA) gene on chromosome 17 with the promyelocytic leukemia (PML) gene on chromosome 15.

A key component of therapy is the use of all-*trans* retinoic acid (ATRA), which promotes the terminal differentiation of malignant promyelocytes to mature neutrophils. Coagulopathy is a common presenting feature and should be corrected with blood products as needed (platelets, fresh frozen plasma, cryoprecipitate) in addition to the administration of ATRA as soon as it is available. Correction of coagulopathy and administration of ATRA should be performed immediately with suspicion of APL and should not be deferred until a firm diagnosis is available.

t(11;14): Overexpression of cyclin D1 in mantle cell lymphomas (MCLs) is strongly associated with the t(11;14)(q13;q32), a translocation between the cyclin D1 locus and the immunoglobulin heavy chain (IgH) locus. Approximately 50% to 65% of MCLs will show the t(11;14) by cytogenetics, but by fluorescence in situ hybridization (FISH), a much higher fraction of cases with cyclin D1 overexpression contain BCL-1/IgH fusion genes.

t(9;22): The vast majority of patients (90%–95%) demonstrate the t(9;22)(q34;q11.2) reciprocal translocation that results in the Ph chromosome-BCR-ABL1 fusion gene or its product, the BCR-ABL1 fusion mRNA. The BCR-ABL1 fusion gene is the target of therapies such as dasatanib, nilotinib, and imatinib.

t(8;14): Burkitt lymphoma is associated with a translocation between the long arm of chromosome 8, the site of the c-MYC oncogene (8q24), and one of three locations on immunoglobulin (Ig) genes. The most common translocation is with the Ig heavy chain gene on chromosome 14 (approximately 80%).

t(14;18): Approximately 85% of patients with follicular lymphoma have t(14;18), which results in the overexpression of B-cell leukemia/lymphoma 2 (BCL2), an oncogene that blocks programmed cell death (apoptosis), leading to prolonged cell survival.

DeAngelo DJ. Tailored approaches to induction therapy for acute promyelocytic leukemia. *J Clin Oncol.* 2017;35(6):583–586.

Adams J, Nassiri M. Acute promyelocytic leukemia: a review and discussion of variant translocations. *Arch Pathol Lab Med.* 2015;139(10):1308–1313.

41. ANSWER: D. Erythropoiesis-stimulating agent (ESA)

The International Prognostic Scoring System (IPSS) is the most widely used prognostic classification system for myelodysplastic syndrome (MDS). The Revised IPSS (IPSS-R) incorporates a larger number of cytogenetic abnormalities, divided into five prognostic categories, a lower cutoff for absolute neutrophil count (<800/μL vs. <1800/μL), and different weights for the clinical parameters to better predict outcomes in newly diagnosed patients. Patients with a low IPSS-R (1.5 to 3) have a median survival of 5.3 years and risk to 25% AML transformation of 10.8 years. The main goals of therapy are to control symptoms due to cytopenias, improve quality of life, and minimize the toxicity of therapy. There is no evidence that the treatment of asymptomatic patients improves long-term survival.

Immediate treatment is indicated for patients with symptomatic anemia or thrombocytopenia or recurrent infections in the setting of neutropenia. This patient is developing worsening dyspnea on exertion as a result of his anemia, so therapy could be considered.

Approximately 15%–25% of unselected patients with MDS have an improvement in hemoglobin when treated with recombinant human erythropoietin. The Nordic MDS Group developed a predictive model for epoetin use in MDS: patients requiring 2 U of PRBCs or more per month and those with serum epoetin level >100 U/L (especially >500 U/L) are less likely to respond.

Allogeneic transplant is the only curative treatment for MDS. Transplant at the time of diagnosis is shown to have the greatest benefit in patients in more advanced IPSS risk groups: intermediate-2 and high risk. Because this patient has low-risk disease, strategies to reduce the need for transfusions is recommended with allogeneic transplant at the time of disease progression.

As is the case with allogeneic hematopoietic stem cell transplant, high-intensity chemotherapy regimens are generally reserved for patients with intermediate-2 or high-risk IPSS scores. This allows for the avoidance of treatment-related morbidity and mortality in most patients with a relatively good prognosis.

Lenalidomide improves anemia in some patients with MDS and a normal marrow karyotype, but this agent is particularly effective in MDS with an interstitial deletion of chromosome 5q. In studies, it has been associated with transfusion independence in 67% of transfusion-dependent patients.

Greenberg PL, Tuechler H, Schanz J, et al. Revised international prognostic scoring system for myelodysplastic syndromes. *Blood.* 2012;120(12):454–465.

42. ANSWER: D. Send peripheral blood for cytogenetics to evaluate for the t(9;22) chromosome translocation.

Chronic myelogenous leukemia (CML) accounts for approximately 15%–20% of leukemias in adults. It has an annual incidence of 1–2 cases per 100,000, with a slight male predominance. The clinical presentation with splenomegaly, immature myeloid forms, and basophilia and eosinophilia is suggestive of CML or another myeloproliferative disorder. The lack of JAK2 and normal Hgb level makes polycythemia vera less likely. Approximately 15%–30% of patients with CML have platelet counts >600,000/μL.

The diagnosis of CML is confirmed by the demonstration of the Philadelphia chromosome t(9;22)(q34;q11.2), the BCR-ABL1 fusion gene, or the BCR-ABL1 fusion mRNA by conventional cytogenetics, fluorescence in situ hybridization (FISH) analysis, or reverse transcription–polymerase chain reaction (RT-PCR).

Hydroxyurea can be used to reduce white blood cell counts while awaiting confirmation of a suspected diagnosis of CML in a patient with significant leukocytosis (e.g., >80 × 10^9 white cells/L). This patient's WBC count is only 60× 10^9 white cells/L, and she is asymptomatic from her disease, so waiting for a diagnosis is appropriate.

This patient is afebrile and has no other symptoms of infection. The relative basophilia is also less consistent with an infectious cause, thus starting empiric antibiotics for a presumed reactive leukocytosis is not needed.

While essential thrombocythemia (ET) is still in the differential diagnosis because 50% of patients with ET do not have the JAK2 mutation, starting high-dose aspirin in this patient is not recommended. Higher doses of aspirin (900 mg/d) have been associated with increased gastrointestinal hemorrhage as compared with low-dose aspirin (75–325 mg/d).

Although morphologically normal, the neutrophils in CML are cytochemically abnormal. Leukocyte alkaline phosphatase (LAP) is typically low in CML. The low LAP score is useful in excluding a reactive leukocytosis, typically due to infection, in which the score is typically elevated or normal, or polycythemia vera, which is also associated with an increased LAP activity. Although the LAP score may provide useful supportive data, it is neither sensitive nor specific for CML.

43. ANSWER: D. Start leukapheresis while establishing diagnosis.

This patient has a WBC count >100,000/μL with anemia and thrombocytopenia. She has a likely diagnosis of leukemia with an elevated WBC count leading to hyperleukocytosis and leukostasis.

Hyperleukocytosis occurs in 10%–20% of patients with AML and more commonly in the monocytic and myelomonocytic variants. Leukostasis results from increased blood viscosity as a direct complication of the presence of large leukemic blasts and the interaction of the blasts with the endothelium to form aggregates, leading to thrombi in the microcirculation. Patients are usually symptomatic when the WBC count reaches levels >100,000. If left untreated, the 1-week mortality rate is approximately 20% to 40%.

In the setting of her WBC count and chest x-ray findings, it is likely that she has pulmonary evidence of leukostasis, presenting with dyspnea, tachypnea, and hypoxemia. Respiratory acidosis and cor pulmonale may also occur. Chest x-ray can show diffuse bilateral infiltrates. Approximately 80% of patients with leukostasis are febrile, usually as a result of associated inflammation. Although starting empiric antibiotics is reasonable, waiting to see if the patient improves would waste valuable time during which the patient can undergo leukapheresis.

Transfusions would increase blood viscosity and increase the risk of worsening the respiratory compromise and intracranial hemorrhage.

Leukapheresis should be initiated while establishing a diagnosis in patients who have symptomatic leukostasis. It is a temporizing measure, thus a diagnosis needs to be made promptly and definitive therapy should be started. Therapy such as hydroxyurea reduces the WBC count by 50% to 80% within 24 to 48 hours and should be used as the sole therapy only in patients with hyperleukocytosis without symptoms of leukostasis. While induction chemotherapy serves to both rapidly decrease the circulating WBC count and target the leukemia cells in the bone marrow, reducing the WBC count within 24 hours of initiation, the patient is rapidly worsening, and it will take time to make the diagnosis.

44. ANSWER: D. von Willebrand factor levels become normal during pregnancy in patients with type I disease.

Approximately 85% of patients with von Willebrand disease (vWD) have type I disease where there is a decrease in the vWF level with no abnormality in vWF function. For reasons that are not well understood, during pregnancy, the vWF levels in type I vWD patients normalize. Thus, it is safe to use an epidural catheter for anesthesia. After delivery of the baby and the placenta, the vWF level returns to the prepregnancy level. Thus, about 25% of women with type I vWD require treatment with DDAVP 2–3 days after delivery but are not at risk for excess bleeding during labor and delivery.

Leebeek FWG, Eikenboom JCJ. Von Willebrand's disease. *N Engl J Med.* 2016;375(21):2067–2080.

45. ANSWER: A. Radiation oncology consultation for consideration of urgent whole-brain radiotherapy (WBRT)

WBRT is a reasonable option for patients with multiple brain lesions not amenable to SRS and/or poor performance status. In patients with good performance status and limited metastatic lesions, SRS is preferred. Although precise guidelines as to size and number of lesions are not agreed upon, most studies consider SRS for one to three lesions (and occasionally more) measuring 3 cm or less per lesion. Although there is a decreased risk of intracranial progression at 1 year with WBRT following SRS, there is no survival benefit. WBRT is associated with potential long-term cognitive impairment, especially in memory and learning. In this patient with good performance status and a limited number of lesions, SRS is the preferred initial approach for management of brain metastases.

Because she has had a seizure, both corticosteroids and anticonvulsant therapy are indicated. In asymptomatic patients with edema, corticosteroids should be considered cautiously. If primary CNS lymphoma is suspected, corticosteroids should be avoided unless clinically necessary. There is no proven role for prophylactic anticonvulsant therapy, but because this patient has had a seizure, treatment should be initiated.

All patients with lung cancer should have their tumors tested for targetable mutations, particularly epidermal growth factor receptor *(EGFR)* and *ALK*. More comprehensive testing may identify additional therapeutic targets as well. However, treatment of symptomatic brain lesions should not be deferred while awaiting molecular testing results.

46. ANSWER: D. A patient with poorly controlled atrial fibrillation and platelets of 20,000/µL

Ibrutinib is a highly effective and generally well-tolerated agent in CLL. It is a potent and irreversible inhibitor of Bruton tyrosine kinase (BTK), which is important in B-cell signaling pathways. BTK inhibition with ibrutinib can lead to decreased proliferation and survival of malignant B cells. Key potential adverse effects include increased risk of atrial fibrillation and bleeding, likely due to ibrutinib-induced platelet dysfunction. In the patient with thrombocytopenia and poorly controlled AF, ibrutinib would be more likely to cause serious adverse events than in the other patients described in the vignette. Ibrutinib is effective in bulky disease, and anemia is not a contraindication. Unlike FCR, ibrutinib is nearly as effective in patients who harbor p53 mutations as compared with those who do not. Ibrutinib is not associated with a significantly increased risk of opportunistic infections or colitis. Idelalisib, an oral kinase inhibitor also used in CLL, is associated with these potential adverse events.

Leong DP, Caron F, Hillis C, et al. The risk of atrial fibrillation with ibrutinib use: a systematic review and meta-analysis. *Blood* 2016;128(1):138–140.

47. ANSWER: B. Referral to medical oncologist for consideration of chemotherapy

This patient has stage III colon cancer. Although proper pathology staging recommends sampling and analysis of at least 12 lymph nodes for ideal staging, it is not going to impact the patient's current management to have more lymph nodes sampled, because the two positive nodes make the patient stage III and guidelines recommend adjuvant chemotherapy. A follow-up colonoscopy in 1 year would be recommended as part of surveillance for this patient, though it is not the next step. Radiation is rarely used in colon cancer, because local recurrence rates are very low; radiation is considered for stages II and III rectal cancer.

Benson AB 3rd, Venook AP, Cederquist L, et al. *Colon cancer*, version 1.2017, NCCN Clinical Practice Guidelines in Oncology. *J Natl Compr Canc Netw.* 2017;15(3):370–398.

48. ANSWER: E. Increase in dose of allopurinol

Tumor lysis syndrome (TLS) is acute cell lysis caused by chemotherapy and radiation therapy. The release of intracellular products (e.g., uric acid, phosphates, calcium, potassium) overwhelms the body's homeostasis mechanism. TLS is more common with hematologic malignancies or cancers with readily growing tumors, particularly acute leukemias and high-grade lymphomas such as Burkitt lymphoma (BL). Patients with BL are at high risk of TLS and uric acid nephropathy, especially during chemotherapy. Prophylactic allopurinol and aggressive hydration should be administered. TLS usually presents with acute kidney injury and metabolic derangements such as hyperphosphatemia, hyperkalemia, and hypocalcemia. Treatment includes inpatient monitoring, vigorous fluid resuscitation, allopurinol or urate oxidase (uricase) therapy to lower uric acid levels, and hemodialysis if renal failure develops. Because the patient is already on allopurinol, it is unlikely that further adjustment of allopurinol dosing will be effective, at least acutely.

Howard SC, Jones DP, Pui CH. The tumor lysis syndrome. *N Engl J Med.* 2011; 364(19):1844–1854.

49. ANSWER: B. Arrange for an urgent MRI of the spine to evaluate for possible cord compression.

This patient likely has epidural spinal cord compression caused by a tumor compressing the dural sac. This can cause permanent neurologic impairment even if treatment is delayed for only a few hours, and therefore it requires attention and treatment with some urgency. Epidural spinal cord compression is associated with renal, prostate, and most commonly breast and lung cancers. The thoracic spine is most often frequently affected, accounting for 70% of patients with the condition. One should suspect an epidural metastasis if the patient complains of new pain that worsens when the patient is lying down or with palpation of vertebral bodies, which is characteristic of this condition. Late neurologic signs such as incontinence and loss of sensory function are associated with permanent paraplegia. MRI has surpassed myelography as the imaging study of choice. If neurologic symptoms are present, the patient should be treated with steroids. This treatment should not be delayed while awaiting diagnostic study results. Use of high-dose dexamethasone (up to 100 mg) is controversial; clinical trials have shown that it has unclear benefits and significantly more serious side effects at higher doses. Most patients with epidural and spinal cord compression need radiation treatment (up to 3000 Gy) or surgery.

50. **ANSWER: A. Establishing a tissue diagnosis is the most important step in management of most patients with SVC syndrome.**

The SVC syndrome is caused by the gradual compression of the superior vena cava, leading to edema and retrograde flow. Lung cancer is the most common malignant cause, although lymphoma, metastatic mediastinal tumors, and indwelling catheters also can cause SVC syndrome. Symptoms may include cough; dyspnea; dysphagia; and swelling or discoloration of the neck, face, or upper extremities. Often, collateral venous circulation causes distention of the superficial veins in the chest wall. Tissue diagnosis (i.e., sputum cytology, thoracentesis, bronchoscopy, or needle aspiration) often is necessary to direct treatment decisions.

Acknowledgment

The authors and editors gratefully acknowledge the contributions of the previous authors—Lawrence Shulman, Wendy Y. Chen, Yuksel Urun, Toni K. Choueiri, Jean M. Connors, Peter Enzinger, Nancy Berliner, Maureen M. Okam, Mark M. Pomerantz, David M. Jackman, Brett E. Glotzbecker, Edwin P. Alyea, Daniel J. DeAngelo, Robert I. Handin, Jeffrey A. Meyerhardt, and Whitney W. Woodmansee

3 Rheumatology

DERRICK J. TODD

1. A 76-year-old woman has been admitted to the hospital for fever, cough, dyspnea, and hypoxemia. She has a history of primary hyperparathyroidism and has refused surgical intervention. Chest radiograph shows a lobar infiltrate, and sputum culture grew *Streptococcus pneumoniae.* She is diagnosed with pneumococcal pneumonia and treated with levofloxacin based on antibiotic sensitivities. Her clinical status improves markedly. On hospital day 4, just prior to discharge, she develops rapid-onset painful swelling in the right wrist associated with redness and warmth. She is afebrile, normotensive, and does not appear to be in a toxic condition. The right wrist is red, warm, swollen, and very painful to active or passive range of motion. Several right metacarpophalangeal (MCP) joints are similarly involved, but the left hand and wrist are completely normal. Blood cultures drawn on the day of admission (prior to antibiotics) have shown no growth. Plain radiograph of the right hand/wrist is as shown in Fig. 3.1.

   What is the most likely diagnosis?
   A. *Streptococcus pneumoniae* septic arthritis
   B. Acute pseudogout arthritis
   C. Seronegative rheumatoid arthritis of the elderly
   D. Wrist osteoarthritis
   E. Wrist fracture

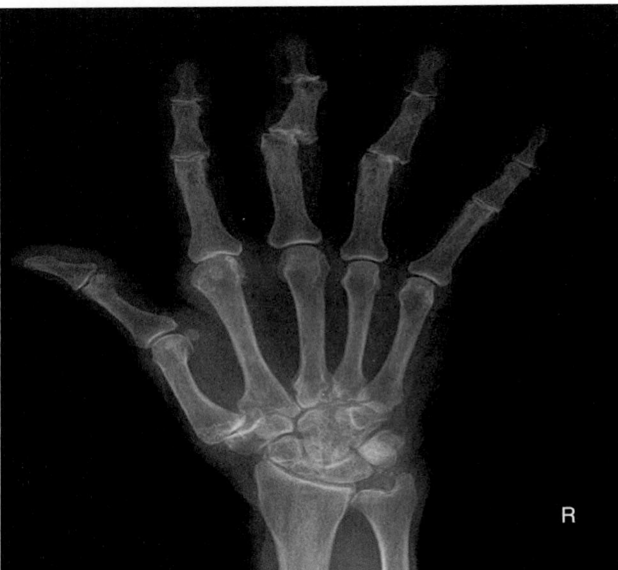

• **Fig. 3.1** Plain radiograph of the right wrist and hand of the patient described in Question 1.

2. A 92-year-old woman has been in the hospital for 3 weeks with unexplained fever, malaise, and weight loss. She reports no other localizing symptoms. Comprehensive physical examination (including pelvic and breast evaluations) has failed to reveal any abnormalities other than generalized muscle wasting and mental lassitude. She has had a battery of laboratory and imaging studies without a specific diagnosis. Complete blood count shows hemoglobin 9.1 g/dL (with normal red blood cell indices), platelets 525 × 10^3 cells/mm^3, and normal white blood count with differential. Erythrocyte sedimentation rate (ESR) is 110 mm/h. Albumin is 2.8 g/dL, and alkaline phosphatase is 250 U/L (normal 40–130). Transaminases, bilirubins, electrolytes, renal parameters, and serum protein electrophoresis (PEP) are all normal. Urinalysis and urine PEP are likewise normal. Cultures of urine and blood have revealed no growth of microorganisms. The patient has no risk factors for tuberculosis infection, and PPD test was negative. Serologic testing for syphilis, Lyme disease, rheumatoid factor, antinuclear antibodies, and antineutrophil cytoplasmic antibodies are all negative. Chest radiographs and computed tomography (CT) scan of the abdomen/pelvis do not demonstrate lymphadenopathy, culprit masses, hemorrhages, or abscesses. Endoscopy and colonoscopy are normal, as are abdominal and transvaginal ultrasound evaluations. Vascular ultrasonographic imaging of the extremities show no evidence of thrombosis.

   Which of the following is the most appropriate next step in trying to identify a source of the patient's fever?
   A. Repeat blood cultures and treat with empiric ceftriaxone.
   B. Interferon-gamma release assay to assess for prior exposure to *Mycobacterium tuberculosis.*
   C. Question family members out of concern for elder abuse.
   D. Liver biopsy
   E. Temporal artery biopsy

3. A 37-year-old previously healthy woman presents to the outpatient clinic with 6 months of progressively achy hands, wrists, elbows, knees, ankles, and feet. Symptoms are worse in the morning and are alleviated by physical activities. Functionally, she is finding it difficult to perform her duties as an orthopedic hand surgeon because of reduced manual strength and dexterity. Naproxen has provided minimal relief. She reports fatigue but no other associated symptoms. Prior history is notable only for uterine fibroids, treated by total hysterectomy at age 35. The patient denies any history of tobacco use, and her alcohol intake is minimal. Physical examination reveals redness, warmth, and swelling of multiple proximal interphalangeal (PIP) joints, metacarpophalangeal (MCP) joints, both wrists, both ankles, and both knees. Her examination is otherwise normal. Laboratory analysis reveals normal comprehensive metabolic profile and normal complete blood count with differential. Rheumatoid factor (RF), anticyclic citrullinated peptide (anti-CCP) antibodies, and antinuclear antibodies (ANA) are not detectable. CRP is 12.5 mg/L (normal <5). Plain film imaging of the hands reveals swelling of the soft tissues around the affected joints but no other abnormalities.

   Which of the following is the most appropriate first step in pharmacologic management of this condition?
   A. Intravenous rituximab 1000 mg for two infusions, given 2 weeks apart
   B. Duloxetine titrated up to 60 mg once daily
   C. Methotrexate titrated up to 25 mg once weekly
   D. Doxycycline 100 mg twice daily
   E. Repeat the RF, anti-CCP antibody, and ANA tests, and consider pharmacologic treatment only if one of the tests is positive.

4. A 39-year-old woman presents to her primary care provider with severe right hip pain. It has come on steadily over the past 6 months in an unrelenting fashion. She is now barely able to walk and uses a wheelchair when in public. Physical examination reveals a woman of average stature in distress when trying to lay supine on the examining table, preferring to keep her right hip slightly flexed. She has good range of motion in the left hip. However, the right hip has severe pain with any degree of extension or internal rotation. She can passively externally rotate only 30 degrees. Hip flexion is preserved. Abdominal and knee exams are normal. Plain film radiography shows complete collapse of the right femoral head with severe "bone-on-bone" osteoarthritis (OA). Magnetic resonance imaging (MRI) of the right hip shows avascular necrosis (AVN) of the femoral head, with trace effusion. There is no pathology of the sacroiliac joints or psoas muscle.

   Which of the following conditions is *not* a risk factor for developing avascular necrosis of the hip?
   A. Antiphospholipid antibody syndrome
   B. Osteoarthritis of the hip
   C. Sickle cell disease
   D. Alcoholism
   E. Gaucher disease

5. A 27-year-old woman is diagnosed with systemic lupus erythematosus (SLE) based on a history that includes the following: 5 months of swollen joints in the hands, photosensitive malar rash, documented pericarditis, lymphopenia, autoimmune hemolytic anemia, and elevated antinuclear antibody (ANA) 1:1280 diffuse pattern. Further serology demonstrates an elevated anti-Smith antibody, but other serologies and complement levels are normal.

   Which of the following therapies for SLE demands regular screening for potential ocular toxicity?
   A. Mycophenolate mofetil
   B. Methotrexate
   C. Cyclophosphamide
   D. Hydroxychloroquine
   E. Belimumab

6. A 46-year-old man presents to the emergency department for his fifth episode of hepatic encephalopathy as a complication of cirrhotic end-stage liver disease. He also has volume overload and episodes of congestive heart failure, with an ejection fraction of 30%. His family is adamant that he has never consumed alcohol excessively. Comorbidities include poorly controlled diabetes mellitus on insulin therapy and osteoporosis. Aspiration of ascites does not suggest spontaneous bacterial peritonitis. He is treated with lactulose and loop diuretics, and his clinical status improves greatly. On hospital day 4, the patient stumbles and reports some pain in the right hand and wrist. It is not red, warm, or swollen, but chronic bony deformities are present in the distal interphalangeal (DIP), proximal interphalangeal (PIP), and metacarpophalangeal (MCP) joints. Plain film imaging is as shown in Fig. 3.2.

   What is the most likely diagnosis?
   A. Rheumatoid arthritis
   B. Fifth metacarpal fracture
   C. Hemochromatosis
   D. Primary osteoarthritis of the hands
   E. Gaucher disease

7. A 49-year-old obese male laborer with a history of prescription drug abuse presents to his primary care provider with low back pain of 4 months' duration. He recalls no specific antecedent injury. Since onset, he has had some degree of constant low back pain, punctuated by exacerbations of pain when he twists or turns awkwardly. Two weeks ago he was instructed to "take some time off" from work, and he has been mostly lying around the house hoping that his back will improve. Over the past 4 months, he has been taking escalating doses of oxycodone (now 15 mg three times daily), obtained from friends or prescribed

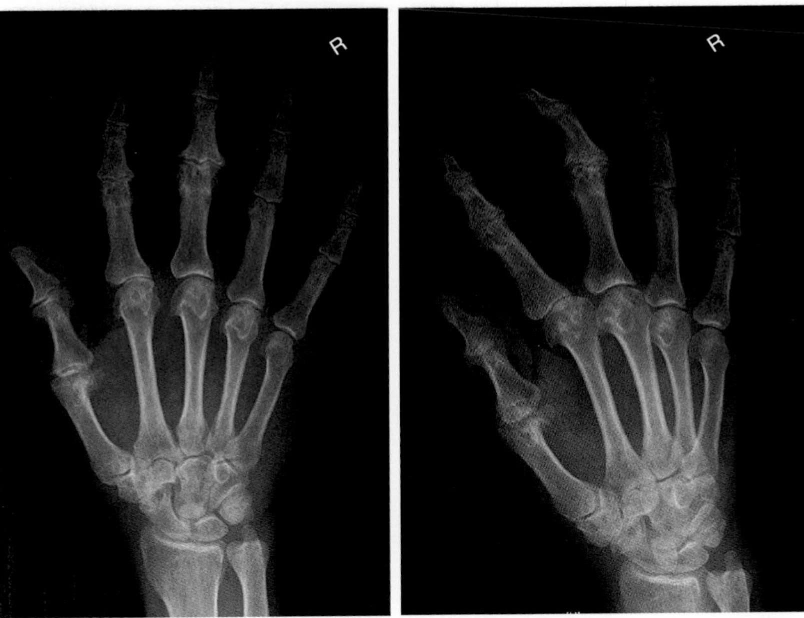

• **Fig. 3.2** Plain radiograph of the right wrist and hand of the patient described in Question 6.

by physicians at nine visits to six different emergency rooms over the past 3 months. Workup available from those evaluations includes normal blood work and normal lumbar spine films. He reports no fever, occult weight loss, bladder or bowel disturbances, or intravenous drug use. Physical examination demonstrates no abnormalities except that he has reduced spine flexion and extension because of pain. He reports that the oxycodone is "not cutting it."

What is the most appropriate next course of action?

A. Reassurance that this will improve
B. Provide a prescription for physical therapy and discuss an "opiate medication contract."
C. Provide a prescription for hydromorphone 2 mg three times daily, with reassurance that this will improve.
D. MRI of the lumbar spine with referral to interventional radiology for any bulging or herniated disc
E. Discharge the patient from your practice for abuse of opiate-based pain medications.

8. A 28-year-old Harvard University geology graduate student presents to student health services with an 8-week history of swelling in her left knee. Her knee is not particularly painful, but the swelling has made it progressively difficult for her to get around. At first, she cut back on mountain climbing and long-distance running. She then had to stop riding her bicycle to class. Now she has difficulty walking more than three city blocks, and she avoids stairs whenever possible. She has no previous medical history and no other joint complaints. Comprehensive review of systems is otherwise unrevealing. She is up to date with immunizations and routine health prevention and maintenance. Physical examination is notable for a swollen, boggy left knee with a massive effusion such that she cannot fully straighten her knee and walks with a limp. There are no other joint abnormalities. Neurologic examination is normal. Laboratory analysis reveals normal comprehensive metabolic profile and complete blood count with differential. Rheumatoid factor (RF) and anticyclic citrullinated peptide (CCP) antibody testing is negative. ESR is 66 mm/h, and CRP is 44.8 mg/L (normal <5). Joint aspiration provides 80 mL of nonbloody, slightly cloudy fluid with white blood cell count 8400 cells/mm^3 (80% lymphocytes). Fluid is negative for crystal analysis, Gram stain, and culture of infectious organisms.

What is the most appropriate next step diagnostic workup or management?

A. Serologic testing for Lyme disease
B. MRI of the left knee
C. Antinuclear antibody (ANA) testing
D. Corticosteroid injection of the left knee
E. Referral to orthopedic surgery for arthroscopic evaluation of the left knee

9. A 39-year-old male kindergarten teacher presents to the emergency department (ED) with severe joint pain "all over." He was in his usual state of good health until 3 days prior, when he started to feel "stiff" in the hands and wrists. Subsequently, he has had progressive pain, redness, and swelling in the hands, wrists, and elbows. He has difficulty moving his shoulders because of pain, and his fiancé sent him to the ED because he could not get out of bed easily in the morning. He reports no other symptoms. He carries sickle cell trait but has an otherwise unremarkable past medical and family history. Physical examination is notable for a generally well-appearing, athletic-appearing man in significant distress during the physical examination because of severe pain in the arms and legs. He has such redness and puffiness in the hands that the assessment of his joints is difficult. His elbows do not extend fully because of joint pain, and he cannot lift his arms or legs off the examination table because of pain in the shoulders and hips, respectively. His knees are tender and slightly swollen. Ankles, feet, and toes have puffy tenderness and are difficult to examine further because of pain. He is afebrile and normotensive. Heart rate is 110 beats per minute but comes down to the 90s with opiate medications for pain control. Remainder of examination is normal. Laboratory analysis reveals hemoglobin 9.4 g/dL, with mean corpuscular volume 71 fL (normal 81–97 fL), and reticulocyte count 0.1%. Platelet count and white blood cell count with differential are normal, as is the comprehensive metabolic profile. ESR is 49 mm/h, and CRP is 251 mg/L (normal <5). Radiographic imaging of the hands and feet demonstrates soft tissue swelling but no other abnormalities.

What is the most likely diagnosis?

A. Septic polyarthritis
B. Viral arthritis
C. Fibromyalgia syndrome
D. Lyme disease
E. Rheumatoid arthritis

10. A 68-year-old woman presents to her primary care provider because of fatigue, malaise, weight loss, and diffuse achiness. Symptoms started insidiously about 4 months ago. She has no other localizing symptoms. Her weight has dropped by 12 pounds since her last visit for annual examination, 9 months previously. Physical examination reveals a frail, fatigued-appearing woman with bitemporal wasting. Her gait is slow and deliberate. She has reduced muscle bulk and strength testing in the proximal arms and legs, mostly due to achiness. Examination is otherwise unrevealing. Laboratory analysis shows normal comprehensive metabolic profile, white blood cell count, and platelet count. Hemoglobin (Hgb) is 10.0 g/dL with normal mean corpuscular volume. ESR is 103 mm/h, and C-reactive protein (CRP) is 2.4 mg/L (normal <5).

Which of the following is the most appropriate next course of action?

A. Antinuclear antibody testing
B. Serum and urine protein electrophoresis
C. Temporal artery biopsy
D. CT scan of the chest, abdomen, and pelvis
E. Prednisone 15 mg daily

11. A 53-year-old man with long-standing scleroderma presents with worsening dyspnea on exertion. Over the past 2 years, he has noticed increasing difficulty climbing stairs and keeping up with his spouse when walking. His scleroderma predominantly affects the hands as sclerodactyly, and it is associated with severe gastroesophageal reflux disease (GERD) and symptomatic Raynaud phenomenon. Vital signs are normal. Physical examination reveals sclerodactyly with acrocyanosis and tightness of the skin on the face. He has multiple matte telangiectasias on the skin and mucosal surfaces. Lungs are clear to auscultation. Cardiac evaluation demonstrates an accentuated paradoxically split P2. Six-minute walk test reveals 98% oxygen saturation at rest, which drops to 92% with ambulation. Chest radiograph is normal.

Which of the following most likely explains the patient's dyspnea?

A. Physical deconditioning
B. Scleroderma cardiomyopathy with congestive heart failure
C. Pulmonary hypertension
D. Occult aspiration from undertreated GERD
E. Pulmonary embolus

12. A 47-year-old man with a history of rheumatoid arthritis (RA) is admitted to the hospital with fever, dyspnea, and chest infiltrate. His RA treatment of methotrexate and etanercept is held. The diagnosis upon admission is presumed community-acquired bacterial pneumonia, and he is treated empirically with a combination of ceftriaxone and azithromycin. However, after 3 days his status has deteriorated such that he is placed on a mechanical ventilator for hypoxemia. Chest CT scan reveals necrotic-appearing pulmonary nodules.

Which of the following is the most appropriate next course of action?

A. Intravenous methylprednisolone 100 mg three times daily for treatment of rheumatoid lung
B. Bronchoscopy with lavage for microscopic organisms
C. Open lung biopsy
D. PET-CT scan to identify source of primary tumor in the setting of pulmonary metastases
E. Switch antibiotic therapy to levofloxacin 750 mg daily

13. A 44-year-old male landscaper presents to his primary care provider because of knee complaints. He has had pain, swelling, and limited motion in the right knee for 5 months. His only other musculoskeletal complaint is nontraumatic swelling of the left fourth finger such that his wedding ring had to be cut off. He is otherwise healthy, except for excessive beer consumption (12 or more per day). Physical examination reveals a massively swollen right knee with near-full extension but only 60 degrees of flexion. His left fourth finger is also swollen and tender, with minimal flexion. Remainder of the joint examination is unrevealing. Laboratory analysis is essentially normal or negative: comprehensive metabolic profile, complete blood count and differential,

CRP, ESR, Lyme disease serology, antinuclear antibody, rheumatoid factor, and anti-CCP antibody. Arthrocentesis yielded 90 mL of nonbloody, cloudy, yellow fluid with 65,000 white blood cells (60% neutrophils). Fluid analysis is negative for polarizable crystals and microbiologic organisms.

Which of the following is most likely to be diagnostic in this case?

A. Detectable anti-Smith antibody
B. A serum uric acid of 11.5 mg/dL
C. Elevated serum angiotensin-converting enzyme (ACE) level
D. Scaly erythematous plaques on the extensor surfaces of the arms and legs
E. Presence of chondrocalcinosis on plain film radiography of the right knee

14. A 21-year-old woman visits her primary care provider because of diffuse joint pains for the past 18 months. They involve her fingers, wrists, elbows, shoulders, hips, knees, ankles, and spine. She has noticed no redness, warmth, or swelling of the joints, nor any muscle pain. She reports that her shoulders and hips feel like they are "popping out of joint" with physical fitness, including during her activities as a semiprofessional ballerina. She reports palpitations and dizziness when sitting upright quickly and states that she has "almost passed out" on several occasions. Comprehensive review of systems is otherwise unremarkable. Physical examination is notable for a thin woman in no acute distress. She has normal seated heart rate and blood pressure, and no chest wall abnormalities. Arms and legs are well proportioned without deformity, and she has no red, warm, swollen joints. She has more than 90 degrees of passive extension at the wrists and metacarpophalangeal (MCP) joints. Elbow and knee joints do not have effusions, and she can extend them 190 degrees voluntarily. Spine and hip motion is excellent; she is able to place her palms flat on the floor without bending her knees. Ocular, skin, cardiopulmonary, and neurologic examinations are normal. Echocardiography for the palpitations reveals only mild mitral valve prolapse.

Which of the following studies is most likely to be abnormal in this patient?

A. Tilt-table test
B. MRI of the left shoulder
C. CT scan of the right hip
D. Serum RF and anti-CCP antibodies
E. Lyme disease serology

15. A 68-year-old woman presents to her primary care provider because of weakness of the shoulders and hips. For 5 weeks, she has noticed progressive difficulty climbing stairs and trouble getting out of a chair. She denies any arthralgias or myalgias, however. She has preexisting chronic dyspnea from various comorbidities that include coronary artery disease, hypertension, atrial fibrillation, type 2 diabetes mellitus, and chronic tobacco use complicated by emphysema. Her only other complaint is a new-onset rash on her face and hands (Fig. 3.3). Physical examination is notable for reduced strength. She is able to get her thighs off the examining table against gravity, but not against mild resistance testing. She has similar weakness in her shoulders. Grip strength is preserved. Lungs have some mild wheezes at the apex but also bibasilar Velcro-type rales. Laboratory testing reveals elevated creatine phosphokinase (CPK) 10,200 U/L, CK-MB 340 ng/mL, aspartate aminotransferase (AST) 348 U/L, and alanine aminotransferase (ALT) 419 U/L. Albumin is 3.1 g/dL. She has otherwise normal comprehensive metabolic profile, complete blood count with differential, and coagulation studies. Electrocardiogram (EKG) does not demonstrate any abnormalities. Chest radiograph demonstrates fibrotic changes at the bibasilar lung fields.

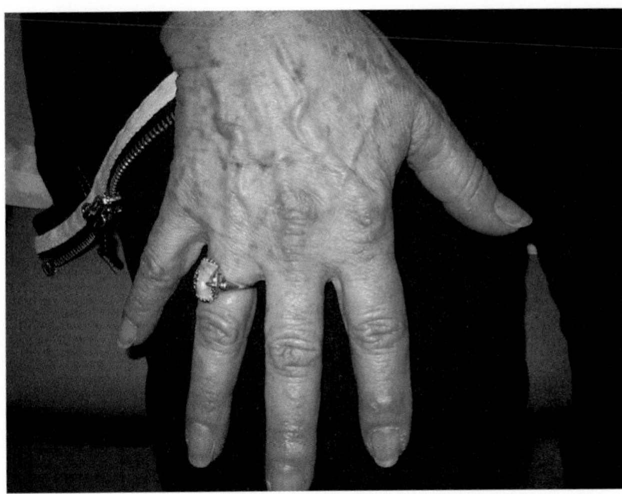

• **Fig. 3.3** Hand of the patient described in Question 15.

Which of the following tests is most likely to be diagnostic for this condition?

A. Liver biopsy
B. Temporal artery biopsy
C. Cardiac MRI
D. Cardiac catheterization
E. Skeletal muscle biopsy

16. A 25-year-old man presents to the emergency department for an episode of acute right lower quadrant abdominal pain, which started abruptly 3 days prior. He has had multiple episodes similar to this in the past, dating back to a bout of appendicitis at age 4. Associated symptoms include fever, nausea, and anorexia. Medical history also includes presumed gout (lacking a crystal-proven diagnosis). Past surgical history includes four separate abdominal surgeries: appendectomy, cholecystectomy, and two exploratory laparoscopies. There is no family history of any similar condition. Physical examination reveals a thin man appearing to be in a toxic condition who is unwilling to maneuver in bed because of abdominal pain. Vital signs include temperature 39.2°C, blood pressure 92/58 mm Hg, heart rate 125 beats per minute, respiratory rate 24 breaths per minute, and 99% oxygen saturation on room air. The abdomen is slightly distended and exquisitely tender to gentle palpation. Bowel sounds are absent. Rectal examination reveals normal tone but no blood. Remainder of examination is unrevealing. Laboratory analysis reveals normal comprehensive metabolic profile except for albumin 2.3 g/dL. Creatinine is 1.0 mg/dL. Uric acid is 4.2 mg/dL. Complete blood count is notable for white blood cell count 21.2 × 10^3 cells/mm^3 (72% neutrophils and 13% bands), hemoglobin 10.4 g/dL (MCV 88 fL), and platelets 630 × 10^3 cells/mm^3. CRP is 310 mg/L and ESR is 107 mm/h. Urinalysis is notable only for 4+ protein, with a spot protein/creatinine ratio of 2.1. CT scan of the abdomen and pelvis demonstrates some free peritoneal fluid, but no free air or other evidence of bowel rupture.

Which of the following studies is most likely to provide the correct diagnosis?

A. *MEFV* genetic testing
B. Endoscopy with biopsy of the duodenum to look for flattened villi and crypts
C. Traditional angiography of the mesenteric vasculature
D. Colonoscopy with biopsy of the terminal ileum
E. Serum antineutrophil cytoplasmic antibody (ANCA) testing

17. A 22-year-old female college student presents to university health services because of bilateral knee pain. She is an avid runner, but she has had to curtail her normal regimen of 30 miles per week because of knee pain. It has come on rather severely over the past 3 weeks, and localizes mostly at the anterior knee. It is exacerbated by rapidly standing from a chair or by descending stairs. She denies knee swelling or lateral thigh discomfort. She has not had morning stiffness or other joint pains. She is tearful because of the severity of the knee pain and the effect it has had on her exercise. She is otherwise healthy. Physical examination reveals a thin, athletic-appearing young woman. She has excellent range of motion in all joints except for the knees, where she has pain with flexion of the knee beyond 110 degrees. She can extend fully. There are no knee effusions. She is tender along the patellar margins, especially if the patella is compressed downward during active knee extension. There is no tenderness along the lateral knees, nor any posterior knee tenderness. She has negative McMurray sign and no instability on varus/valgus stress maneuvers or anterior/posterior drawer sign testing.

Which of the following is the most likely diagnosis?

A. Patellofemoral syndrome
B. Iliotibial band syndrome
C. Tear of the medial meniscus
D. Tear of the anterior cruciate ligament (ACL)
E. Popliteal (Baker) cyst

18. A 21-year-old female college student presents to the emergency department with new-onset fever, headache, dyspnea, and weight gain. She was in her usual state of excellent health until 6 weeks prior, when her current symptoms started. She has noticed puffiness around her eyes and swelling in her ankles. Associated symptoms include cold fingers and toes with blue discoloration. She takes no medications regularly. Vital signs were notable for temperature 37.9°C, blood pressure 192/110 mm Hg, heart rate 108 beats per minute, respiratory rate 22 breaths per minute, and oxygen saturation 92% on room air. She is ill appearing, with periorbital and lower-extremity edema. Other notable features of the physical examination include lungs with bibasilar wet rales and acrocyanosis with digital ulcerations. There is no sclerodactyly. Laboratory analysis includes blood urea nitrogen (BUN) 82 mg/dL, creatinine 5.2 mg/dL, albumin 1.9 g/dL, Hgb 8.4 g/dL with MCV 82 fL, platelet count 74 × 10^3 cells/mm^3, and white blood cell count 2.5 × 10^3 cells/mm^3 with 80% neutrophils, 10% lymphocytes, 6% monocytes, and 3% eosinophils. Urinalysis demonstrates 50–100 RBCs with casts, +++ protein, and no leukocytes. ESR is 110 mm/h, CRP is 12.9 mg/L (normal <5), and antinuclear antibody is 1:5120 speckled pattern. Blood cultures are normal. EKG is normal. Chest radiograph demonstrates fluffy vascular congestion and trace bibasilar effusions.

Which of the following additional test results would be most consistent with her presentation?

A. p-ANCA–positive, antimyeloperoxidase (MPO) antibody–negative, and antiproteinase-3 (PR3) antibody–negative
B. Uric acid 13.5 mg/dL and bone marrow biopsy with 75% clonal promyelocytes
C. Anti–double-stranded DNA antibody 522 U/mL (normal <5), C3 complement 52 mg/dL (normal 75–175), C4 complement 8 mg/dL (normal 14–40)
D. CPK 8600 U/mL, anti-Jo1 antibody 82 U/mL (normal <5)
E. HLA-B27–positive, sacroiliac joint fusion on plain radiography, and renal biopsy showing changes most consistent with IgA nephropathy

19. A 58-year-old man presents to the outpatient clinic with 3 days of an excruciatingly painful, red, warm, swollen left great toe. He has had to use crutches and been unable to sleep because of the severity of pain. He has had episodes similar to this in the past, and on one occasion he had an arthrocentesis that provided a "crystal-proven" diagnosis of gout. Relevant comorbidities include stage IV chronic kidney disease (glomerular filtration rate 19 mL/min) as a complication of hypertension. He has never had nephrolithiasis. Physical examination reveals a red, warm, very tender left first metatarsal phalangeal joint. There are no other active joints. The bilateral olecranon bursae have large tophi.

What is the most appropriate next course of action?

A. Check a serum uric acid (sUA) level and initiate allopurinol if the sUA is >6 mg/dL.
B. Check a 24-hour urine uric acid and initiate probenecid 500 mg twice daily if the patient is an "under-excretor."
C. Treat with colchicine 0.6-mg tablets: 2 tablets to start and 1–2 tablets per day for the next 5 days.
D. Treat with naproxen 500 mg twice daily with food.
E. Treat with intramuscular methylprednisolone 80 mg ×1.

20. A 50-year-old man presents to his primary care provider because of rapid-onset right shoulder pain of 3 days' duration. He was previously healthy, recalls no antecedent injury or trauma, and has never experienced shoulder pain of this severity before. On physical examination, the shoulder is not visibly red, warm, or swollen. He experiences significant discomfort on active abduction and forward flexion (against resistance) until he reaches 90 degrees horizontal, at which point pain limits further motion. Passive range of motion testing achieves an additional 30 degrees in these planes. He does not tolerate resisted internal or external rotation, nor resisted abduction with his arm held slightly in front of his body in internal rotation.

What is the most likely diagnosis?

A. Biceps tendonitis
B. Septic arthritis
C. Acute calcific tendonitis
D. Glenohumeral osteoarthritis
E. Complete tear of the supraspinatus

21. An 84-year-old generally healthy man calls his primary care provider (PCP) on a Saturday afternoon to report 3 weeks of unilateral headache, scalp tenderness, and achiness in the jaw when chewing a bagel. He has had no visual disturbances and denies any head trauma. Two nights prior, he went to a local emergency department (ED) for these same symptoms, where he was diagnosed with a new migraine headache, given acetaminophen 1000 mg three times daily, and instructed to call his PCP in the event that his symptoms failed to improve. Laboratory testing from the ED revealed ESR 110 mm/h, normal cerebrospinal fluid analysis, and a head CT scan that did not show any evidence of intracerebral hemorrhage.

What is the most appropriate next step in management?

A. Reassure the patient that his symptoms are a common complication of lumbar puncture. He should remain supine as much as possible for 48 hours and touch base on Monday morning if his symptoms persist.
B. Arrange for an expedited temporal artery biopsy first thing Monday morning. In the meantime, inform the patient to call back in the event of any vision loss.
C. Prescribe prednisone 1 mg/kg. Instruct the patient to start it immediately and to call with any new visual disturbances. Arrange for an expedited temporal artery biopsy first thing Monday morning.
D. Inform the patient that he likely has viral meningitis and should return to the ED for treatment.
E. Inform the patient that he may have a cerebral aneurysm and refer him back the ED for magnetic resonance angiography of the brain.

22. A 66-year-old obese woman with a history of chronic back pain presents for an initial evaluation of left lateral hip discomfort of 5 weeks' duration. She reports no antecedent injury, but it hurts to sleep on that side at night. Symptoms do not radiate to the groin. On physical examination, she has an antalgic waddling gait but demonstrates good active and passive range of motion in the left hip. Passive adduction reproduces her lateral hip pain, as does palpation over the lateral hip.

Which of the following is an appropriate next step in diagnosis or management of this condition?

A. Reassurance and physical therapy, focusing on posture, core muscle tone, and hip range of motion
B. MRI of the left hip
C. Methylprednisolone taper from 24 mg down to 0 over 6 days (dropping the dose by 4 mg each day)
D. Whole-body bone scan
E. Bone mineral densitometry

23. A 59-year-old woman with long-standing destructive rheumatoid arthritis (RA) has recently moved to the area and is scheduled to undergo revision total hip arthroplasty because of refractory pain and functional limitations. She is seeing you for preoperative clearance evaluation. Her primary complaint is gait instability, urinary incontinence, and paresthesias in the bilateral arms. Prior records are not immediately available, but you know that she has already had multiple previous orthopedic procedures, including bilateral hip and knee arthroplasties, bilateral wrist fusion surgeries, and a left elbow arthroplasty. For her RA, she is taking etanercept and methotrexate, which will be stopped by her rheumatologist 2 weeks prior to surgery. She has no history of heart disease or identifiable risk factors other than the RA. Physical examination reveals general muscle atrophy and multiple joint deformities. There are no red, warm, or swollen joints. Neurologic testing reveals hyperreflexivity of the bilateral upper extremities and positive Hoffman sign. Gait cannot be tested because of instability.

What is the most important preoperative testing to be done in this patient?

A. Rheumatoid factor (RF) and anticyclic citrullinated peptide (CCP) antibody testing
B. ESR and CRP testing
C. Cardiac exercise stress testing with sestamibi-enhanced nuclear imaging
D. Lateral cervical spine x-ray imaging, with flexion and extension views
E. Lumbar spine MRI

24. A 48-year-old man with a history of alcoholism and cirrhosis presents to urgent care because he has been tripping over his own feet. He describes an inability to get his toes off the ground when walking. He has not had any change in his baseline cirrhosis, and his mental status is lucid. He describes general arthralgias with some morning stiffness. Physical examination reveals stigmata of cirrhosis with scleral icterus, jaundice, and abdominal ascites. Gait is altered by left-leg toe drag that occurs throughout stride, and he lacks strength in the tibialis anterior muscle. Lower-extremity reflexes are otherwise intact. He has a painless rash on the legs as shown in Fig. 3.4. He has diffuse tenderness of muscles and joints but no red, warm, or swollen joints. Laboratory testing reveals the following: serum sodium 129 mEq/L, serum creatinine 1.4 mg/dL, normal complete blood count with differential, CRP 88.1 mg/L, ESR 99 mm/h, rheumatoid factor 110 U/mL (normal <15), C3 complement 112 mg/dL (normal 75–175), and C4 complement 5 mg/dL (normal 14–40). Urinalysis has 100–200 RBC per high-power field, with some dysmorphia. There is +++ protein.

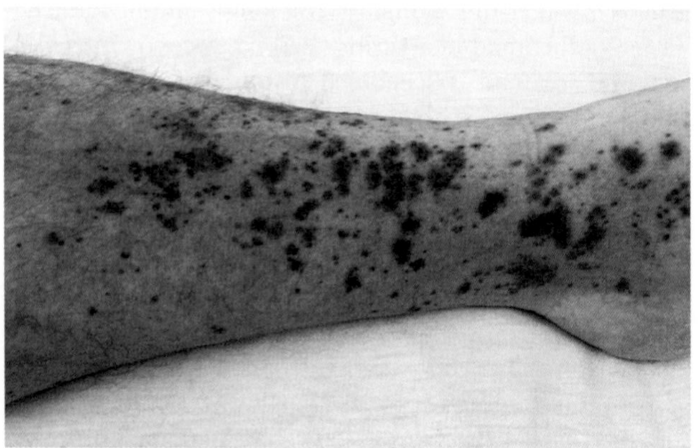

• **Fig. 3.4** Leg of the patient described in Question 24.

Which of the following serologic tests, if positive, would best explain the above clinical scenario?

A. Antinuclear antibody
B. Hepatitis C antibody
C. Anti-CCP antibody
D. Heterophile antibody testing (monospot)
E. Lyme disease serology

25. A 68-year-old man is seen by his primary care provider for osteoarthritic right knee pain of 12 years' duration. He initially had pain only when running, but this progressed to pain on ambulation. Currently, he reports pain when walking more than two city blocks, standing for more than 20 minutes, and nocturnal knee pain. He reports no knee swelling, locking, or instability. When out with friends, he cannot keep up with them and frequently has to sit because of his knee pain. Physical therapy and naproxen 500 mg twice daily have not adequately relieved his pain. He has derived only 2 weeks of relief from each of three prior corticosteroid injections into the right knee joint. Comorbidities include type 2 diabetes mellitus, cerebrovascular disease with mild carotid stenosis, hypertension, hyperlipidemia, and obesity (body mass index 34.2 kg/m^2). On physical examination, he has good range of motion in the bilateral hips, left knee, and bilateral ankles. Both knees have hypertrophic osteoarthritic changes, crepitus, mild effusions, full extension, and only 90 degrees of flexion. He has genu valgus deformity of both knees and no instability on varus/valgus stress maneuvers or anterior/posterior drawer sign testing. There is minimal tenderness on the left but diffuse joint-line tenderness on the right. Previous right knee aspiration has yielded 25 mL of fluid with 288 white blood cells per mm^3. Plain film radiography shows tricompartmental osteoarthritic change of both knees with significant joint space narrowing medially.

What is the most appropriate next course of action?

A. Inject the right knee with triamcinolone 40 mg, prescribe physical therapy, and advise weight loss.
B. Switch naproxen to oxycodone 5 mg three times daily. Reassess in 1 year.
C. MRI of the right knee
D. Refer to orthopedics for arthroscopic debridement of loose cartilage.
E. Refer to orthopedics for consideration of right total knee arthroplasty.

26. A 28-year-old woman presents to her primary care provider with numbness and paresthesias in the first three fingers of both hands. Symptoms are worst when she first awakens in the morning, and they impact her profession as a hairstylist. Physical examination reveals no redness, warmth, or swelling of the fingers, thumbs, or wrists. She has preserved thenar muscle strength and no atrophy. Passive forced flexion of the wrist reproduces her symptoms after 30 seconds. There is no swelling of the wrist, and range of motion is intact. She is diagnosed with carpal tunnel syndrome (CTS).

Which of the following conditions is not associated with CTS?

A. Acromegaly
B. Scleroderma
C. Chondrocalcinosis of the wrist
D. Rheumatoid arthritis
E. Hypothyroidism

27. A 51-year-old morbidly obese man presents to his primary care provider with paresthesias and painless numbness of the anterior left thigh. Symptoms are best when he first awakens in the morning and progressively worsen over the course of a day. He has noticed this coming on over the previous 3 weeks. Comorbidities include diabetes mellitus. Physical examination reveals clearly demarcated absence of sensation overlying the anterior thigh. There are no motor deficits. Lower-extremity reflexes are intact. Hip range of motion is normal.

Which of the following explains the most likely diagnosis?

A. Diabetic amyotrophy
B. Avascular necrosis of the left femoral head
C. Entrapment neuropathy of the left lateral femoral cutaneous nerve
D. Irritation of the gluteus medius and gluteus minimus muscles at their tendon insertion on the left greater trochanter
E. Degenerative arthritis of the left hip

28. A 49-year-old woman presents to a new primary care provider with complaints of diffuse joint and muscle pains that have been present for over 20 years. The pain has escalated over the past 18 months to the point where she has stopped working as a cashier and is applying for disability. She is no longer able to derive enjoyment from her young grandchildren, because she is always in pain. When asked about red, warm, or swollen joints, she reports a severe burning pain in her arms, legs, and back. She has no significant comorbidities other than obesity (body mass index 41.1 kg/m^2) and chronic back pain. Review of systems is notable for fatigue, weight gain, and poor sleep. She does not smoke or drink excessive alcohol, but she describes a lot of stress related to the loss of her job and prolonged divorce proceedings over the past 2 years. Physical examination is notable for an obese woman who is tearful throughout the musculoskeletal exam. She has diffuse tenderness in the arms, legs, and thorax. There are no obviously warm, swollen, or tender joints, but the assessment is partly limited by obesity and her distress even with light touch. Neurologic examination reveals reduced effort at strength testing but normal when distracted. Laboratory analysis is normal: comprehensive metabolic profile, complete blood count and differential, thyroid-stimulating hormone (TSH), creatine kinase, and C-reactive protein.

What is the next most appropriate step in diagnostic testing or management?

A. Electromyogram (EMG) with nerve conduction studies (NCS) of all four extremities
B. Test antinuclear antibody (ANA) and rheumatoid factor (RF).
C. Serology testing for Lyme disease
D. Recommend combination of physical therapy, sleep routine, weight loss, and psychiatric counseling.
E. Initiate oxycodone 5 mg twice daily, with dose escalation as needed.

29. A 24-year-old woman presents to her primary care provider with discomfort in her fingers and toes. Symptoms have been present for 4 years and are distinctly worse in the winter. Cold exposure causes white and blue color changes, leading to numbness and stiffness in the involved digits. Symptoms are alleviated by rewarming the fingers, but they are accompanied by fiery red erythema and discomfort. Medical history is notable only for attention-deficit/hyperactivity disorder, treated with dextroamphetamine. On physical examination, there is no erythema, warmth, or swelling in the fingers or wrists. There is no sclerodactyly or periungual erythema. Digital nailfold capillaroscopy reveals mild tortuosity of capillaries without microaneurysms, hemorrhage, or dropout. Radial and ulnar pulses are brisk, and Allen test is normal bilaterally.

Which of the following is the most appropriate next step in diagnostic workup?

A. Test for antinuclear antibodies, anti-dsDNA, anti-Ro, anti-La, anti-Smith, and anti-RNP antibodies.
B. Test for antinuclear antibodies, anti-SCL70, and anticentromere antibodies.
C. Test for antinuclear antibodies, antiphospholipid antibodies, and lupus anticoagulant.
D. Magnetic resonance angiography of the bilateral upper extremities
E. No additional workup necessary

30. A 46-year-old woman with systemic sclerosis (scleroderma) presents to the emergency department because of headache, dyspnea, and lower-extremity edema. She has had recent complications of her scleroderma, including Raynaud crisis with gangrene of the left fourth finger, interstitial pulmonary fibrosis, and pericardial effusion. Vital signs include temperature 36.8°C, blood pressure 140/95 mm Hg in both arms, heart rate 72 beats per minute, respiratory rate 24 breaths per minute, and oxygen saturation 94% on room air. Physical examination reveals an ill-appearing individual with scleroderma involving the hands, arms, face, trunk, legs, and feet. She has scattered cutaneous telangiectasia. She has dry gangrenous changes of the left fourth finger distal to the distal interphalangeal joint. Lungs have bibasilar Velcro rales. Cardiac examination is unrevealing. Laboratory analysis reveals BUN 40 mg/dL, creatinine 3.2 mg/dL, white blood cell count 7.2 × 10^3 cells/mm^3, hemoglobin 8.9 g/dL, and platelet count 85 × 10^3/mm^3. Blood smear demonstrates schistocytes. Prothrombin time and partial thromboplastin time are normal. Liver function studies are normal. Urinalysis shows ++++ protein and >100 RBC per high-power field. Chest radiograph is consistent with pulmonary edema. There is no cardiomegaly. EKG is unrevealing.

Which of the following must be included in the next steps of managing this patient?

A. Plasma exchange therapy
B. Captopril 25 mg orally three times daily, with dose escalation to control blood pressure
C. Labetalol 100 mg orally twice daily, with dose escalation to control blood pressure
D. Amlodipine 5 mg orally once daily, with dose escalation to control blood pressure
E. Methylprednisolone 250 mg intravenously every 12 hours

31. A 68-year-old diabetic man presents to the emergency department because of right ankle pain and altered gait. On physical examination, the ankle is swollen posteriorly but has full passive range of motion. Squeezing of the calf with the patient seated does not result in dorsiflexion of the ankle. Two weeks ago he had been admitted to the hospital with pneumococcal pneumonia.

What was the most likely agent used to treat his pneumonia?

A. Imipenem
B. Trimethoprim/sulfamethoxazole
C. Cefpodoxime
D. Levofloxacin
E. Azathioprine

32. A 77-year-old man is recovering in the surgical intensive care unit from coronary artery bypass graft surgery. On postoperative day 3, he develops severe pain of the anterior aspect of the right knee with focal erythema, warmth, and swelling. On physical examination, he keeps his right leg fully extended and yells in pain if the knee is flexed actively or passively. The knee is exquisitely tender over the patella. Examination does not demonstrate any perceivable knee fluid for aspiration.

Which of the following is the most likely diagnosis?

A. Gouty bursitis of the right prepatellar bursa
B. Gouty arthritis of the right knee
C. Septic arthritis of the right knee
D. Right knee meniscal injury from unintended intraoperative injury
E. Quadriceps tendon rupture

33. A 28-year-old woman presents to the emergency department because of severe pain and swelling in multiple joints. Two weeks ago she was admitted with severe gastrointestinal dysentery, from which she has recovered. Ibuprofen has offered little relief. Physical examination reveals overt erythema, warmth, and swelling of the fingers, hands, wrists, and elbows. She has a swollen left knee. Laboratory testing reveals an ESR 88 mm/h and CRP 182 mg/L (normal <5).

Which of the following microorganisms is not associated with reactive arthritis?

A. *Staphylococcus aureus*
B. *Streptococcus pyogenes*
C. *Chlamydia trachomatis*
D. *Yersinia pestis*
E. *Salmonella enteritidis*

34. A 52-year-old obese woman presents with bilateral foot pain of 3 weeks' duration. Symptoms localize to the plantar aspect of the foot and are worse first thing in the morning when she steps out of bed, lasting for at least 2 hours. She has not noticed any redness, warmth, or swelling of the feet, nor in any other joints. Other medical conditions include osteoporosis secondary to surgical menopause at age 31. Physical examination demonstrates no redness, warmth, or swelling of the feet and no tenderness on squeeze of the metatarsophalangeal joints. She has focal tenderness to palpation at the plantar aspect of the calcaneus bones. Plain film radiography of the feet is normal.

Which of the following is the most likely diagnosis?

A. Occult stress fracture of the fifth metatarsal bone
B. Plantar fasciitis
C. Acute gouty arthritis of the talonavicular joint
D. Charcot arthropathy
E. Occult injury of the anterior talofibular ligament

35. A 28-year-old woman has rheumatoid arthritis (RA) that is well controlled on a combination of methotrexate and adalimumab (anti-TNF-α monoclonal antibody). She will be traveling to the Brazilian Amazon rain forest as part of a graduate school degree program in anthropology. She has never been agreeable to immunizations in the past, but she is requesting whatever the travel clinic advises.

In addition to malaria prophylaxis and education about appropriate use of insect repellant to avoid dengue and Zika virus infections, which of the following vaccine regimens should she receive?

A. Hepatitis A vaccine, oral typhoid vaccine, yellow fever vaccine, and MMR booster
B. Hepatitis A vaccine, injectable typhoid vaccine, and yellow fever vaccine
C. Hepatitis A vaccine, injectable typhoid vaccine, and a letter of exemption from yellow fever vaccine

D. Hepatitis A vaccine, injectable typhoid vaccine, and a letter of exemption from yellow fever and MMR vaccines

36. A 25-year-old previously healthy woman presents to her primary care provider with bilateral ankle pain and a rash. Symptoms started 2 weeks ago as pain, swelling, and tenderness in the bilateral ankles. Her feet are swollen to the point that she cannot wear her regular shoes and it hurts to walk. No other joints are involved. Ten days ago, she began to notice tender erythematous "lumps" on her anterior shins. Physical examination confirms the history. She has swelling around both ankles and reduced active range of motion because of pain. Passive range of motion is preserved, however, including flexion/extension and inversion/eversion at the ankle. The Achilles tendon is unaffected. The shins have fewer than a dozen scattered tender erythematous nodules of varying size, none larger than 1 cm. There is no overlying skin breakdown.

Which of the following tests would be expected to show an abnormality that would aid in the diagnosis of her condition?

A. Ankle film
B. Chest radiograph
C. Rheumatoid factor and anti-CCP antibody
D. Serum uric acid level
E. Serum Lyme disease serologies

37. A 32-year-old man presents with low back pain and leg numbness. Three weeks ago, he was lifting window air-conditioning units when he felt a "pop" in his low back associated with severe pain. He rested his back for 1 week and has been using a friend's prescription for hydrocodone. With this, the pain has improved slightly. Two weeks ago, however, he began to notice constipation such that he has not had a bowel movement in 8 days. He has also had new-onset impotence and reports increased urinary urgency with frequent dribbling of only small volumes of urine. This is associated with paresthesias down the right posterior leg and numbness in the perineum. Physical examination reveals a man who does not appear to be in a toxic condition and who has trouble finding a comfortable position on the examination table. Back range of motion is limited to 30 degrees of forward flexion because of lumbar spine pain, and there is associated spasm of paraspinous muscles. Neurologic examination is entirely normal in the upper extremities. Assessment of lower extremities reveals weakness of ankle plantar flexion on the right with intact ankle dorsiflexion and hip flexion. His gait is altered in that he shortens the length of stride during the "push-off" phase on the right leg and cannot stand on his toes on the right because of weakness. Reflexes are normal at the bilateral patellae, diminished at the left Achilles, and absent at the right Achilles. Cremasteric reflex is intact. Sensory examination reveals reduced detection of pin prick and proprioception in the posterior right thigh and lateral toes of the right foot.

Which of the following is the most appropriate next step in evaluation and management of this patient?

A. Physical therapy and reassurance. Reassess in 4 weeks.
B. Plain film radiography of the back. If normal, then offer physical therapy and reassurance. Reassess in 4 weeks.
C. Schedule nonurgent MRI of the lumbar spine. If there is a herniated disc, then offer physical therapy and reassurance. Reassess in 4 weeks.
D. Schedule nonurgent MRI of the lumbar spine. If there is a herniated disc, then refer to interventional radiology for corticosteroid injection.
E. Referral to emergency department for urgent MRI of the lumbar spine

38. A 50-year-old woman has had chronic systemic sarcoidosis for 4 years. She has had involvement of the heart, liver, lungs, skeletal muscle, and joints. Despite aggressive immunosuppressive measures with methotrexate and infliximab, she has continued to require chronic corticosteroid therapy with daily prednisone. The prednisone dose is currently 40 mg daily. It has fluctuated between 20 and 60 mg daily with disease activity, and has been no less than 20 mg daily for 3 years. On physical examination, she is obese with cushingoid features. Blood pressure is 150/95 mm Hg, and body mass index is 39.5 kg/m^2. Comorbidities include steroid-induced diabetes mellitus.

Which of the following conditions is not a direct side effect of chronic corticosteroid therapy?

A. Increased risk of infectious illnesses
B. Accelerated cataract formation
C. Hyperuricemia
D. Avascular necrosis of bone
E. Proximal muscle weakness

39. A 74-year-old woman presents to the outpatient clinic reporting 8 weeks of sudden-onset fatigue and achiness in the shoulders and hips. Two weeks ago she saw an orthopedic surgeon, who diagnosed rotator cuff tendonitis and injected 40 mg of triamcinolone into the left subacromial bursa. She reports that, following the injection, "everything went away and I felt great." However, this benefit only lasted 3 days, and all of her symptoms have returned. She has no other medical illnesses. She has not had any red, warm, or swollen joints. She denies any headaches, visual disturbances, scalp tenderness, or jaw achiness after chewing. Laboratory analysis reveals ESR 64 mm/h and CRP 76.2 mg/L (normal <5.0).

Which of the following features also typically characterizes the condition most likely affecting this patient?

A. Morning stiffness
B. Blindness

C. Elevated rheumatoid factor
D. Chondrocalcinosis
E. Joint space narrowing on plain films of shoulders and hips

40. A 35-year-old woman presents to urgent care for fever, rash, and joint pain. She was in her usual state of health until 3 weeks ago, when she experienced a severe sore throat. She was seen by her primary care provider. Testing for strep throat by rapid testing and culture was negative, but she was treated with empiric amoxicillin, without improvement (completed 10 days ago). She has subsequently developed pain and swelling in the wrists and high daily fevers that are accompanied by a generalized rash. She feels generally well between attacks but has not had any relief of episodes with naproxen 500 mg twice daily. Physical examination is notable for a woman of average stature who is uncomfortable but does not appear to be in a toxic condition. Temperature is 38.9°C, blood pressure is 110/72 mm Hg, heart rate is 110 beats per minute, respiratory rate is 18 breaths per minute, and oxygen saturation is 98% on room air. Neck is supple, but she has cervical and axillary adenopathy. She has redness, warmth, and swelling of the bilateral wrists and metacarpophalangeal joints. Skin shows a salmon-pink maculopapular rash involving mostly her trunk. Laboratory analysis is notable for a normal comprehensive metabolic profile. Complete blood count reveals white blood cell count 18.5×10^3 cells per mm^3 (70% neutrophils and 15% bands), Hgb 11.1 g/dL, and platelet count $772 \times 10^3/mm^3$. CRP is 199 mg/L (normal <5), and ESR is 92 mm/h. Blood cultures obtained 5 days prior have demonstrated no growth. ANA, RF, and anti-CCP antibodies are all negative. CT scan of the abdomen, chest, and pelvis reveals some mild hepatosplenomegaly and diffuse adenopathy. Peripheral blood flow cytometry does not reveal any hematologic malignancy. Excisional biopsy of an axillary lymph node excludes a malignancy and demonstrates "reactive lymphadenitis."

Which of the following is the most likely diagnosis?
A. Lyme disease
B. Adult-onset Still disease
C. Systemic lupus erythematosus
D. Acute bacterial endocarditis
E. Behçet disease

41. A 32-year-old woman gives birth to a baby girl at 34 weeks of gestation because of fetal distress. The newborn becomes cyanotic shortly after delivery. Rapid assessment identifies a heart rate of 50 beats per minute and complete heart block. With pacemaker support, the infant's status improves quickly, and the cyanosis resolves. The newborn develops infantile jaundice starting on day 5 of life, and is treated with phototherapy. On day 9 of life, the infant develops a patchy, well-circumscribed maculopapular rash.

Which of the following conditions in the mother might explain the newborn's condition?
A. Sjögren syndrome
B. Lyme disease
C. Marfan syndrome
D. Acute rheumatic fever
E. Maternal methotrexate exposure during pregnancy

42. A 75-year-old man presents to his primary care provider for an annual physical examination. He has relatively few comorbidities, but he reports ongoing chronic daily low back pain that radiates into the buttocks. He reports morning stiffness and progressive pain over the course of the day. He describes difficulty in standing for more than 10 minutes, and he has to lean on a walker or shopping cart when trying to get out and about during the day. For his back pain, he has (1) taken tramadol 50 mg three times daily and acetaminophen 1000 mg three times daily, (2) engaged in regular physical therapy, and (3) received multiple epidural corticosteroid injections and facet joint injections over the past 12 months. None of these approaches has provided adequate relief. Physical examination is largely unrevealing except for weakness of hip flexor strength and reduced flexion and extension of the lumbar spine. His gait is slow and deliberate, but steady. Plain film radiography and MRI from 1 year ago have revealed multilevel degenerative changes with disc desiccation, nerve impingement, facet joint arthropathy, and central spinal stenosis.

Which of the following is the next most appropriate next course of action?
A. Reassurance and change tramadol to oxycodone 5 mg three times daily
B. Reassurance and another prescription for physical therapy
C. Repeat MRI of the lumbar spine
D. Referral to interventional radiology for corticosteroid injection into an involved facet joint
E. Referral to spine surgery for decompressive laminectomy

43. A 72-year-old woman presents to her primary care physician with 3 weeks of declining health because of fatigue, cough, and dyspnea. She has a history of atrial fibrillation, for which she takes warfarin and atenolol. She has no other significant medical comorbidities. During the appointment, she coughs up scant amounts of fresh blood. Vital signs include temperature 37.2°C, heart rate 62 beats per minute (irregular), blood pressure 162/90 mm Hg, respiratory rate 25 breaths per minute, and oxygen saturation 91% on room air. Physical examination shows a fatigued-appearing woman in some moderate amount of respiratory distress, using accessory muscles. Lungs have diffuse rales. She has mild periorbital edema and pitting leg edema to the upper shins. Urgent chest radiograph is obtained that shows patchy infiltrates in bilateral lung fields. Initial laboratory assessment includes the following: BUN 82 mg/dL, creatinine 4.1 mg/dL (baseline normal), white blood cell count 13.2 × 10^3 cells/mm^3 with normal differential, hemoglobin 9.2 g/dL, and platelet count 622 × 10^3 cells/mm^3, ESR 104 mm/h, and CRP 301 mg/L (normal <5). Urinalysis reveals +++ protein and 75–100 red blood cells per high-power field.

Which of the following findings would not adequately explain this patient's current presentation?

A. Antinuclear antibody 1:2560 speckled pattern, anti–double-stranded DNA antibody 721 U/mL (normal <5), C3 complement 57 mg/dL (normal 75–175), and C4 complement 9 mg/dL (normal 14–40)
B. Detectable antiglomerular basement membrane antibody
C. Detectable antineutrophil cytoplasmic antibody with cytoplasmic pattern and antiproteinase-3 antibody positivity
D. Temporal artery biopsy showing granulomatous arteritis
E. Urine toxicology positive for cocaine

44. A 39-year-old man presents to the outpatient clinic having noticed the slow accumulation of chalky white material in many fingers and toes (Fig. 3.5). He reports that they have occasionally become inflamed, but are not painful. He has a history of end-stage renal disease from Alport syndrome, and he received a cadaveric renal transplant 2 years ago (functioning well with serum creatinine 1.2 mg/dL). Four years ago, he had an episode of acute monoarthritis of the left knee, and arthrocentesis showed negatively birefringent needle-shaped crystals with no growth in fluid culture. Current medications include prednisone 5.0 mg daily and azathioprine 150 mg daily. Serum uric acid is 11.4 mg/dL.

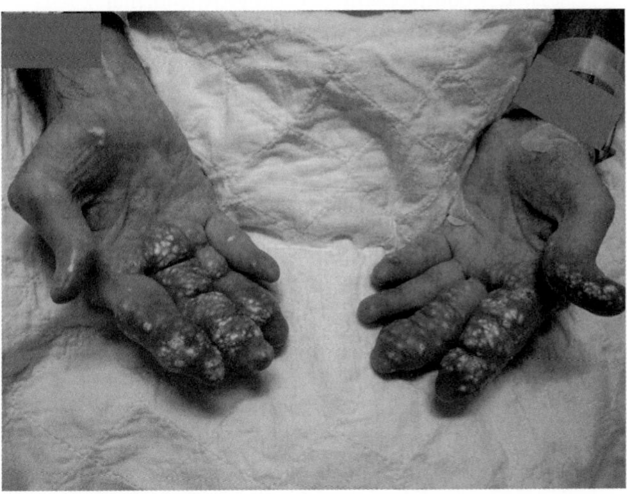

• **Fig. 3.5** Hands of the patient described in Question 44.

What is the most appropriate next course of action?

A. Initiate allopurinol 300 mg daily and treat any flares of gouty arthritis with higher doses of prednisone "as needed."
B. Check a 24-hour urine uric acid, and initiate probenecid 500 mg twice daily if the patient is an "under-excretor."
C. Discuss with patient's nephrologist about alternative immunosuppressive therapies for the renal graft.
D. Increase prednisone to 15 mg daily.
E. Initiate febuxostat 80 mg daily, and treat any flares of gouty arthritis with higher doses of prednisone "as needed."

45. A 48-year-old man with rheumatoid arthritis (RA) for 4 years presents to his primary care physician with 5 days of severe right knee pain and swelling. His RA has been well controlled for 2 years on a combination of disease-modifying antirheumatic drugs (DMARDs): methotrexate and adalimumab (an injectable TNF-α antagonist). He has no prosthetic joints and no other comorbidities. His joint examination reveals no abnormalities of the upper extremities or left leg. His right hip and ankle move well, but the right knee is red, warm, and swollen with a modest side effusion. He has a 20-degree flexion contracture of the knee and pain when trying to extend it fully or flex it more than 45 degrees. He has no fevers and does not appear to be in a toxic condition. Laboratory analysis is notable for ESR 48 mm/h and CRP 119.1 mg/L (normal <5). Plain film radiography of the right knee reveals an effusion but no other abnormalities.

What is the most appropriate next step?

A. MRI of the right knee
B. Aspiration of the right knee for fluid analysis
C. Aspiration of the right knee for symptomatic relief, followed by corticosteroid injection
D. Touch base with his rheumatologist to discuss a change in the DMARD regimen.
E. Prescribe a course of oral corticosteroids tapered over 1 week for treatment of an RA flare.

46. A 33-year-old woman is brought to the emergency department (ED) by ambulance. She reports fever and progressively severe dyspnea but no cough, hemoptysis, or chest pain. She has a 9-month history of severe systemic lupus erythematosus (SLE) complicated by nonhemolytic anemia, thrombocytopenia, and class IV lupus nephritis. Baseline laboratory tests from 3 weeks ago showed creatinine 2.8 mg/dL, hemoglobin 10.2 g/dL, and platelet count 95 × 10^3 cells/mm^3. For her SLE, she is being treated aggressively with monthly intravenous cyclophosphamide 750 mg/m^2, prednisone 60 mg daily, and hydroxychloroquine 400 mg daily. In the ED, initial vital signs show temperature 37.8°C, blood pressure 90/48 mm Hg, heart rate 122 beats per minute, respiratory rate 28 breaths per minute, and oxygen saturation 88% on room air. Within minutes of arrival, she exhibits increased work of breathing and has respiratory arrest, prompting intubation. Mechanical ventilation improves oxygenation saturation (94%) on 60% inhaled oxygen. Initial admission blood work shows BUN 42 mg/dL, creatinine 3.1 mg/dL, hemoglobin 7.7 g/dL, white blood cell count 9.2 × 10^3 cells/mm^3 (normal differential), and platelet count 88 × 10^3 cells/mm^3. Toxicology tests are negative for illicit drugs. Blood cultures are drawn and are pending. EKG demonstrates no abnormalities. Chest radiograph is as shown in Fig. 3.6.

Besides stabilizing the patient for her acute critical illness, which of the following is also indicated as the next most appropriate step in diagnosing this patient's illness?

A. Chest CT angiogram with iodinated contrast
B. Pulmonary function testing with corrected carbon monoxide diffusion capacity in the lungs (DLCO) measurement
C. Lumbar puncture
D. Cardiac MRI with gadolinium contrast
E. Flexible bronchoscopy

47. A 42-year-old man presents to his outpatient primary care provider with back stiffness. He has had these symptoms for as long as he can remember. Initially, his stiffness was limited to the lumbar spine, but he now reports stiffness in the thoracic and cervical spine, accompanied by pleuritic chest discomfort. He has difficulty turning his head to look in the side mirrors when driving. His symptoms are worse in the morning and abate over the course of the day. His medical history is notable only for episodic redness in the left eye accompanied by pain and photophobia (last episode 12 months ago). Physical examination reveals a generally healthy individual with limited motion of the spine and reduced chest excursion. Laboratory analysis reveals CRP 22.8 mg/L (normal <5). Radiographic imaging demonstrates ankylosis of the sacroiliac joints. A diagnosis of ankylosing spondylitis is made.

Which of the following will most likely to lead to symptomatic improvement by treating the underlying condition?

A. HLA-B27 testing
B. Prednisone 20 mg daily
C. Methotrexate 25 mg once weekly
D. Oxycodone 5 mg three times daily
E. Adalimumab 40 mg every other week

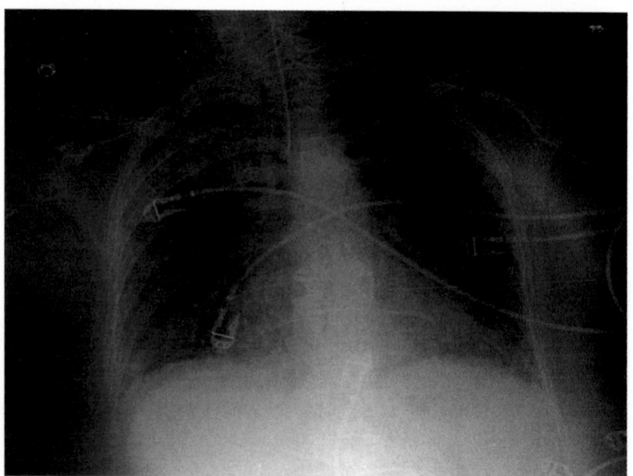

• **Fig. 3.6** Chest radiograph of the patient described in Question 46.

48. A 67-year-old woman with long-standing Sjögren syndrome (SjS) presents with painless firm swelling of the left cheek of 4 months' duration. She has had years of dry eyes and dry mouth due to SjS, leading to corneal abrasions and multiple dental caries. She also has SjS-associated interstitial lung disease, for which she has been on chronic prednisone 5–10 mg daily and azathioprine 2 mg/kg for 14 years. She has osteoporosis, for which she has been on alendronate 70 mg weekly for 10 years. Historically, her serologic workup has included an antinuclear antibody (ANA) 1:1280 speckled pattern, high-titer anti-Ro and anti-La antibodies, rheumatoid factor (RF) at 145 U/mL (normal <15), and polyclonal hypergammaglobulinemia. She has had normal complement levels and negative anti-dsDNA, anti-Smith, and anti-RNP antibodies. Physical examination reveals asymmetric swelling of the left cheek overlying the masseter muscle. It is firm, nontender, and has poorly defined borders. She has dry mucous membranes and lacks salivary pooling on oral inspection. She has had extensive dental work. There is no exposed bone, but she still has multiple caries. She has palpable purpuric lesions on the legs. Laboratory analysis reveals normal comprehensive metabolic profile and complete blood count. ESR is 68 mm/h, CRP is 119 mg/L (normal <5), C3 complement is 66 mg/dL (normal 75–175), and C4 complement is 3 mg/dL (normal 14–40). RF is now normal for the first time on record.

Which of the following is the most likely diagnosis?

A. Parotid lymphoma
B. Sarcoidosis
C. Sialolithiasis
D. Suppurative bacterial sialadenitis
E. Osteonecrosis of the jaw

49. A 48-year-old woman from Guatemala presents to the emergency department of a tertiary care center in the United States in search of an opinion regarding her poor health. She has been receiving hemodialysis for 12 years because of end-stage renal disease as a complication of type 1 diabetes mellitus. Nine months ago, while living in Guatemala, she experienced a generalized seizure. Part of the workup included magnetic resonance angiography, which revealed no intracranial structural or vascular abnormalities other than moderate cerebrovascular disease. It was concluded that her seizure was the result of an otherwise asymptomatic episode of hypoglycemia. She has not had any further seizures. However, in the past 6 months, she has noticed thickening and hardening of the skin associated with progressive immobility. Symptoms started in her legs but have progressed to involve her arms. She does not describe Raynaud phenomenon. On physical examination, she has tightness and hardening of the skin of her calves, thighs, and forearms. There is a brawny discoloration of the skin, which is tethered down on deeper tissues such that she has flexion contractures of the ankles, knees, fingers, and elbows. Her face and torso are not affected, but there is a yellowish discoloration of the sclera of both eyes.

Which of the following is the most likely diagnosis?

A. Scleroderma
B. Lipodermatosclerosis
C. Scleredema diabeticorum
D. Eosinophilic fasciitis
E. Nephrogenic systemic fibrosis

50. A 62-year-old male laborer presents to a new primary care provider (PCP) with 3 years of persistent stiffness and achiness in many joints, including the hands, wrists, elbows, shoulders, hips, and knees. His shoulders and hips bother him more than anything else. At the end of a long shift, his joints feel somewhat better than at the beginning of the day. He was told by his previous PCP that he has "arthritis" related to his job in construction, and he had been managed primarily with escalating doses of oxycodone for symptoms. Comorbidities include chronic obstructive pulmonary disease from years of cigarette smoking, type 2 diabetes mellitus, hypertension, hypercholesterolemia, and Hashimoto thyroiditis. Physical examination reveals "beefy hands" with boggy changes in the metacarpophalangeal (MCP) and wrist joints. His wrists are somewhat fused, with very limited range of motion. He is unable to extend his elbows fully because of 5-degree flexion contractures. Both knees have modest-sized knee effusions, but he can extend them fully. Laboratory analysis reveals a normal comprehensive metabolic profile and normal complete blood count with differential. Serum uric acid is 4.0 mg/dL. Rheumatoid factor (RF), anticyclic citrullinated (CCP) antibodies, and antinuclear antibodies (ANA) are not detectable. CRP is 42.0 mg/L (normal <5). Aspiration of the right knee obtains 45 mL of nonbloody, cloudy, yellow fluid with a white blood cell count 35,000 cells/mm^3 (60% neutrophils). No organisms are identified upon fluid Gram stain or culture, and compensated polarized light microscopy does not reveal any birefringent crystals. Plain film imaging of the hands shows erosions and joint space narrowing in multiple MCP joints and wrists.

What is the most likely diagnosis?

A. Rheumatoid arthritis
B. Chronic gouty arthropathy
C. Primary osteoarthritis of the involved joints
D. Rheumatic fever
E. Polymyalgia rheumatic

Chapter 3 Answers

1. ANSWER: B. Acute pseudogout arthritis

This patient has experienced an acute inflammatory arthritis of the right wrist and several MCP joints, as evidenced by the sudden onset of redness, warmth, and swelling, as described. Osteoarthritis (Answer D) rarely affects the wrist and is considered mostly noninflammatory. Rheumatoid arthritis (Answer C) is unlikely to come on in such an abrupt manner with unilateral findings. Although occult injury should always be considered, there is no history of fracture, and the plain radiograph does not support the diagnosis of fracture (Answer E). Septic arthritis (Answer A) is not the most likely answer for several reasons. Most important, this patient would have to have polyarticular septic arthritis of the wrist and several MCP joints, a very unlikely scenario when considering her negative blood cultures, appropriate antibiotic therapy, and general improvement in all other clinical parameters. Septic arthritis is often the result of hematogenous seeding of a joint from bacteremia rather than transcutaneous inoculation of a joint. Polyarticular septic arthritis would indicate a high-grade bacteremia. Although larger joints such as the knees, hips, and shoulders are more likely to be affected by septic arthritis, any joint can become infected. The most likely answer is pseudogout arthritis (Answer B) based on the clinical presentation of acute arthritis of the MCP and wrist joints. Supporting evidence includes the chondrocalcinosis on plain film, more commonly found in patients with hyperparathyroidism. Arthrocentesis of joint fluid would likely reveal elevated fluid white blood cells (>2000/mm^3), negative cultures, and positively birefringent rhomboid-shaped crystals consistent with calcium pyrophosphate dihydrate (Fig. 3.1).

2. ANSWER: E. Temporal artery biopsy

Giant cell arteritis (GCA) is not an uncommon cause for "fever of unknown origin" (FUO) in elderly patients, accounting for about 17% of FUOs in this demographic group. Many of the features described in this case can be found in patients with unrecognized

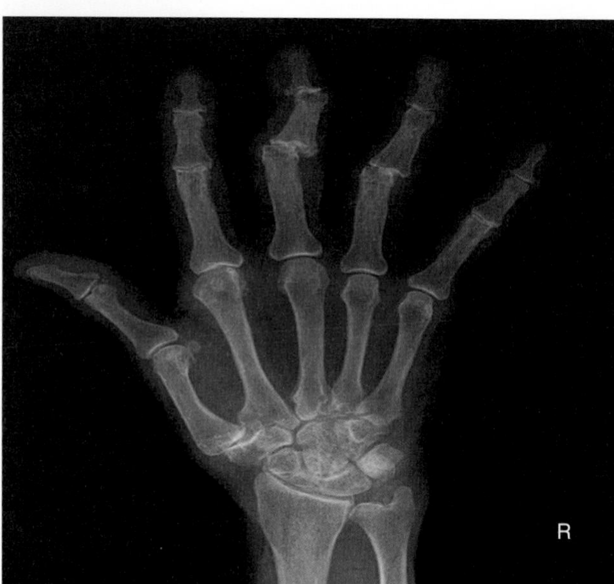

• **Fig. 3.1** Calcium pyrophosphate dihydrate and chondrocalcinosis of the hands/wrists for patient in Question 1.

GCA: anemia of chronic disease, reactive thrombocytosis, elevated inflammatory indices, hypoalbuminemia, and elevated alkaline phosphatase. Most important, infectious and malignant etiologies have been largely ruled out. There is no microbiologic evidence to warrant empiric levofloxacin (Answer A) or localizing features to suggest tuberculosis infection (Answer B). Elder abuse (Answer C) should always be considered in elderly patients with "failure to thrive" but would not explain the fevers or elevated inflammatory indices. The elevated alkaline phosphatase and hypoalbuminemia may be enough to warrant liver biopsy, but one might expect some sort of abnormalities in abdominal/pelvic CT imaging or ultrasound studies if liver disease was the source of fever. In this case, the abnormalities are secondary to GCA and will likely correct with corticosteroid treatment.

Mourad O, Palda V, Detsky AS. A comprehensive evidence-based approach to fever of unknown origin. *Arch Intern Med.* 2003;163(5):545–551.

3. **ANSWER: C. Methotrexate titrated up to 25 mg once weekly**

This patient likely has a new diagnosis of rheumatoid arthritis (RA). RA is the most common cause of a chronic inflammatory polyarthritis, defined as having symptoms of >6 weeks' duration. Her history, physical examination, and inflammatory indices suggest an inflammatory process. When detectable, anti-CCP antibodies have high specificity for RA (>90%), which is even better than RF. Even though her anti-CCP antibody test is negative, RA remains the most likely diagnosis. Up to 25% of patients with RA remain seronegative for the duration of their condition. Weekly low-dose methotrexate (Answer C) is the most appropriate and most commonly prescribed first-line pharmacologic agent for the majority of patients with RA. Methotrexate is one of many disease-modifying antirheumatic drugs (DMARDs) available for the treatment of RA. DMARDs reduce the signs and symptoms of RA, and most DMARDs reduce progression of structural joint damage and preserve physical function in patients with RA. Methotrexate is highly teratogenic and contraindicated in patients desiring pregnancy (not an issue in this patient). Risk of hepatotoxicity and cirrhosis make methotrexate relatively contraindicated in patients with excessive alcohol consumption. Rituximab (Answer A) is a biologic DMARD that is approved to treat RA. However, it is rarely prescribed as a first-line DMARD, and efficacy tends to be limited to patients with "seropositive" disease (i.e., in those patients with detectable RF and/or anti-CCP antibodies). The other answer options are not appropriate for this patient and unnecessarily delay therapy. Duloxetine (Answer B) is sometimes helpful in the management of chronic noninflammatory musculoskeletal pain in patients with fibromyalgia syndrome. This patient's inflammatory features are incongruent with a diagnosis of fibromyalgia. Doxycycline (Answer D) might be used to treat Lyme arthritis or other manifestation of Lyme disease. However, this patient's chronic polyarticular presentation is inconsistent with late Lyme arthritis, which usually affects only one joint. There is no reason to repeat the RF, anti-CCP antibody, or ANA tests (Answer E), and delaying treatment risks continued symptoms and onset of irreversible joint damage.

Singh JA, Saag KG, Bridges Jr SL, et al. 2015 American College of Rheumatology guideline for the treatment of rheumatoid arthritis. *Arthritis Rheumatol.* 2016;68(1):1–26.

4. **ANSWER: B. Osteoarthritis of the hip**

Avascular necrosis (AVN) can affect almost any bone, but the head of the femur is by far the most commonly involved site. AVN can lead to cortical collapse of bone, with resultant accelerated osteoarthritis (OA) of the adjoining joint. Thus OA is the result (not a cause) of AVN (Answer B). Pain is almost always the presenting complaint, but many cases can be entirely asymptomatic and discovered incidentally. For patients with unrelenting pain, total joint arthroplasty should be considered. The other conditions listed all increase the risk of AVN. Additional risk factors include high-dose corticosteroid therapy, radiation, trauma, systemic lupus erythematosus (SLE), HIV infection, decompression (caisson) disease, transplant, Legg-Calvé-Perthes disease, and slipped capital femoral epiphysis (SCFE) syndrome.

5. **ANSWER: D. Hydroxychloroquine**

Hydroxychloroquine is a generally safe and well-tolerated agent for the treatment of SLE. Rarely, however, it can cause pigment to deposit in the retina, which can lead to permanently impaired vision. Thus regular ophthalmologic screening for potential toxicity is very important. Chloroquine, a related agent, carries a higher risk for retinal toxicity and therefore is used less commonly. None of the other agents (Answers A–C and E) causes direct visual toxicity, although each of these is immunosuppressive and could increase the risk of ocular infections (e.g., zoster, toxoplasmosis). It is important to bear in mind the late-onset complications of cyclophosphamide: sterility, lymphoma, and malignancies of the urinary tract. These might not manifest until decades after a drug exposure. Belimumab is a recently approved biologic treatment for SLE. It is a monoclonal antibody directed against B lymphocyte stimulator. Belimumab has shown evidence of benefit in mostly cutaneous, hematologic, and articular manifestations of SLE.

6. **ANSWER: C. Hemochromatosis**

Hemochromatosis (Fig. 3.2) has many clinical manifestations related to iron accumulation in target organs: cirrhotic liver disease, congestive heart failure, hypogonadism, diabetes mellitus, bronzing of the skin, and accelerated degenerative arthritis. Many of these are present in this case. Hemochromatosis-related arthropathy is one of several causes of secondary osteoarthritis (OA), and it classically affects the MCP joints. This patient's hand radiographs show some characteristic changes of hemochromatosis arthropathy, including aggressive osteoarthritis changes and "hooked osteophytes" of the MCP joints. Although hemochromatosis arthropathy is largely a noninflammatory process, it is associated with chondrocalcinosis (as seen in the radiograph in Fig. 3.2) and episodes of pseudogout. Involvement of MCP and wrist joints argues against primary OA (Answer D), which very rarely affects these joints. Primary OA tends to be limited to DIP and PIP joints and the base of the thumb. There are no clinical features of inflammation to suggest rheumatoid arthritis (Answer A). Metacarpal fracture (Answer B) is not present in this radiograph. Gaucher disease (Answer E) is associated with cirrhosis, osteoporosis, and joint pain. However, this condition mostly involves large joints (hips and knees) and is associated with avascular necrosis, not accelerated osteoarthritis of the hands.

Sahinbegovic E, Dallos T, Aigner E, et al. Musculoskeletal disease burden of hereditary hemochromatosis. *Arthritis Rheum.* 2010;62(12):3792–3798.

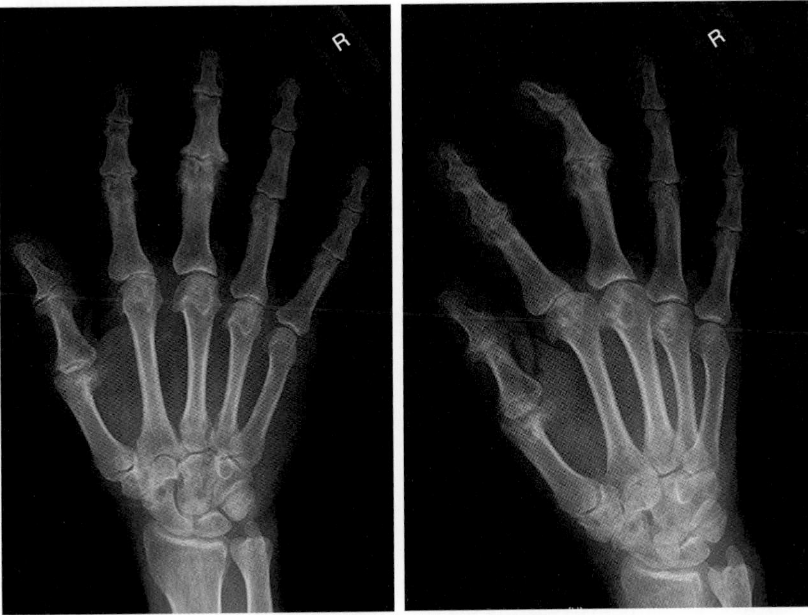

• **Fig. 3.2** Hemochromatosis arthropathy (right hand/wrist) for patient in Question 6.

7. **ANSWER: B. Provide a prescription for physical therapy and discuss an "opiate medication contract."**

This patient describes lumbago—musculoskeletal low back pain without evidence of any "red flags": fever, occult weight loss, numbness in the perineum, new-onset impotence, bowel or bladder retention, history of malignancy, and recent intravenous drug abuse. The presence of these findings would prompt consideration of further imaging to assess for inflammatory, infectious, or neoplastic origin, such as epidural or paraspinous abscess, compressive mass, or cauda equina syndrome. This patient should first engage in physical therapy to improve core muscle strength, conditioning, and range of motion. Weight loss is advisable. This patient also demonstrates misuse of oxycodone. Thus discussions of an opiate medication contract are indicated. It is unlikely that reassurance alone (Answer A) will satisfy this patient, and it will be unlikely to change his current pattern of opiate use. Switching oxycodone to the more potent hydromorphone will likely only compound what appears to be opiate misuse. MRI of the lumbar spine (Answer D) might be appropriate if he reported any "red flags" or failed a concerted effort at physical therapy. It is inappropriate to discharge this patient from your practice (Answer E) until you can demonstrate that the patient intentionally misconstrues facts or misrepresents himself to obtain opiate-based medications, or if there is redirection of his prescription medications to other individuals in exchange for money or favors. An opiate medication contract would clearly indicate appropriate use and misuse of opiates, such that violation of the contract could provide supporting evidence to discharge the patient from your practice. Many states mandate that prescribers review an opiate prescription database prior to dispensing an opiate prescription to a patient. The purpose of these databases is to track patients' opiate prescription, prescribing physicians, and dispensing pharmacies in an effort to detect patients who "doctor hop" to receive multiple opiate prescriptions from multiple providers.

Dowell D, Haegerich TM, Chou R. CDC guideline for prescribing opioids for chronic pain—United States, 2016. *MMWR Recomm Rep.* 2016;65(1):1–49.

8. ANSWER: A. Serologic testing for Lyme disease

The patient presents with a chronic inflammatory monoarthritis. While unlikely to be suppurative septic arthritis of 8 weeks' duration (e.g., from *Staphylococcus aureus*), chronic infectious processes must be considered. In patients living in certain parts of the United States, such as New England and parts of the upper Midwest and Pacific Northwest, infection by the tick-borne spirochete *Borrelia burgdorferi* causes Lyme disease. One late-onset manifestation of Lyme disease is joint infection, occurring weeks or typically months after exposure to the culprit tick. Lyme arthritis is almost invariably a chronic inflammatory monoarthritis, most often of the knee. Patients do not necessarily recall the initial tick bite or any classic "bull's-eye rash" of early Lyme disease. Lyme arthritis is not to be confused with "chronic Lyme disease," a nebulous condition that is likely not related to active Lyme disease and encompasses a constellation of somatic complaints that linger after standard treatment for Lyme disease: chronic pain, fatigue, impaired cognition, and other manifestations. Long-term antibiotic therapy for "chronic Lyme disease" is highly controversial and has not been proven to result in improved symptoms in multiple clinical trials. Still, some patients and advocacy groups insist that chronic antibiotics result in a positive response. The other answer options could be appropriate next steps in the event that Lyme arthritis was ruled out by negative serologic testing. Note that most patients with ANA-associated connective tissue diseases such as systemic lupus erythematosus do not experience chronic inflammatory monoarthritis of this nature. Although rheumatoid arthritis can occasionally present as a chronic inflammatory monoarthritis, this presentation would be more typical of a spondyloarthritis condition: psoriatic arthritis, ankylosing spondylitis, reactive arthritis, or the arthropathy of inflammatory bowel disease (IBD arthropathy).

Berende A, ter Hofstede HJ, Vos FJ, et al. Randomized trial of longer-term therapy for symptoms attributed to Lyme disease. *N Engl J Med.* 2016;374(13):1209–1220.

Melia MT, Auwaerter PG. Time for a different approach to Lyme disease and long-term symptoms. *N Engl J Med.* 2016;374(13):1277–1278.

Wormser GP, Dattwyler RJ, Shapiro ED, et al. The clinical assessment, treatment, and prevention of Lyme disease, human granulocytic anaplasmosis, and babesiosis: clinical practice guidelines by the Infectious Diseases Society of America. *Clin Infect Dis.* 2006;43(9):1089–1134.

9. ANSWER: B. Viral arthritis

This patient likely has acute viral polyarthritis (Answer B) due to parvovirus B19. In children, this virus is the cause of Fifth disease, characterized by fever, rash, and occasional joint pains. In adults, however, inflammatory joint disease may be the only manifestation. The condition is too recent in onset to be diagnosed as rheumatoid arthritis (Answer E). The arthritis of Lyme disease is most often a chronic inflammatory monoarthritis, and therefore Answer D is not correct. Everything about his presentation suggests an inflammatory process, and thus fibromyalgia syndrome (Answer C) is incorrect. Septic polyarthritis (Answer A) is unlikely because patients are often much sicker than this patient. Septic joints are seeded hematogenously, and thus septic polyarthritis indicates a very high level of bacteremia. Another notable feature of parvoviral arthritis is the impairment of red blood cell (RBC) production (hence the inappropriately low reticulocyte count). In patients with sickle cell disease or other states of high RBC turnover, parvoviral infection can cause an aplastic crisis. Diagnosis of parvoviral infection is confirmed by serologic or PCR-based testing; an elevated parvovirus IgM or parvovirus PCR indicates recent infection. Treatment of parvoviral arthritis is supportive: pain relief with nonsteroidal antiinflammatory drugs (NSAIDs) or low-dose systemic corticosteroids until the viral process abates.

Young NS, Brown KE. Parvovirus B19. *N Engl J Med.* 2004;350(6):586–597.

10. ANSWER: B. Serum and urine protein electrophoresis

This patient presents with nonspecific symptoms, anemia, and an elevated ESR. Although these symptoms might represent polymyalgia rheumatica (PMR), the discrepantly low CRP warrants consideration of other processes. CRP is a nonspecific indicator of inflammation that can be elevated because of inflammation, infection, and some malignancies. In this case, factors other than inflammation have led to an increased ESR; an immunoglobulin paraproteinemia increases the ESR without affecting the CRP because positively charged immunoglobulin promotes electrostatic adhesion of negatively charged red blood cells such that they settle out of suspension faster. In this case, the patient has multiple myeloma, which would be detected by serum or urine protein electrophoresis (SPEP/UPEP). There is nothing to suggest systemic lupus erythematosus or other connective tissue disorder, so an antinuclear antibody is unnecessary (Answer A). Temporal artery biopsy (Answer C) is used to diagnose giant cell arteritis (GCA). Sometimes GCA can present as fever, malaise, and weight loss of unknown origin. CT scanning (Answer D) can reveal occult abscess or solid organ malignancy. Prior to temporal artery biopsy or CT scanning, however, the discrepancy in ESR and CRP first should be assessed with the much less invasive and more cost-effective SPEP/UPEP. Finally, it is inappropriate to treat the patient empirically with low-dose corticosteroids (Answer E) for something such as polymyalgia rheumatic (PMR) until one has ruled out other explanations for the patient's complaints and laboratory abnormalities. PMR should always be considered a diagnosis of exclusion.

11. **ANSWER: C. Pulmonary hypertension**

The patient has pulmonary hypertension (pHTN) as a complication of scleroderma. Features associated with pHTN include CREST-variant scleroderma and anticentromere antibodies. This condition is suggested by abnormalities in echocardiography and pulmonary function testing (isolated low carbon monoxide diffusion capacity in the lungs [DLCO]). It is confirmed by direct measurement of pulmonary artery pressures by right heart catheterization. Treatment options include endothelin antagonist agents (e.g., ambrisentan), phosphodiesterase inhibitors (e.g., tadalafil), and prostacyclin analogues. Scleroderma cardiomyopathy is a fibrotic complication of scleroderma, associated with anti-SCL70 antibodies and diffuse fibrotic disease.

12. **ANSWER: B. Bronchoscopy with lavage for microscopic organisms**

This patient is immune suppressed secondary to his RA therapy. Based on his deteriorating clinical status, further investigation is warranted to assess for atypical infectious source. This patient could have pulmonary abscess, fungal pneumonia, or tuberculoma. Bronchoscopy with lavage (Answer B) is the least invasive test that will still yield clinically important information. Lung biopsy (Answer C) might be necessary if bronchoscopy fails to yield a diagnosis, but it is more invasive than bronchoscopy and carries greater risk of morbidity. Switching antibiotics (Answer E) might lead to clinical improvement if this was simply bacterial pneumonia resistant to the initial choice of antibiotics. If incorrect, however, this would delay diagnosis and treatment. PET-CT scan (Answer D) is not yet indicated, because malignancy has not been shown (and indeed infection is more likely and of greater immediate concern). Finally, RA can cause necrotic pulmonary nodules, but empiric treatment for rheumatoid lung (Answer A) is inappropriate until infectious processes have been ruled out.

13. **ANSWER: D. Scaly erythematous plaques on the extensor surfaces of the arms and legs**

This answer describes a patient with psoriasis, which can also involve the scalp, external auditory canal, supragluteal cleft, and umbilicus. Nail pitting and other nail abnormalities can also be present. In patients with psoriasis, unexplained inflammatory joint disease often indicates the presence of psoriatic arthritis. This can take on several forms: inflammatory monoarthritis or oligoarthritis typically of the lower extremities (as in this case), dactylitis of fingers or toes (as in this case), a rheumatoid-pattern polyarthritis, inflammatory spondyloarthritis of the spine, accelerated osteoarthritis of the distal interphalangeal (DIP) joints, and inflammatory enthesitis of the tendon–bone interface. In this patient, septic arthritis and crystalline arthritides are much less likely based on arthrocentesis results, which show inflammatory fluid that lacks crystals and microorganisms. Serum uric acid (Answer B), serum ACE level (Answer C), and radiographic evidence of chondrocalcinosis (Answer E) are associated with gout, sarcoid arthritis, and pseudogout, respectively, but none of these are diagnostic for their respective conditions. Anti-Smith antibodies are a specific autoantibody sometimes found in patients with systemic lupus erythematosus (SLE). However, SLE is unlikely in this patient clinical based on the negative ANA and monoarticular joint involvement.

14. **ANSWER: A. Tilt-table test**

The patient demonstrates evidence of a joint hypermobility syndrome (HMS). Several rare genetic disorders can lead to HMS (e.g., Marfan syndrome and genetically definable Ehlers-Danlos syndrome [EDS]). However, this patient demonstrates none of the characteristic nonarticular features of these rare syndromes, and thus she most likely has benign joint HMS. Formerly termed *type 3 Ehlers-Danlos syndrome*, a genetic basis for benign joint HMS is not as well established as in the other forms of EDS. Thus benign joint HMS remains primarily a clinical diagnosis, and no further testing for genetics or other causes of joint pain is necessary (Answers B–E). Benign joint HMS is associated with dysautonomia features, such as postural orthostatic tachycardia syndrome (POTS). The presence of this condition would be supported by a positive tilt-table test (Answer E). Treatment of joint complaints in patients with benign joint HMS is challenging, but it should include primarily physical therapy to improve muscle tone and fitness while limiting extreme range-of-motion exercises. Immunosuppressive and antiinflammatory therapies are of no value. Narcotics are counterproductive and can lead to tolerance, dependency, and addiction. Psychological support is often indicated for patients with refractory symptoms.

15. ANSWER: E. Skeletal muscle biopsy

The patient has dermatomyositis (DM; Fig. 3.3). This patient's painless proximal muscle weakness and characteristic rash are classic for DM. The CPK, CK-MB, AST, and ALT are all of skeletal muscle origin, so testing other targets is unlikely to yield a diagnosis (Answers A–D). She also likely has interstitial lung disease (ILD), which is commonly associated with DM. DM is one of several idiopathic inflammatory myopathies (IIMs). Others include polymyositis (PM), malignancy-associated myositis, inclusion body myositis (IBM), and juvenile dermatomyositis (J-DM). In patients with some forms of IIM, autoantibody testing can reveal an elevated antinuclear antibody (ANA) titer. A subset of patients with DM will have more specific myositis-associated autoantibodies such as anti-Jo-1, and these patients have higher rates of DM-associated ILD. Patients with J-DM can experience bowel vasculitis and subcutaneous calcifications (calcinosis cutis). The diagnosis of the various IIMs is confirmed by skeletal muscle biopsy (Answer E). Electron microscopy is advisable if IBM is being considered to visualize classic vacuolar changes in diseased muscle. Unlike the other IIMs, however, IBM usually includes chronic distal muscle weakness and atrophy. Because muscle involvement in any of the IIMs can be patchy, EMG or MRI is often used to identify a muscle suitable for biopsy. There is an association between IIMs and malignancies, typically of the lung, GI tract, and female reproductive tract. Although all patients should have age-appropriate cancer screening, it is not be unreasonable to perform additional imaging to assess for occult cancer (especially in this patient): CT scan of the chest, abdomen, and pelvis, as well as consideration of transvaginal pelvic ultrasound. Treatment of most forms of IIM initially involves corticosteroids, often in high doses (1 mg/kg) with a long and slow taper. Methotrexate is the most commonly used nonsteroid-based immunosuppressive agent. Unfortunately, there are no effective therapies for IBM, which carries a dismal prognosis.

Dalakas MC. Inflammatory muscle diseases. *N Engl J Med* 2015; 372(18):1734–1747.

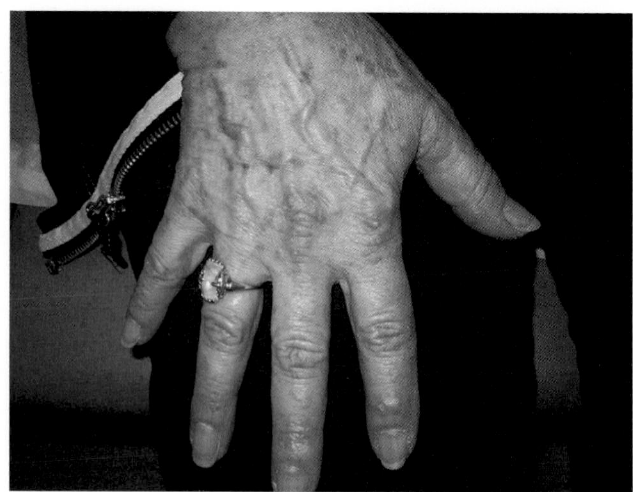

• **Fig. 3.3** Dermatomyositis rash.

16. ANSWER: A. *MEFV* genetic testing

The patient has familial Mediterranean fever (FMF), one of several hereditary periodic fever syndromes. FMF most often results from a homozygous mutation of the *MEFV* gene. This gene encodes the pyrin protein, which is involved with leukocyte function. FMF is an autosomal recessive disorder, so a family history may or may not be present. Clinical features of FMF include recurrent attacks characterized by fever and abdominal pain. Accompanying features can include leukocytosis, thrombocytosis, rash, and inflammatory joint pain (hence this patient's questionable history of "gout"). Inflammatory markers are elevated during attacks but relatively normal when asymptomatic. An important complication of FMF is secondary amyloidosis, which this patient may have, based on a history of chronic untreated inflammation and unexplained proteinuria. Secondary renal amyloidosis can be prevented (and to some degree reversed) by treatment with daily colchicine. The patient does not have features of celiac disease or Crohn disease; hence, endoscopy and colonoscopy are not relevant (Answers B and D). He is not experiencing recurrent mesenteric ischemia from vasculitis, and there is nothing specifically suggesting systemic vasculitis, so workup for these conditions (Answers C and E) delays proper diagnosis.

Ozen S, Bilginer Y. A clinical guide to autoinflammatory diseases: familial Mediterranean fever and next-of-kin. *Nat Rev Rheumatol.* 2014;10(3):135–147.

17. ANSWER: A. Patellofemoral syndrome

This case describes a classical presentation for patellofemoral syndrome (PFS), a common mechanical disorder of young, active adults. One would expect the pain of iliotibial (IT) band syndrome to be lateral. Physical examination testing does not suggest the other options (Answers C–E). McMurray test assesses for tear of the medial meniscus. Anterior drawer sign testing assesses for tear of the ACL. Baker cyst should be suspected in patients with posterior fullness and pain with knee flexion.

18. ANSWER: C. Anti–double-stranded DNA antibody 522 U/mL (normal <5), C3 complement 52 mg/dL (normal 75–175), C4 complement 8 mg/dL (normal 14–40)

The patient has systemic lupus erythematosus (SLE) complicated by lupus nephritis (LN), with associated symptoms and findings of renal failure (peripheral edema and congestive heart failure). This is supported by the presence of aggressive Raynaud phenomenon, leukopenia (and lymphopenia), thrombocytopenia, hematuria, proteinuria, and elevated ANA. SLE has myriad clinical features, and LN is an important one to recognize. The serologic workup of SLE includes more than just the ANA, which is itself a nonspecific test. In addition to hematuria and proteinuria, patients with LN often (but not always) will have elevated anti-dsDNA antibodies and hypocomplementemia. Anti-Smith antibody is a test specific for SLE. Anti-Ro and anti-La antibodies are associated with SLE and Sjögren syndrome. Anti-RNP antibody is associated with an overlap condition sometimes termed *mixed connective tissue disease* (MCTD), in which there are features of SLE, scleroderma, dermatomyositis, Sjögren syndrome, and/or rheumatoid arthritis. The patient does not have other features to suggest an ANCA-associated vasculitis. Further, Answer A indicates only a nonspecific p-ANCA pattern and lacks the autoantibodies associated with ANCA vasculitis (anti-MPO and anti-PR3). Answer B would be seen in a patient with acute promyelocytic leukemia, which would not be consistent with this patient's presentation or complete blood count. The patient does not have features of dermatomyositis (Answer D), which largely spares the kidney. Longstanding ankylosing spondylitis (Answer E) is associated with IgA nephropathy, but the remainder of her clinical presentation does not suggest this diagnosis. Diagnosis of LN is confirmed by kidney biopsy. Treatment of lupus nephritis includes high-dose corticosteroids (1 mg/kg slowly tapered over months) plus an immunosuppressive or cytotoxic agent such as mycophenolate mofetil (MMF) or intravenous cyclophosphamide. Recent studies indicate that MMF is as effective as cyclophosphamide for the treatment of LN. MMF has a more favorable side effect profile than cyclophosphamide, which carries a risk of sterility (especially in women aged >30).

Hanh BH, McMahon MA, Wilkinson A, et al. American College of Rheumatology guidelines for screening, treatment, and management of lupus nephritis. *Arthritis Care Res.* 2012;64(6):797–808.

19. ANSWER: E. Treat with intramuscular methylprednisolone 80 mg ×1.

The patient is experiencing an attack of acute gouty arthritis. Although the presence of tophi would be an indication for antihyperuricemic therapy in the future, it is inappropriate to initiate it at the time of an acute attack (at least as monotherapy) because sudden drops in uric acid often exacerbate gouty inflammation. Thus Answers A and B are not the next most appropriate course of action at this time. Three classes of medications are traditionally used to treat the inflammation of acute gouty arthritis: colchicine, nonsteroidal antiinflammatory drugs (NSAIDs), and corticosteroids. The indicated course of colchicine in Answer C is inappropriate for a patient with marginal renal function. Very low doses of colchicine (0.3 mg every other day) might be tolerated as a prophylactic dose against attacks, but this is unlikely to be very effective in an attack of acute gout such as this one. Answer D is inappropriate because NSAIDS are highly nephrotoxic in patients with marginal renal function. Answer E is the correct answer because corticosteroids provide rapid relief of inflammatory pain in patients with acute gouty arthritis. Appropriate routes of administration include intramuscular, intraarticular, intravenous, and oral. Recent studies have shown that a short course of the interleukin-1 receptor antagonist (IL-Ra) anakinra is highly effective in treating acute gouty arthritis. Factors that limit its use include a lack of familiarity, insurance barriers, and concerns of immunosuppression.

20. ANSWER: C. Acute calcific tendonitis

The patient describes rapid onset of rotator cuff pain in the absence of antecedent symptoms or injury. Acute calcific tendonitis is a common condition in which basic calcium phosphate crystals deposited along a tendon trigger an immune response, with resultant acute inflammation and pain. It is often unheralded by any specific antecedent injury of overuse. The physical examination does not suggest biceps tendonitis (Answer A), because more than just forward flexion of the shoulder is affected. Septic arthritis (Answer B) would likely cause a patient to appear in a toxic condition, with severe pain. Further, the examination would be limited on active and passive range of motion. Likewise, glenohumeral arthritis (Answer D) would limit shoulder motion actively and passively. Finally, although the examination suggests involvement of the supraspinatus tendon, complete tear is unlikely to explain acute-onset symptoms in the absence of antecedent injury. If there is clinical uncertainty about the presence of a complete rotator cuff tear, the clinician can inject 3 mL of 2% lidocaine into the subacromial space. If this completely corrects the shoulder pain and functional deficit, then complete rotator cuff tear is unlikely, as is septic arthritis or significant glenohumeral arthritis.

21. ANSWER: C. Prescribe prednisone 1 mg/kg. Instruct the patient to start it immediately and to call with any new visual disturbances. Arrange

for an expedited temporal artery biopsy first thing Monday morning.

The patient describes symptoms consistent with giant cell arteritis (GCA). A dreaded complication of GCA is blindness, which results from ischemic optic neuropathy from vasculitis involving branches of the ophthalmic and retinal arteries. If blindness develops, it is often irreversible. Thus empiric treatment with high-dose corticosteroids is indicated in patients with possible GCA while arrangements are made for expedited temporal artery (TA) biopsy to confirm the diagnosis. Only Answer C addresses these issues fully. All other answers risk irreversible blindness. Of note, once empiric corticosteroids are started for suspected GCA, a TA biopsy should be performed within 7–10 days if possible to avoid a "false-negative" biopsy. Regardless, 10%–15% of patients with GCA will still have a negative TA biopsy. In these cases, one should consider alternative diagnoses or even contralateral TA biopsy, which will pick up another 5%–10% of cases of GCA. Finally, it is important to remember that GCA rarely if ever affects individuals younger than age 50, and other explanations for headache and scalp tenderness should be sought in these patients.

Weyand CM, Goronzy JJ. Giant-cell arteritis and polymyalgia rheumatica. *N Engl J Med.* 2014;371(17):50–57.

22. **ANSWER: A. Reassurance and physical therapy, focusing on posture, core muscle tone, and hip range of motion**

The patient has a greater trochanteric pain syndrome, based on clinical evaluation. Formerly, the term *trochanteric bursitis* was used to describe this condition, but there is greater evidence that the term is inaccurate. In patients with greater trochanteric pain syndrome, there is often evidence of tendinopathy of the gluteus medius and gluteus minimus tendons rather than overt trochanteric bursitis. Further diagnostic imaging studies (Answers B, D, and E) are not necessary upon initial evaluation of this condition. Physical therapy is appropriate (Answer A), and corticosteroid injection can be considered. There is little role for systemic corticosteroid treatment (Answer C).

Blankenbaker DG, Ullrick SR, Davis KW, et al. Correlation of MRI findings with clinical findings of trochanteric pain syndrome. *Skeletal Radiol.* 2008;37(10):903–909.

23. **ANSWER: D. Lateral cervical spine x-ray imaging, with flexion and extension views**

This patient is demonstrating signs and symptoms of cervical myelopathy, likely as a complication of RA affecting the cervical spine. Atlantoaxial instability is a rare but serious complication of RA, most often occurring in patients with long-standing deforming disease. The best initial assessment for this is lateral cervical spine x-ray imaging, with flexion and extension views (Answer D). MRI and/or CT scans of the cervical spine might also be indicated. Testing for RF and anti-CCP antibodies (Answer A) is part of the diagnostic workup of inflammatory arthritis and unnecessary in this case. ESR and CRP can correlate with RA disease activity, but these do little to clarify the patient's clinical presentation. It is unlikely that the patient would tolerate exercise stress testing (Answer C). RA generally spares the lumbar spine, and lumbar spine disease would not explain the patient's upper-extremity symptoms. Hence, lumbar spine MRI (Answer E) is not indicated.

24. **ANSWER: B. Hepatitis C antibody**

In addition to alcoholic cirrhosis, the patient has chronic hepatitis C infection complicated by cryoglobulinemic vasculitis. As in this case, cryoglobulinemic vasculitis can cause palpable purpura (Fig. 3.4), glomerulonephritis, and mononeuritis multiplex (the foot drop). Bowel vasculitis, pulmonary hemorrhage, and cerebral vasculitis are rare complications. Immunologic disturbances in patients with hepatitis C include detectable rheumatoid factor (RF) and disproportionately low C4 complement (compared with normal C3 complement). The patient does not describe or have symptoms of rheumatoid arthritis (RA); hence, testing for anti-CCP antibodies (Answer E) is unnecessary at this time. The remaining tests (Answers A, D, and E) do not address the clinical scenario and are notoriously nonspecific, with many "false-positive" tests.

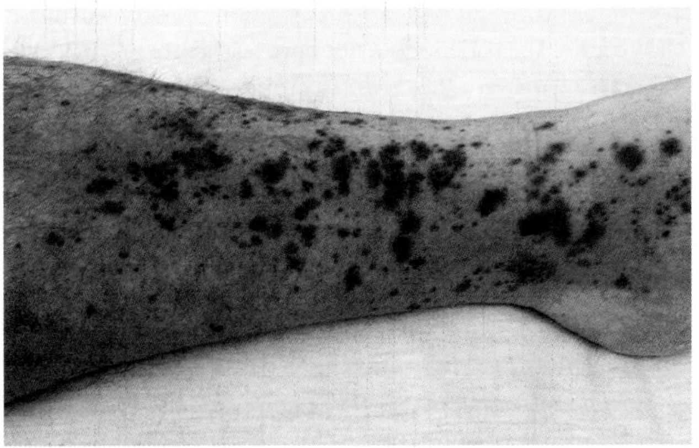

• **Fig. 3.4** Lower-extremity petechiae.

25. **ANSWER: E. Referral to orthopedics for consideration of right total knee arthroplasty**

This patient has end-stage osteoarthritis (OA) of the right knee. He would benefit from consideration of right total knee arthroplasty (TKA). He has already attempted conservative measures, including physical therapy and corticosteroid injections, without much benefit. Thus advising him to do this again (Answer

A) will likely be of little benefit. Narcotic-based therapies (Answer B) might be useful for a short-term bridge to get him to orthopedics, but not as a standalone treatment. There is little role for MRI of the knee or arthroscopic debridement in patients with advanced knee OA (Answers C and D); these choices do not change the ultimate need for TKA. Decision making for timing of TKA is done on a case-by-case basis. Pain and functional limitation are the driving forces behind optimal timing of referral to orthopedics. Physical therapy and weight loss remain an important part of preoperative management. Patients undergoing TKA should experience severe enough pain that they will derive benefit from joint replacement, but they should not be so debilitated that they might miss a window within which optimal recovery is possible. Indeed, patients who are wheelchair bound or similarly disabled will not typically derive the same benefit as patients able to maintain muscle mass through active participation in perioperative physical therapy.

26. ANSWER: C. Chondrocalcinosis of the wrist

Carpal tunnel syndrome (CTS) is most commonly the result of an overuse syndrome of the fingers. Flexor tendons swell slightly in response to overuse. This compresses the median nerve in the carpal tunnel, resulting in a median nerve neuropathy. Severe cases can lead to thenar muscle atrophy. Electromyogram with nerve conduction studies can be used to determine the severity of median nerve deficit. Other conditions that cause swelling of wrist flexor tendons (or the median nerve itself) can increase the risk of carpal tunnel syndrome: acromegaly, hypothyroidism, scleroderma, rheumatoid arthritis, other inflammatory arthritides (e.g., psoriatic arthritis), and pregnancy. Chondrocalcinosis commonly affects the wrists in older individuals, but it is not associated with CTS. It can lead to (1) acute flares of pseudogout arthritis, (2) chronic inflammatory "pseudo-rheumatoid" arthritis, or (3) accelerated degenerative "pseudo-osteoarthritis."

27. ANSWER: C. Entrapment neuropathy of the left lateral femoral cutaneous nerve

This patient is experiencing meralgia paresthetica—an entrapment neuropathy of the lateral femoral cutaneous nerve. Risk factors include abdominal obesity and tight-fitting belts/corsets. Diabetic amyotrophy (Answer A) is a lumbosacral plexopathy that occurs in patients with diabetes even with good blood sugar control. It causes pain, weakness, and muscle atrophy of the anterior thigh. Avascular necrosis (AVN) and degenerative arthritis (osteoarthritis) of the hip joint usually localizes as pain in the groin or deep buttock. Hip range of motion is often impaired. Trochanteric bursitis (Answer D) causes pain overlying the trochanteric bursa at the lateral hip. It does not impair passive hip range of motion, but it is not associated with paresthesias or numbness.

28. ANSWER: D. Recommend combination of physical therapy, sleep routine, weight loss, and psychiatric counseling.

The patient has fibromyalgia syndrome (FMS), a noninflammatory, nonstructural chronic dysfunctional pain syndrome of muscles, bones, and joints. Her history, examination, and laboratory results are not consistent with an inflammatory joint disorder. With more than 20 years of symptoms, one would expect significant abnormalities if she had an inflammatory, infectious, or neuromuscular process present. Thus EMG/NCS and serologic testing for connective tissue diseases (Answers A and B) are inappropriate. Likewise, tick-borne illnesses such as Lyme disease (Answer C) do not explain her constellation of symptoms. The history and examination describe hyperesthesia with allodynia (tenderness to normally nonpainful stimulus), common features in patients with FMS. For the most part, narcotic-based therapies are inappropriate with patients with FMS. They can lead to tolerance, dependency, dose escalation, and sometimes frank addiction. Rather, patients should be encouraged to address lifestyle issues that are often associated with FMS: physical inactivity, obesity, sleep disturbances, and underlying depression and anxiety (Answer D). It would be appropriate to consider pharmacotherapy for FMS if a patient is unable to address these issues.

Clauw DJ. Fibromyalgia: a clinical review. *JAMA.* 2014; 311(15):1547–1555.

29. ANSWER: E. No additional workup necessary

This patient describes Raynaud phenomenon: cold-induced vasospasm of the digits with triphasic color changes. Most patients, including this one, have *primary* Raynaud phenomenon, indicating an absence of any underlying connective tissue disorder (CTD). Patients have benign symptoms and findings, and no further workup is indicated (Answer E). *Secondary* Raynaud phenomenon is the term used to describe Raynaud phenomenon occurring secondary to another condition. These include vascular trauma or malformation (Answer D); microangiopathic injury from antiphospholipid syndrome (Answer B), chemotherapy, or other cause; and the various CTDs: systemic lupus erythematosus (Answer A), scleroderma (Answer B), Sjögren syndrome, rheumatoid arthritis, dermatomyositis, and mixed connective tissue disorders. In this case, the patient describes no symptoms of these other disorders, and the examination does not suggest them. Thus an exhaustive serologic and imaging workup for benign primary Raynaud syndrome is unnecessary and not cost effective. Factors that can exacerbate primary or secondary Raynaud attacks include caffeine ingestion, amphetamine use, anxiety, over-the-counter cold medications containing pseudoephedrine, and cocaine abuse.

Wigley FM, Flavahan NA. Raynaud's phenomenon. *N Engl J Med.* 2016; 375(6):556–565.

30. ANSWER: B. Captopril 25 mg orally three times daily, with dose escalation to control blood pressure

This patient is experiencing a scleroderma renal crisis (SRC). Evidence for this is the presence of scleroderma, hypertension, renal dysfunction, and evidence of microangiopathic hemolytic anemia (MAHA). Other causes of MAHA include antiphospholipid antibody syndrome, disseminated intravascular coagulation (DIC), hemolytic-uremic syndrome (HUS), thrombotic thrombocytopenic purpura (TTP), hypertensive emergency, hemolytic anemia/elevated liver studies/low platelets (HELLP) syndrome of pregnancy, certain malignancies, and graft-versus-host disease. SCR affects only a subset of patients with scleroderma, and highest-risk patients include those with rapidly progressive skin disease and anti-RNA polymerase III antibody (a laboratory test that is commercially available). SRC represents a hyper-renin state, leading to ischemic injury to the nephron. Even modest degrees of hypertension (as in this case) can lead to rapid renal demise. Thus despite rising creatinine levels, treatment with angiotensin-converting enzyme inhibitors (ACEi) must be rapidly initiated, with the goal of normalizing blood pressure. Prior to the recognition of ACEi therapy for SRC, this condition carried a grim prognosis, accounting for a sizable fraction of mortality in patients with scleroderma. Other antihypertensive agents (Answers C and D) might actually mask the renal injury and are inappropriate. Plasma exchange (Answer A) would be indicated for patients with TTP, but it is ineffective in SRC. Corticosteroids (Answer E) are used for treatment of glomerulonephritis. They are counterproductive and potentially catastrophic in patients with SRC.

31. ANSWER: D. Levofloxacin

The patient has experienced quinolone-associated rupture of the Achilles tendon. This is a rare but serious adverse reaction to fluoroquinolone-class antibiotics. Classic features include altered gait because of impaired plantar flexion from Achilles tendon rupture. The Achilles tendon is intact with a normal Thompson test; squeezing the calf should normally cause dorsiflexion at the ankle. The other antibiotics are not associated with this complication.

32. ANSWER: A. Gouty bursitis of the right prepatellar bursa

The physical examination suggests an acute inflammatory bursitis of the prepatellar bursa. With this condition, knee flexion will cause excruciating pain because of increased pressure within the inflamed bursa. There is nothing to suggest active inflammation of the knee from gout or sepsis (Answers B or C). Typically, patients with these conditions will have buildup of inflammatory fluid, and the joint will be partly flexed to alleviate buildup of intraarticular pressure. The examination also does not suggest meniscal injury (reproduced with a positive McMurray test) or quadriceps tendon rupture (which prevents extension of the knee against resistance).

33. ANSWER: A. *Staphylococcus aureus*

Reactive arthritis typically presents as abrupt-onset pain and swelling in multiple small joints. It is associated with various infectious agents, including *Streptococcus pyogenes, Clostridium difficile, Chlamydia trachomatis, Yersinia pestis, Salmonella* species, *Campylobacter* species, and *Shigella* species. *Staphylococcus aureus* is a common infectious agent, but it is not associated with reactive arthritis.

34. ANSWER: B. Plantar fasciitis

This patient has a clinical presentation consistent with plantar fasciitis. This condition causes focal pain at the origin of the plantar fascia as it comes off of the plantar calcaneus. Obesity is a risk factor. Stress fracture (Answer A) could still be present even with normal radiographs, but this patient's examination does not suggest involvement of the fifth metatarsal bone, and bilateral simultaneous stress fracture would be unusual. Acute gouty arthritis (Answer C) would be associated with inflammatory findings of erythema, warmth, and swelling. Charcot arthropathy (Answer D) is a complication of sensory deprivation of the extremity, such as occurs in diabetic neuropathy or tabes dorsalis (syphilis). The anterior talofibular ligament (ATFL) is commonly injured in forced inversion injury of the ankle. Pain localizes laterally and not to the plantar foot. Treatment of plantar fasciitis is first conservative, with stretching, weight loss, and nonsteroidal antiinflammatory drugs. If these fail, one could consider corticosteroid injection.

35. ANSWER: C. Hepatitis A vaccine, injectable typhoid vaccine, and a letter of exemption from yellow fever vaccine

This patient is immune suppressed because of her disease-modifying antirheumatic drug (DMARD) therapy. The yellow fever, MMR, and oral typhoid vaccines are all live vaccines and are therefore contraindicated in patients on biologic DMARDs. Administering the yellow fever vaccine in particular can be dangerous because life-threatening visceral infection due to the vaccine has been reported in this population. Proof of yellow fever vaccination is required for entry into many countries where yellow fever is endemic. Therefore it is prudent in advance to provide patients who cannot be vaccinated with a letter that excuses them from vaccination. In addition, patients should be carefully educated about the risks of yellow fever and how to avoid mosquito bites that could lead to yellow fever. MMR booster would be reasonable to give to an immunocompetent traveler to the Amazon, but it is not indicated here, because it is a live vaccine. This vaccine is not a requirement for entry into countries, so a letter of excuse is not needed for this vaccine for international travel. Hepatitis A and the injectable typhoid vaccines are both inactivated vaccines and are indicated for travelers to Brazil based on Centers for Disease Control and Prevention guidance.

Mota LM, Oliveira AC, Lima RA, et al. Vaccination against yellow fever among patients on immunosuppressors with diagnoses of rheumatic diseases [in Portuguese]. *Rev Soc Bras Med Trop.* 2009;42(1):23–27.

Rubin LG, Levin MJ, Ljungman P, et al. 2013 IDSA clinical practice guideline for vaccination of the immunocompromised host. *Clin Infect Dis.* 2014;58(3):309–318.

36. ANSWER: B. Chest radiograph

This patient describes classic features of Lofgren syndrome: ankle periarthritis and erythema nodosum. Chest radiograph will often demonstrate hilar adenopathy, and biopsy of one of these lymph nodes will show noncaseating granulomatous inflammation consistent with sarcoidosis. This variant of sarcoidosis has an excellent prognosis. Patients will almost universally recover fully and not experience other organ-specific manifestations of sarcoid disease. Associated features include oral contraceptive pill use, antecedent streptococcal pharyngitis, inflammatory bowel disease, and gastrointestinal dysentery (specifically *Yersinia* species). Ankle film (Answer A) will not add to the clinical impression that there is ankle swelling. Serologic testing for RA or Lyme disease (Answers C or E) is not necessary, because the clinical assessment does not suggest inflammatory arthritis of the ankles; normal passive range of motion of the joint argues for a periarticular process and not articular disease. Further, Lyme arthritis is normally monoarticular. Finally, the clinical assessment is not consistent with gouty arthritis (Answer D), a condition unlikely to affect a premenopausal woman without any specific risk factors.

37. ANSWER: E. Referral to the emergency department for urgent MRI of the lumbar spine

This patient is experiencing cauda equina syndrome: compression of the cauda equina from a paraspinal source. In this case, an intervertebral disc has herniated into the spinal canal, impairing function of sacral nerves. The patient reports symptoms that could be mistaken for an S1 radiculopathy alone: loss of plantar flexion, absent Achilles reflex, and reduced posterior thigh sensation. However, he also has "red flag" features of back pain to prompt evaluation for cauda equina syndrome: sensory loss in the perineum, impotence, urinary retention, and bowel retention. If not identified and corrected urgently, sacral nerve deficits can become long standing. The remaining options (Answers A–D) delay the diagnosis of this neurosurgical emergency. Other "red flags" for low back pain not present in this case include fever, occult weight loss, history of malignancy, and recent intravenous drug abuse. These findings should prompt consideration of inflammatory, infectious, or malignant etiologies of back pain.

Gardner A, Gardner E, Morley T, et al. Cauda equina syndrome: a review of the current clinical and medico-legal position. *Eur Spine J.* 2011; 20(5):690–697.

38. ANSWER: C. Hyperuricemia

Hyperuricemia is not a direct consequence of corticosteroid use. Obesity, diabetes mellitus, and hypertension are all side effects of corticosteroids that are themselves risk factors for hyperuricemia. Corticosteroids impair the immune system (Answer A), are a cause of cataracts even in young patients (Answer B), can precipitate avascular necrosis of bone (Answer D), and can cause a wasting steroid myopathy that typically presents as leg weakness in the hip flexors (Answer E).

39. ANSWER: A. Morning stiffness

The most likely diagnosis is polymyalgia rheumatica (PMR), without features to suggest giant cell arteritis (GCA). Morning stiffness (Answer A) is commonly reported in patients with PMR. Elderly patients can have incidental findings of rheumatoid factor, chondrocalcinosis, and joint space narrowing (Answers C–E), but these are not features of PMR. Blindness is a feared complication of GCA, but the patient denies other symptoms of GCA: headaches, visual disturbances, scalp tenderness, and jaw achiness after chewing (jaw claudication).

Weyand CM, Goronzy JJ. Giant-cell arteritis and polymyalgia rheumatica. *N Engl J Med.* 2014;371(1):50–57.

40. ANSWER: B. Adult-onset Still disease

This patient demonstrates many criteria that support a diagnosis of adult-onset Still disease (AOSD): pharyngitis, fever, rash, inflammatory arthritis, leukocytosis, thrombocytosis, hepatosplenomegaly, lymphadenopathy, and elevated inflammatory indices. Most important, an extensive workup for other potential etiologies for her condition has been negative, including serologic studies. One additional useful test is the serum ferritin level, which can sometimes be strikingly elevated (>10,000 μg/mL). The clinical scenario is not that of Lyme disease infection (Answer A). Behçet disease (Answer E) is a syndrome that includes oral ulcers, genital ulcers, and uveitis. Associated features include fever, pyoderma gangrenosum, vasculitis, and pathergy (neutrophilic pustule formation at the site of innocuous skin perforation such as a sterile needle).

Acute bacterial endocarditis (Answer D) is excluded by the negative blood cultures, nontoxic appearance, and time course of 3 weeks' duration. Systemic lupus erythematosus (SLE; Answer C) could explain her clinical presentation. However, it is essentially ruled out by the negative ANA test, which has excellent negative predictive value. Unlike this case, SLE is more often associated with leukopenia and thrombocytopenia.

Efthimiou P, Paik PK, Bielory L. Diagnosis and management of adult onset Still's disease. *Ann Rheum Dis.* 2006;65(5): 564–572.

41. ANSWER: A. Sjögren syndrome

The mother likely has circulating anti-Ro (anti-SSA) antibodies, which can cross the placenta and cause a neonatal "anti-Ro syndrome" characterized by fetal heart block and photosensitive rash (similar to subacute cutaneous lupus of adults). Besides Sjögren syndrome, this antibody can be found in patients with systemic lupus erythematosus (SLE) or very rarely as an incidental finding in healthy mothers. The rash is self-limited and only of cosmetic concern. The congenital heart block, however, is often irreversible. It represents failure of formation of the conductive system of the heart during the early second trimester of pregnancy. Thus careful monitoring should be performed starting around week 15 for any pregnant woman with known anti-Ro antibody positivity, including careful monitoring of fetal heart rate. Affected patients would benefit from having high-risk obstetrics follow the pregnancy. Primigravida women with anti-Ro antibodies carry an approximately 5% chance of the first pregnancy being affected by congenital heart block. In subsequent pregnancies, this risk is near zero for women who had unaffected first pregnancies. However, the risk is much higher for those women in whom their first pregnancy was affected by fetal heart block. Hydroxychloroquine appears to be effective in reducing the rate of fetal heart block in at-risk mothers. Once detected, however, fetal heart block is not always reversible; no treatments have been shown to be highly effective for reversing conductive abnormalities. Treatment options include high-dose betamethasone or intravenous immunoglobulin. None of the other answers are associated with fetal heart block. Both Lyme disease (Answer A) and acute rheumatic fever (Answer D) can cause heart block in the affected individual. Marfan syndrome (Answer C) can complicate pregnancies because of maternal aortic dissection. Methotrexate (Answer E) is highly teratogenic to the growing fetus, which often does not survive in utero exposure. Many severe birth defects are described (including neural tube defects), but not congenital heart block.

42. ANSWER: E. Referral to spine surgery for decompressive laminectomy

The patient has lumbar spinal stenosis that is refractory to conservative interventions of physical therapy, analgesics, and corticosteroid injections. His physical function is compromised, and he is experiencing weakness of hip flexor muscles. Repeating these interventions (Answers A, B, and D) is unlikely to provide much relief. Repeat MRI of the lumbar spine (Answer C) is unlikely to reveal any new pathology, and he does not describe any "red flags" of back pain that would prompt workup for inflammatory, infectious, or neoplastic processes. Referral to spine surgery is appropriate because decompressive laminectomy can alleviate symptoms and improve leg weakness.

43. ANSWER: D. Temporal artery biopsy showing granulomatous arteritis

The patient is experiencing a "pulmonary-renal syndrome": pulmonary hemorrhage from diffuse aveolitis and crescentic glomerulonephritis. These syndromes result from small-vessel vasculitis in the lung and kidney. Inflammatory indices are elevated ESR and CRP, thrombocytosis, and anemia of chronic disease. Of all answers, only giant cell arteritis/temporal arteritis (Answer D) is not associated with small-vessel vasculitis of this nature. The serologic studies indicate systemic lupus erythematosus (SLE) (Answer A), Goodpasture syndrome (Answer B), and ANCA-associated vasculitis (Answer C). Levamisole is an antihelminthic agent used to "cut" cocaine. In some individuals, it can induce an ANCA-associated vasculitic condition clinically indistinguishable from granulomatosis with polyangiitis (GPA), formerly Wegener granulomatosis.

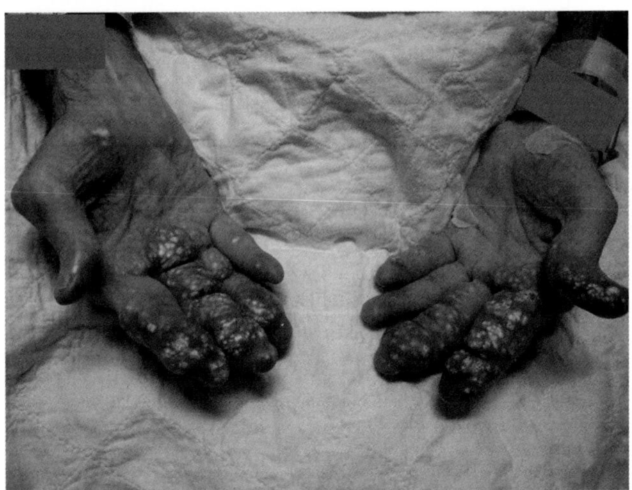

• **Fig. 3.5** Tophaceous gout picture.

44. ANSWER: C. Discuss with patient's nephrologist about alternative immunosuppressive therapies for the renal graft.

The patient is currently taking azathioprine (AZA), an inhibitor of purine synthesis. AZA metabolites are further metabolized by xanthine oxidase (XO), which normally converts purine metabolites into uric acid.

Although XO inhibitors such as allopurinol and febuxostat normally reduce uric acid formation, they also lead to accumulation of AZA (and toxicity), unless the AZA dose is very much reduced. Thus Answers A and E are incorrect in this patient because of concurrent azathioprine use. Answer B is incorrect because probenecid increases the risk of nephrolithiasis, a potentially devastating complication in patients with a single functioning kidney or transplanted kidney. Answer D is not correct, because the patient does not describe symptoms of acute gout, and corticosteroids do not solve the underlying problem of hyperuricemia with tophaceous gouty deposits (Fig. 3.5). This patient is young and likely to experience complications of the numerous tophi, such as a destructive arthropathy or skin breakdown complicated by infections like osteomyelitis. Thus the best answer is C, with a discussion about alternatives to AZA so that the patient might benefit from the addition of allopurinol or febuxostat to prevent long-term complications of gouty tophi. Alternatively, although not typically advised, the azathioprine dose could be very much reduced, and a very low dose XO inhibitor could be added, with careful dose titration and monitoring of blood counts. Note that calcineurin inhibitors such as cyclosporine increase serum uric acid levels but are not contraindicated in conjunction with XO inhibitors.

45. ANSWER: B. Aspiration of the right knee for fluid analysis

The patient may have septic arthritis of the right knee. Aspiration with fluid analysis (Answer B) is the only option that can address that concern properly. In patients who present with an acute inflammatory monoarthritis, septic arthritis should always be high in the differential diagnosis. This is particularly true when a patient with RA under good control presents with a single inflamed joint. Patients with RA are at increased risk for septic arthritis for many reasons: increased vascularity of inflamed joints, immunosuppressive qualities of DMARD therapies, underlying structural joint disease, and frequent presence of prosthetic joints. Septic arthritis occurs most commonly from hematogenous seeding of the joint from bacteremia, thus a source of infection must be sought in any patient with joint infection. Joint aspiration with steroid injection (Answer C) misses that this is a potential joint infection and delays diagnosis. Likewise, the other answers delay diagnosis of a potentially serious septic arthritis.

46. ANSWER: E. Flexible bronchoscopy

This patient is presenting with features of diffuse alveolar hemorrhage (DAH), a potentially life-threatening complication of SLE (Fig. 3.6). Diagnosis is made by flexible bronchoscopy (Answer E), which also allows for bronchial lavage to test for infectious microorganisms (an alternative explanation for her presentation). The most common features of DAH are dyspnea, hypoxemia, and unexplained rapid drop in hemoglobin (>2 g/dL). Fever is common, but hemoptysis is reported in only 50% of cases. Thus as in this case, the absence of hemoptysis does not exclude DAH. Missing DAH can have dire consequences; the mortality rate of SLE-related DAH approaches 50%. CT angiogram with iodinated contrast (Answer A) risks contrast-induced nephropathy, and MRI with gadolinium contrast (Answer D) risks nephrogenic systemic fibrosis. Neither imaging study accurately permits a diagnosis of DAH. Although pulmonary function tests (PFTs) might show elevated DLCO in the presence of alveolar blood (Answer B), the patient will be unable to comply with PFTs while intubated. Lumbar puncture to exclude various causes of meningitis and meningoencephalitis (Answer C) would be indicated in a patient such as this whose primary complaint is delirium without identifiable cause, because immunosuppression raises the risk for infection, and SLE can cause vasculitis and meningoencephalitis of the central nervous system.

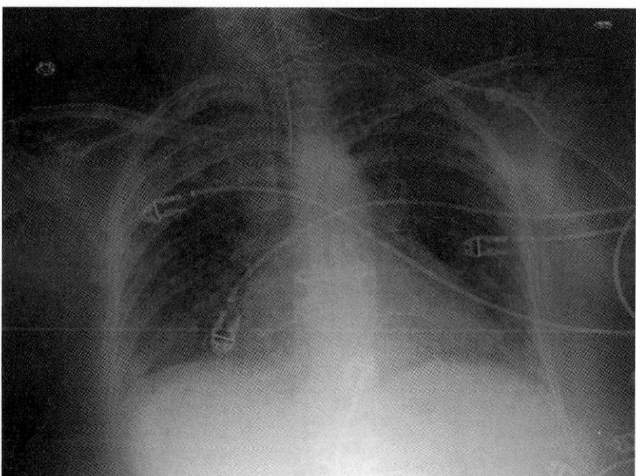

• **Fig. 3.6** Systemic lupus erythematosus diffuse alveolar hemorrhage chest radiograph.

47. ANSWER: E. Adalimumab 40 mg every other week

Ankylosing spondylitis (AS) is one of several spondyloarthritides, a category of disorders that also includes psoriatic arthritis, reactive arthritis, and the arthropathy of inflammatory bowel disease (IBD arthropathy). This patient describes years of inflammatory back pain, worse in the morning and improved with activity. Symptoms of AS usually start in the area of the sacroiliac joints (deep buttocks and low back) and slowly progress up the spine. Thoracic spine involvement can cause thoracic wall pain and affect chest expansion. AS is associated with episodes of unilateral anterior uveitis. Inflammatory markers are often (but not always) elevated. The diagnosis is made based on symptoms of inflammatory back pain and supportive imaging. Plain film radiographic changes are described in this case. MRI is more sensitive and specific for sacroiliitis, but it is unnecessary in this case. Testing for HLA-B27 haplotype (Answer A) is sometimes used to stratify the likelihood of AS, but it is not diagnostic. Upward of 8%–10% of white individuals carry HLA-B27, and >95% of these people do not have AS. For years, treatment of patients with AS with inflammatory spine pain was limited to cyclooxygenase (COX) inhibitors: nonsteroidal antiinflammatory drugs (NSAIDs). Corticosteroids, methotrexate, and even opiate-based therapies (Answers B–D) are relatively ineffective or not sustainable for the long term. Sulfasalazine has a role in the treatment of peripheral arthritis, but it is of no value in relieving spine pain. Antagonists of tumor necrosis factor alpha (TNF-α) have been available since the late 1990s and are extremely effective in relieving the symptoms of inflammatory back pain in patients with AS and other types of spondyloarthritis. Five TNF-α antagonists are currently available: adalimumab, certolizumab, etanercept, golimumab, and infliximab.

Taurog JD, Chhabra A, Colbert RA, et al. Ankylosing spondylitis and axial spondyloarthritis. *N Engl J Med.* 2016;374(26):2563–2574.

48. ANSWER: A. Parotid lymphoma

Patients with Sjögren syndrome (SjS) have a very high risk of developing lymphoma in the mucosa-associated lymphoid tissue (MALT) of the parotid and submandibular glands, upward of 50–100 times the normal population. One potential etiology is that chronic inflammation in these tissues may lead to malignant degeneration of abnormal autoimmune lymphocytes. Knowing this risk is important when evaluating asymmetric glandular swelling in a patient with SjS. Laboratory features associated with the presence of these lymphomas include vasculitic rash, falling complement levels, and normalization of a previously abnormal RF. Imaging and surgical referral for biopsy are indicated. Sarcoidosis (Answer B) can affect the lacrimal and salivary glands, often in association with fever (uveoparotid fever or Heerfordt syndrome). Sialolithiasis and suppurative bacterial sialadenitis (Answers C and D) can both occur in patients with SjS, but these conditions are almost always acute and associated with pain. Ten years of bisphosphonate therapy increases this patient's risk for osteonecrosis of the jaw (Answer E). However, that condition is not suggested by the history or physical examination, which describes extraoral swelling of the parotid gland and associated changes in serologic tests.

49. ANSWER: E. Nephrogenic systemic fibrosis

Nephrogenic systemic fibrosis (NSF) is a complication of gadolinium exposure that occurs in patients with severely compromised renal function: severe acute kidney injury, stage 4 or 5 chronic kidney disease, or dialysis therapy. Retained gadolinium induces a fibrotic reaction in deep dermal tissues and sometimes in internal organs. This case describes a classic presentation of NSF, including the yellowish scleral plaques and joint contractures from fibrosis of periarticular tissues. Scleroderma (Answer A) is highly associated with Raynaud phenomenon and often affects the face, which is spared in NSF. Lipodermatosclerosis (Answer B) is a gravity-dependent complication of chronic venous stasis that affects the lower extremities only and usually does not cause joint contractures. Scleredema diabeticorum (Answer C) is a fibrotic reaction of dermal tissue that occurs in patients with diabetes. Unlike NSF, it predominantly affects parts of the upper torso, such as the shoulder and upper back. Eosinophilic fasciitis is an inflammatory disorder of fascia (not dermis) caused by aberrant eosinophilic infiltration, leading to edema of the affected extremity. It is not associated with renal dysfunction, but patients may have an underlying myelodysplastic syndrome.

Todd DJ, Kay J. Gadolinium-induced fibrosis. *Annu Rev Med.* 2016;67:273–291.

50. ANSWER: A. Rheumatoid arthritis

Rheumatoid arthritis (RA) is the most common chronic inflammatory polyarthritis affecting either gender or any age group. It is characterized by redness, warmth, and swelling of the joints, often accompanied by morning stiffness. Almost any joint can be involved, with the general exception of the thoracolumbar spine and distal interphalangeal (DIP) joints. Approximately 25% of patients with RA do not have detectable RF or anti-CCP antibodies at any point in their disease course (as in this case). Although these patients (termed *seronegative RA*) often have a less severe disease course, they can still develop joint damage and erosions (as noted in the films in this case). Inflammatory indices are often elevated, but these are nonspecific. Several features of this case argue against chronic gouty arthritis (Answer B). He reports no history of episodic acute gouty arthritis, and crystals were not observed in the joint fluid aspirate. The relatively normal uric acid does not completely exclude gout, but the value of 4.0 mg/dL makes it unlikely that the patient has a chronic, erosive gouty arthropathy. Primary osteoarthritis (Answer C) rarely affects the MCP, wrist, or elbow joints. Rheumatic fever (Answer D) can cause arthralgia and lead to joint deformities. Patients can experience a noninflammatory joint laxity (Jaccoud arthropathy) similar to that found in patients with systemic lupus erythematosus.

However, the patient also lacks the other clinical features of rheumatic fever, including the fever, rash, pharyngitis, and cardiac complications. Finally, polymyalgia rheumatic (PMR) is a seronegative inflammatory disorder of individuals >50 years old (Answer E). It primarily affects the shoulders and hips, as in this case. However, PMR is not considered a cause of erosive inflammatory polyarthritis of the extremities, as in this case. Thus although in some ways a diagnosis of exclusion, seronegative RA is the most appropriate diagnosis in this case.

Acknowledgment

The author and editors gratefully acknowledge the contributions of the previous author, Dr. Jonathan S. Coblyn.

4

Pulmonary and Critical Care Medicine

SCOTT L. SCHISSEL AND ELIZABETH GAY

1. A 67-year-old woman presents to clinic to establish care for asthma. She has been followed for many years at another facility. She has moderate persistent disease, with several exacerbations per year. Her current medications include theophylline, salmeterol inhaler twice daily, and albuterol inhaler as needed.

   Which of the following serious adverse outcomes led to a black-box warning regarding the use of long-acting inhaled beta-agonist bronchodilators in the treatment of asthma?

   A. Atrial fibrillation and flutter
   B. Ventricular tachycardia and fibrillation
   C. Myocardial infarction and stroke
   D. Respiratory failure and death
   E. Angioedema and anaphylaxis

2. A 72-year-old man presents to the clinic for evaluation of dyspnea. He notes a 5-year history of slowly progressive dyspnea on exertion. He has a chronic cough with white to yellow phlegm, most bothersome in the morning. He also notes some wheezing with exertion. He smokes one pack of cigarettes per day, down from two packs per day a few years ago. He started smoking at age 16. He worked in a beer factory, with some exposure to dust. Physical examination shows the following vital signs: temperature 37°C, heart rate 94 beats per minute, blood pressure 145/80 mm Hg, respiratory rate 20 breaths per minute, and Sao_2 94% on room air. Generally, he was alert and had no respiratory distress. The oropharynx was clear with poor dentition. No jugular venous distention was present. His chest had diminished breath sounds with scattered end-expiratory wheezes. His cardiovascular presentation was regular rhythm and rate, distant S1 and S2, with no murmurs. His extremities were warm with no clubbing, cyanosis, or edema.

   Which of the following pulmonary function test results would you expect for this patient?

   A. FEV_1 2.0 L (66% of predicted), FVC 4.0 L (100% of predicted), FEV_1/FVC 0.5 (66% of predicted)
   B. FEV_1 1.0 L (33% of predicted), FVC 1.25 L (31% of predicted), FEV_1/FVC 0.8 (107% of predicted)
   C. FEV_1 3.0 L (100% of predicted), FVC 4.0 L (100% of predicted), FEV_1/FVC 0.75 (100% of predicted)
   D. FEV_1 2.0 L (66% of predicted), FVC 2.67 L (67% of predicted), FEV_1/FVC 0.75 (100% of predicted)

3. A 43-year-old man presents with several years of dyspnea on exertion. He also has exertional chest tightness and has been told he has exercise-induced asthma. He uses albuterol before exercise, but he has not noticed any improvement in his symptoms. He undergoes spirometry, which reveals moderate fixed obstruction, with an FEV_1 of 65% of predicted. Chest CT scan is obtained and shows widespread emphysema.

   Which of the following is the most accurate statement about the most likely diagnosis?

   A. The diagnosis is established by a blood test.
   B. All patients with this disease develop obstructive lung disease.
   C. The majority of persons develop clinically significant liver disease at some point during their lifetime.
   D. A characteristic feature is a preserved diffusion capacity of the lung for carbon monoxide (DLCO) on pulmonary function testing.

4. A 45-year-old woman with asthma reports that she has experienced chest tightness and wheezing approximately 30 minutes after ingestion of aspirin 81 mg.

   Which of the following is the most appropriate response?

   A. "Your symptoms are not likely to have been caused by aspirin at this low dose."
   B. "You are allergic to aspirin and should instead use ibuprofen or naproxen for pain relief with antiinflammatory activity."
   C. "Because cross-sensitization is common, you should avoid peanuts and tree nuts such as cashews and almonds."
   D. "Given your history, a leukotriene modifier such as montelukast, zafirlukast, or zileuton might be particularly helpful as treatment for your asthma."
   E. "Given your history, a long-acting beta-agonist bronchodilator such as formoterol or salmeterol might be particularly harmful as treatment for your asthma."

5. A 68-year-old man with an 80-pack-year history of tobacco use has mild shortness of breath only while climbing "steep hills," but he has required treatment two times in 1 year for acute exacerbations of chronic obstructive pulmonary disease (COPD). Spirometry reveals an FEV_1 of 2.2 L, 80% of predicted, and an FEV_1/FVC ratio of 60%.

Which of the following best describes this patient's Global Initiative for Chronic Obstructive Lung Disease (GOLD) stage of COPD?

A. Stage 1A
B. Stage 1C
C. Stage 2A
D. Stage 2C
E. Stage 3A

6. A 45-year-old man presents with a productive cough, fever, and left-sided chest pain of approximately 1 week's duration. Physical examination reveals dullness to percussion and decreased breath sounds throughout the lower half of the left chest posteriorly. His white blood cell count is 17,500/μL with 85% polymorphonuclear leukocytes and 6% band forms. A chest x-ray shows a moderate to large left pleural effusion. Sputum Gram stain shows many neutrophils with mixed flora, including gram-positive cocci, gram-positive rods, and gram-negative rods. Sputum culture grows only "normal oral flora" after 48 hours. Thoracentesis succeeds in withdrawing only 60 mL of serous fluid. Pleural fluid analysis reveals a high total protein concentration (4 g/dL), white blood cells 6,500/μL with 80% polymorphonuclear cells, and no organisms on Gram stain or bacterial culture. Pleural fluid pH is 7.10; pleural fluid amylase is low. The patient is started on azithromycin and cefotaxime in the emergency department but fails to improve.

Which of the following is the next best step in management?

A. Discontinuation of azithromycin and cefotaxime and initiation of levofloxacin
B. Chest tube drainage of pleural space, with thoracoscopic lysis of pleural adhesions if necessary
C. Pleural biopsy
D. Barium swallow to evaluate for esophageal rupture (Boerhaave syndrome)
E. Systemic corticosteroids for probable inflammatory pleuritis related to collagen vascular disease

7. A 51-year-old woman presents with the gradual onset of dyspnea. She denies any infectious symptoms. Her past medical history is notable for a "kidney tumor." Chest x-ray shows a moderate-sized right pleural effusion. Thoracentesis reveals 600 mL of milky-appearing fluid with a triglyceride concentration of 145 mg/dL.

Which of the following is the most likely cause of the pleural effusion?

A. Lymphangioleiomyomatosis (LAM)
B. Pneumonia
C. Malignancy
D. Pulmonary infarction
E. Sarcoidosis

8. An 82-year-old man presents with a 6-month history of nonproductive cough and gradually increasing exertional dyspnea, but no fever, chest pain, or hemoptysis. He has no history of collagen vascular disease. He continues to work as an accountant and has had no unusual exposures in his home or work environments. He takes hydrochlorothiazide for hypertension, aspirin 81 mg, and a multivitamin. On examination, he has early clubbing and high-pitched inspiratory crackles throughout the lower lung zones posteriorly. Chest x-ray reveals linear and small nodular opacities ("reticulonodular pattern"), predominantly in the lower lung zones. Spirometry suggests a moderate restrictive pattern. Chest CT with high-resolution images reveals linear opacities, most prominent in the lung periphery, with traction bronchiectasis and areas of "honeycombing" at the lung bases; there are no areas with "ground-glass" opacities (Fig. 4.1). Fiberoptic bronchoscopy is performed with normal visualized tracheobronchial mucosa. Analysis of bronchoalveolar lavage fluid shows no malignant cells and no organisms. Transbronchial lung biopsies reveal minimal and nonspecific inflammatory changes in the interstitium, with collagen deposition (fibrosis) and increased numbers of alveolar macrophages.

Based on this clinical information, what is the most likely diagnosis?

A. Sarcoidosis
B. Nonspecific interstitial pneumonia
C. Idiopathic pulmonary fibrosis
D. Cryptogenic organizing pneumonia (COP)
E. Langerhans cell histiocytosis

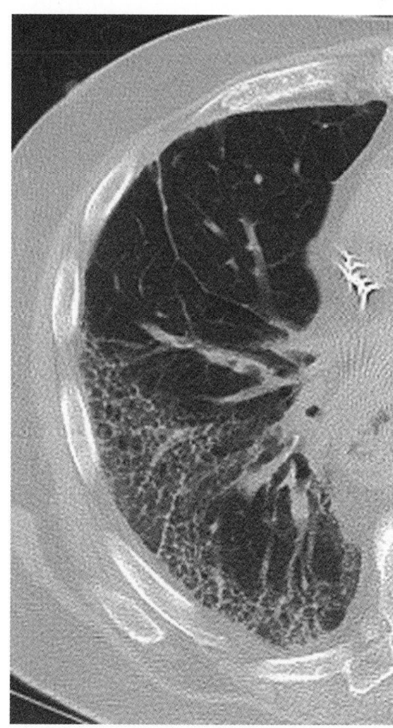

• **Fig. 4.1** Chest CT scan showing linear opacities with traction bronchiectasis and areas of "honeycombing" for patient in Question 8.

9. A 63-year-old man presents to the pulmonary clinic with a chronic cough and dyspnea on exertion. His exam is notable for basilar inspiratory crackles. His social history is notable for 30 years of employment in a shipyard. Chest CT shows basilar linear opacities and areas of "honeycombing."

Which of the following test results would be expected in this patient?

A. Normal oxygen saturation at rest that falls to 82% with exertion
B. Normal oxygen saturation at rest without change with exertion
C. Normal DLCO (diffusion capacity of the lung for carbon monoxide)
D. Increased lung static compliance
E. Increased total lung capacity (TLC), functional residual capacity (FRC), and residual volume (RV) on full measurement of lung volumes

10. A 67-year-old man with a diagnosis of idiopathic pulmonary fibrosis presents to discuss treatment options. Over the past 2 years, his FVC has declined from 75% of predicted to 60% of predicted. He has noticed increased dry cough and dyspnea on exertion.

Which of the following therapies would be most likely to prevent further lung function decline in this patient?

A. High-dose oral steroids
B. High-dose oral steroids plus azathioprine
C. Rituximab
D. Hydroxychloroquine
E. Pirfenidone

11. A 47-year-old man with a history of asthma and nasal polyps presents for evaluation of daytime sleepiness. He also has history of hypertension and retrognathia as well as chronic insomnia and poor sleep quality. On examination, you note a height of 62 inches but a normal BMI. His neck circumference is 15 inches.

Which of the following attributes is a risk factor for obstructive sleep apnea?

A. Retrognathia
B. Dress shirt neck circumference >15 inches
C. Nasal polyps with complete nasal airflow obstruction
D. Short stature (<60 inches tall in women, <65 inches tall in men)
E. Insomnia

12. A 52-year-old woman with known obstructive sleep apnea and an apnea-hypopnea index of 62 presents to the clinic for follow-up. She reports inability to tolerate prescribed continuous positive airway pressure (CPAP) because she feels claustrophobic.

She is at increased risk of death resulting from which of the following?

A. Aspiration
B. Laryngospasm
C. Diabetic ketoacidosis
D. Motor vehicle accidents
E. Hypoxemic respiratory failure

13. A 52-year-old man with no history of smoking presents with a history of frequent episodes of bronchitis. He has a chronic barking cough that has not improved with steroid inhalers or bronchodilators. He has a history of arthritis but no history of gastroesophageal reflux disease (GERD), rashes, or exertional dyspnea. Pulmonary function tests show mild fixed obstruction and no restriction.

Which of the following is the most likely diagnosis?

A. Scleroderma
B. Polymyositis
C. Relapsing polychondritis
D. Systemic lupus erythematosus
E. Mixed connective tissue disease

14. A 30-year-old man presents for evaluation of polycythemia. He is found to have resting hypoxemia (Sao_2 = 87%) and signs of right heart failure, with jugular venous distention and peripheral edema. He reports excessive daytime sleepiness. His examination is remarkable for morbid obesity (body mass index [BMI] = 42 kg/m^2), narrowed posterior pharyngeal opening, and clear chest on auscultation. His hematocrit is 52%. Chest x-ray is normal. Spirometry identifies a pattern suggesting mild restriction. Arterial blood gases reveal Po_2 55 mm Hg, Pco_2 72 mm Hg, and pH 7.32. Continuous positive airway pressure (CPAP) fails to correct his nocturnal hypoxemia and daytime hypersomnolence.

Which of the following would be an expected finding in his evaluation?

A. Normal ventilatory response to carbon dioxide
B. Orthodeoxia
C. Central apneas
D. Restless legs syndrome
E. Prolonged sleep latency period

15. A 52-year-old woman presents for evaluation of dyspnea and fatigue. Her medical history is notable for obesity, hypertension, and type 2 diabetes. She has no history of smoking, but she was placed on oxygen a few years ago for hypoxemia. On exam, she has a room air oxygen saturation of 88%. Her lungs are clear, and cardiac exam shows no murmurs, with a normal S1 and S2. She has trace lower extremity edema. Her pulmonary function tests show mild restriction but no evidence of obstruction. Polysomnography shows severe obstructive sleep apnea, with an apnea-hypopnea index of 43.

Which of the following tests represents the next best diagnostic step?

A. Chest x-ray
B. Blood gas on room air
C. CBC with differential
D. Chest CT
E. Six-minute walk test

16. A 62-year-old man presents with a history of wheezing and dyspnea. The wheezing has been refractory to all inhalers and to a course of oral prednisone. Chest CT shows a tracheal tumor. He undergoes pulmonary function testing.

Which of the following images represents the most likely flow–volume loop?

A. Fig. 4.2 Flow–volume loop
B. Fig. 4.3 Flow–volume loop
C. Fig. 4.4 Flow–volume loop
D. Fig. 4.5 Flow–volume loop
E. Fig. 4.6 Flow–volume loop

17. A 43-year-old woman with a history of frequent sinusitis and pneumonia presents for evaluation. Imaging is obtained, which shows bilateral lower lobe bronchiectasis.

Which of the following tests is most likely to identify an etiology of bronchiectasis for which a specific therapy is available?

A. Antinuclear cytoplasmic antibody (ANCA)
B. Serum immunoglobulin G
C. Gluten autoantibodies (serum endomysial and antitissue transglutaminase antibodies)
D. Bronchial biopsy examined by electron microscopy
E. Full pulmonary function tests, including measurement of lung volumes and diffusion capacity of the lung for carbon monoxide

18. A 68-year-old woman presents for evaluation of chronic cough and fatigue. She describes 1 year of cough productive of yellow sputum. The cough failed to improve with empiric antibiotic courses, inhalers, and therapy for

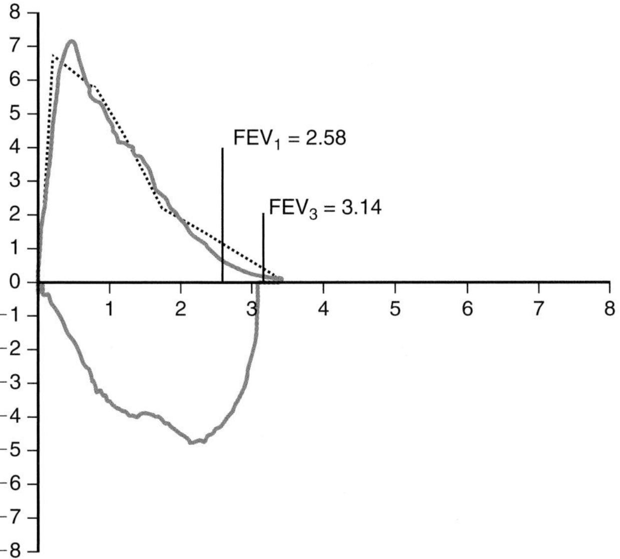

• **Fig. 4.2** A. Flow–volume loop for patient in Question 16.

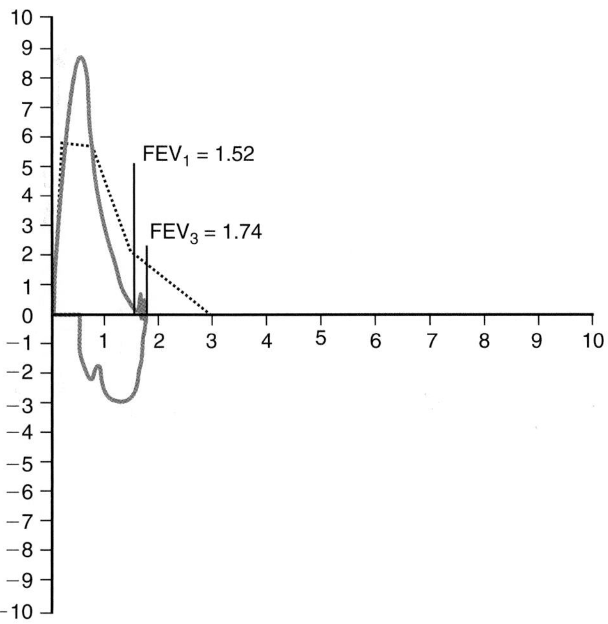

• **Fig. 4.3** B. Flow–volume loop for patient in Question 16.

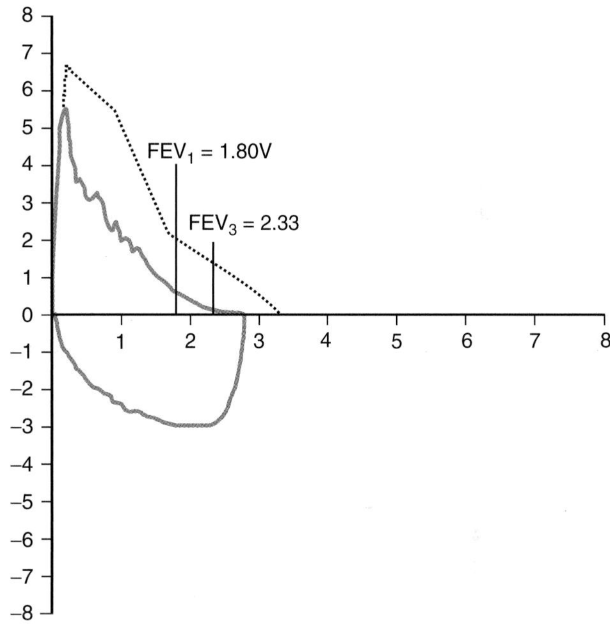

• **Fig. 4.4** C. Flow–volume loop for patient in Question 16.

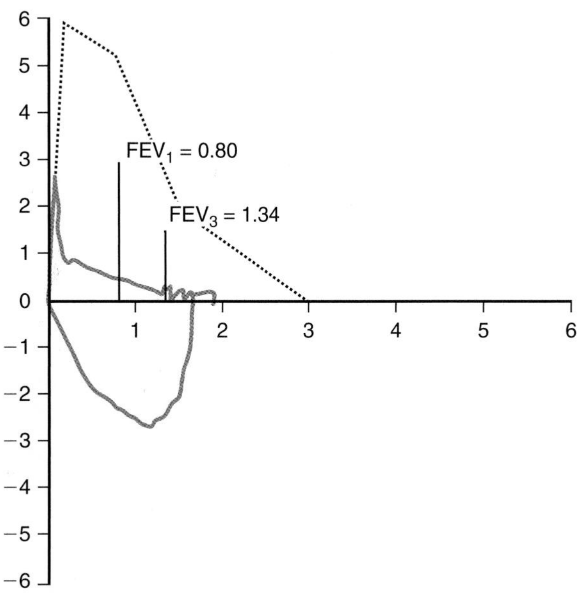

• **Fig. 4.5** D. Flow–volume loop for patient in Question 16.

reflux. Physical exam is notable for a thin, elderly woman in no distress, with clear lung fields. Pulmonary function testing reveals normal spirometry and diffusion.

Which of the following findings would you expect on chest CT (Fig. 4.7)?

A. Ground-glass opacity
B. Consolidation with air bronchograms
C. Honeycombing
D. Tree-in-bud nodules
E. Atelectasis

19. The accompanying chest x-ray (Fig. 4.8) is most likely from a patient with which of the following diagnoses?

A. Alpha-1 antitrypsin deficiency
B. Ankylosing spondylitis
C. Bronchiectasis due to cystic fibrosis
D. Granulomatosis with polyangiitis (Wegener granulomatosis)
E. Lymphangioleiomyomatosis (LAM)

20. A 55-year-old cigarette-smoking man born and reared in New York City is found to have a round, noncalcified right lower lobe nodule 1.8 cm in diameter, new since a prior chest x-ray obtained 1 year ago. Other than his usual "smoker's cough," he has been free of respiratory symptoms. His physical examination is normal. Positron emission tomography (PET) scan reveals increased uptake of radiolabeled glucose within the lung nodule but at no other sites. Spirometry indicates mild airflow obstruction; a cardiac stress test shows no evidence of myocardial ischemia.

Which of the following would be the next best step in management?

A. Measurement of prostate-specific antigen (PSA), upper gastrointestinal series, and colonoscopy
B. Fiberoptic bronchoscopy and transbronchial lung biopsy
C. Transthoracic needle aspirate/biopsy
D. Surgical resection of the lung nodule
E. Repeat chest imaging in 3 months to assess for growth of the nodule

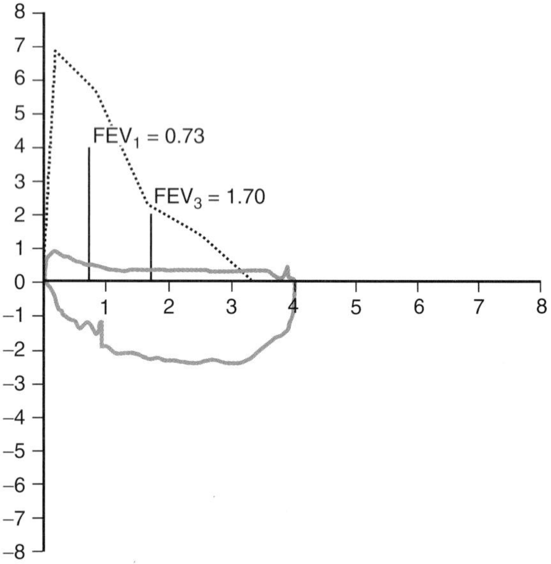

• **Fig. 4.6** E. Flow–volume loop for patient in Question 16.

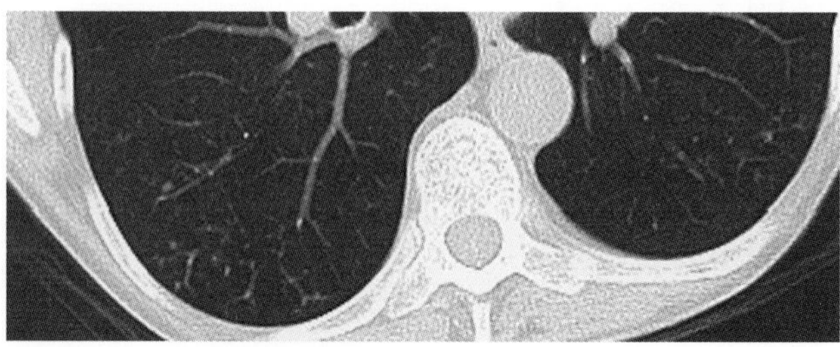

• **Fig. 4.7** CT for patient in Question 18.

21. A 53-year-old woman with a history of chronic obstructive pulmonary disease presents for routine follow-up. She is doing well from a respiratory standpoint but notes hoarseness. The hoarse voice comes and goes, but she is concerned about it.

Which one of the following medications is the most likely cause of her hoarseness?

A. Salmeterol
B. Fluticasone
C. Tiotropium
D. Albuterol
E. Ipratropium

22. A 43-year-old woman presents with exertional dyspnea, progressive over the past few years. She is now breathless climbing one flight of stairs. She is a lifelong nonsmoker without a history of asthma. Her chest x-ray shows mild hyperinflation. Spirometry and lung volumes indicate severe airflow obstruction without significant improvement following bronchodilator. Alpha-1 antitrypsin level is normal.

Which of the following is the most likely explanation for her lung disease?

A. She works in an old office building with central ventilation and without windows that can be opened.
B. She owns four large parrots.
C. She has ulcerative colitis.
D. She has mixed connective tissue disease.
E. She has a history of breast cancer treated with lumpectomy and postsurgical radiation therapy to the breast.

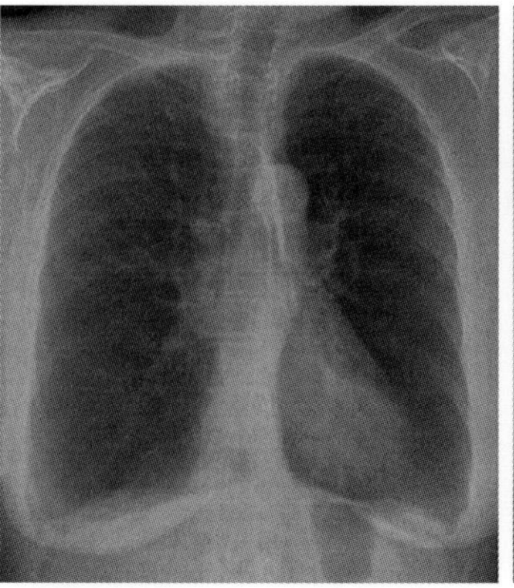

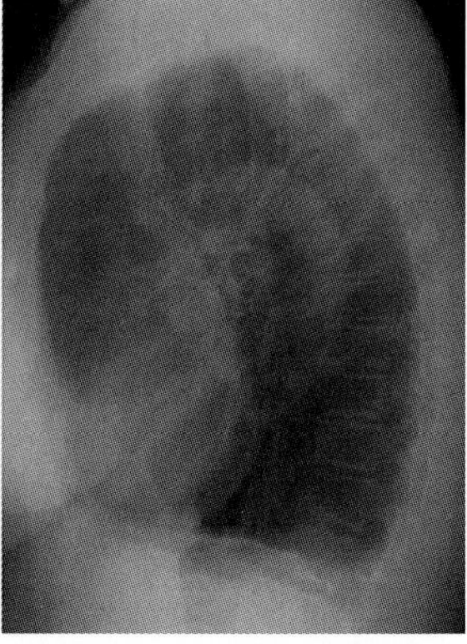

• **Fig. 4.8** Posteroanterior and lateral chest x-ray for patient in Question 19.

23. A 72-year-old woman with an 80-pack-year history of tobacco use and severe, GOLD stage D COPD with FEV_1 0.7 L, 38% of predicted is admitted to the hospital with 4 days of shortness of breath at rest, increased cough, and cough productive of yellow sputum. A chest x-ray reveals no pulmonary infiltrates. Her arterial blood gas on room air shows the following values: pH 7.30, $Paco_2$ 55 mm Hg, and Pao_2 58 mm Hg.

Which of the following is the best recommendation about treatment for this patient?

A. Start an 8-week course of oral steroids because it is associated with fewer relapses than a 2-week course of treatment.
B. Use intravenous corticosteroids because they are more effective and have fewer gastrointestinal side effects than oral corticosteroids.
C. Avoid bilevel positive airway pressure ventilation because it may cause hyperinflation and auto–positive end-expiratory pressure (auto-PEEP).
D. Start antibiotics because the patient has a change in sputum quantity and character.
E. Send for a sputum Gram stain and culture because these can often guide the choice of antibiotics.

24. A 24-year-old man is found to have bilateral hilar and mediastinal lymphadenopathy on a routine preemployment chest x-ray (Fig. 4.9). He has a mild, dry cough but no other respiratory or systemic symptoms. He was born and raised in New England, with no history of tuberculosis or exposure to anyone with known tuberculosis. Physical examination is normal, as are routine blood studies (complete blood count and comprehensive metabolic profile). Mediastinoscopy with right paratracheal lymph node biopsy reveals noncaseating granulomas. Stains for organisms are negative.

Which of the following is the most appropriate treatment at this time?

A. Low-dose oral steroids (prednisone 10 mg/day, with dose adjusted according to his response to treatment)
B. Initial high-dose steroids (prednisone 40–60 mg/day), tapered and then discontinued over approximately 6 months

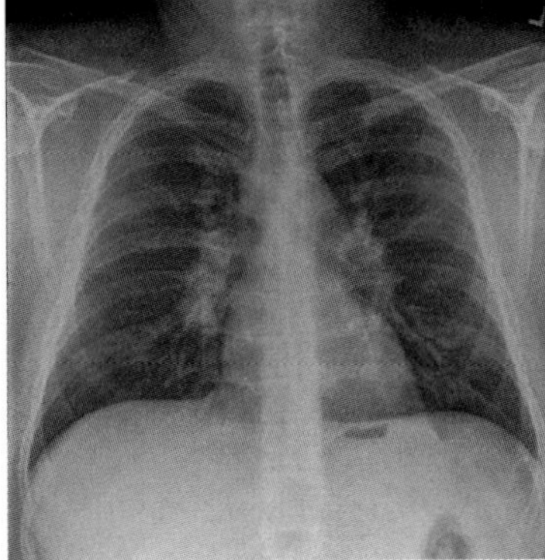
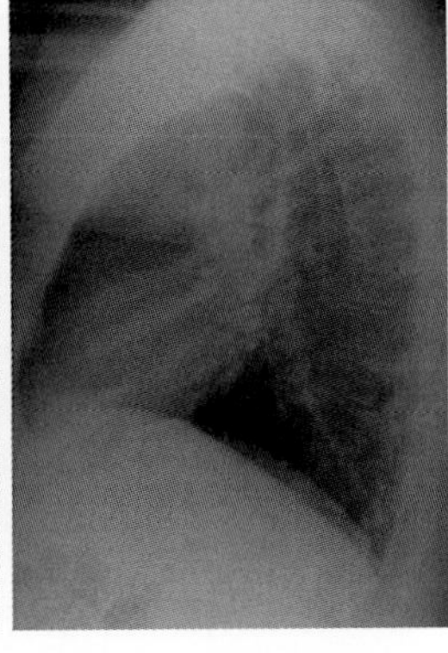

• **Fig. 4.9** Posteroanterior and lateral chest x-ray for patient in Question 24.

C. Hydroxychloroquine (Plaquenil) 200 mg PO twice daily
D. Methotrexate 15 mg PO once per week
E. No therapy

25. A 72-year-old man with COPD and severe chronic airflow obstruction presents to the emergency department with shortness of breath, productive cough, and wheezing. His medications at home include tiotropium, fluticasone-salmeterol combination, albuterol by metered-dose inhaler, aspirin (for primary prevention of cardiovascular events), and lisinopril for hypertension. His chest x-ray is normal; oxygen saturation on 6 L/min oxygen by nasal prongs is 90%. Despite frequent nebulized bronchodilators and systemic steroids, he has worsening respiratory distress and hypoxemia and is intubated and begun on mechanical ventilation. Ventilator settings are as follows: volume-cycled ventilation in assist-control mode at 18 breaths per minute, 600 mL/breath, with positive end-expiratory pressure at 5 cm H_2O and 40% inspired oxygen. After approximately 30 minutes, he develops new-onset ventricular arrhythmias. He remains afebrile and normotensive. Arterial blood gases reveal the following: Po_2 195 mm Hg, Pco_2 36 mm Hg, pH 7.56, and measured bicarbonate 30 mEq/L.

Which of the following is a potential cause of his arrhythmia?

A. Sudden reversal of chronic hypoxemia (acute hyperoxia)
B. Acute metabolic alkalemia due to "unmasking" of compensatory chronic metabolic alkalosis
C. Auto-PEEP with high intrathoracic pressures and inadequate minute ventilation
D. Acute-on-chronic respiratory acidosis due to refractory exacerbation of COPD
E. Hypochloremic, hypokalemic metabolic alkalosis induced by combination of beta-agonists and corticosteroids

26. A 67-year-old man presents to the emergency department with fever and cough. Chest x-ray demonstrates a dense right lower lobe consolidation, and he is started on antibiotics. While awaiting admission to the medical floor, he becomes hypotensive and is unresponsive to several liters of intravenous fluid. A central line is placed.

Which of the following statements is true regarding the choice of norepinephrine versus dopamine as treatment for his hypotension?

A. Dopamine is more likely to protect renal function.
B. Dopamine is more likely to cause cardiac arrhythmias.
C. Norepinephrine results in more overall adverse events.
D. Norepinephrine results in higher mortality in cardiogenic shock.
E. Evidence for comparison of these vasopressors is limited by lack of randomized control trials.

27. A 45-year-old man is admitted with severe bilateral pneumonia. He is intubated and placed on assist-control ventilation with low tidal volumes, but the fraction of inspired oxygen (Fio_2) cannot be decreased below 0.9 despite optimal PEEP.

Paralysis for 48 hours in this setting is most likely to result in which of the following?

A. An increase in neuromuscular weakness
B. A reduction in mortality
C. An increase in lung injury
D. A decrease in sedation requirements
E. An increase in organ failure

28. A 65-year-old man with no significant past medical history is admitted with septic shock due to a left lower lobe pneumonia. He rapidly decompensates and requires vasopressors and intubation. A chest x-ray following intubation demonstrates diffuse bilateral airspace opacities. His oxygen saturation is 95% with a Pao_2 of 75 mm Hg on an Fio_2 of 1.0 and PEEP of 7.5 cm H_2O. He is 5 feet, 8 inches tall and weighs 100 kg, with a predicted body weight of 68.4 kg.

Which of the following mandatory (assist-control) ventilator modes would be best for managing this patient's condition?

A. Volume targeted, tidal volume 800 mL
B. Volume targeted, tidal volume 700 mL
C. Volume targeted, tidal volume 650 mL
D. Volume targeted, tidal volume 410 mL
E. Pressure targeted, peak pressure 25 cm H_2O

29. An 87-year-old woman with severe COPD remains in respiratory distress despite noninvasive ventilation. Preparations are made to proceed with rapid-sequence intubation using propofol and succinylcholine.

Which of the following conditions is a potential contraindication to these medications?

A. Neuroleptic malignant syndrome
B. Chronic corticosteroid use
C. Hypernatremia
D. Hypertension
E. Hyperkalemia

30. A 45-year-old man is admitted to the ICU with severe pancreatitis. Over the first 24 hours he develops hypotension requiring vasopressors, respiratory failure requiring intubation, and renal failure. Over the last several hours, his urine output has decreased, his vasopressor requirement has increased, and his abdomen has become progressively distended.

Which of the following is the best next step in his management?

A. Abdominal CT
B. Empiric antibiotics
C. Abdominal ultrasound
D. Measurement of bladder pressure
E. Abdominal plain film

31. A 39-year-old woman with depression is admitted after being found intoxicated next to an empty bottle of acetaminophen. Her laboratory results are notable for an alanine aminotransferase (ALT) of 55 U/L and an aspartate aminotransferase (AST) of 34 U/L. Serum and urine drug screens are pending.

Which of the following is the best next step in her management?

A. Toxicology screen before providing further therapy
B. Sodium bicarbonate
C. Activated charcoal
D. *N*-acetylcysteine
E. Gastric lavage

32. A 76-year-old woman with severe COPD is admitted with 2 days of dyspnea and cough. She is alert, in moderate respiratory distress, and has an oxygen saturation of 93% on 3 L/min supplemental oxygen delivered by nasal cannulae. A chest x-ray demonstrates no abnormal pulmonary opacities. She receives intensive bronchodilator therapy and systemic steroids. Arterial blood gases demonstrate pH 7.27, Pco_2 66 mm Hg, and Pao_2 74 mm Hg.

Which of the following is the best next step in her care?

A. Increase supplemental oxygen
B. Intubation and mechanical ventilation
C. Noninvasive ventilation
D. Decrease supplemental oxygen
E. Initiate antibiotics

33. A 78-year-old man with severe Parkinson disease was admitted 3 days ago with an aspiration pneumonia and required intubation for respiratory failure. His fevers have resolved and his oxygenation has improved. His current ventilator settings are volume-cycled ventilation, assist-control mode, tidal volume 400 mL, PEEP 5 cm H_2O, and Fio_2 0.4. His oxygen saturation is 95%.

Which of the following is the best next step in care?

A. Extubation
B. Spontaneous breathing trial
C. Pressure support weaning
D. Decrease PEEP and Fio_2
E. Synchronized intermittent mandatory ventilation (SIMV)

34. A 55-year-old woman is admitted with severe sepsis and renal failure. Her hemodynamics improve, and she is weaned off vasopressors. Her fever and leukocytosis also resolve. However, she remains oliguric, and her creatinine continues to rise.

Which of the following statements about renal replacement therapy in this setting is most accurate?

A. Continuous renal replacement therapy (CRRT) does not have a mortality benefit compared with intermittent hemodialysis (IHD).
B. High-intensity renal replacement therapy (either CRRT or IHD) has consistently been demonstrated to improve mortality.

C. CRRT reduces mortality, but only in patients on vasopressors.
D. CRRT reduces mortality, but only in patients on mechanical ventilation.
E. IHD is contraindicated in patients on vasopressors.

35. A 45-year-old obese woman with Crohn disease complicated by multiple flares is admitted with fever, abdominal pain, diarrhea, and hypotension. In the emergency department, she receives 2.5 L of intravenous fluid, but her systolic blood pressure remains in the range of 70 mm Hg, and a central venous catheter is placed. Her central venous pressure (CVP) is 6 mm Hg with significant respiratory variation. Vasopressors are initiated, and her mean arterial pressure is currently 55 mm Hg. Laboratory values are notable for a leukocytosis and a hematocrit of 27%; her albumin is 2.8 g/dL.

Which of the following is the best next step in management?
A. Increase vasopressor dose
B. Intravenous crystalloid drip, at a rate of 200 mL/h
C. Intravenous administration of colloid
D. Red blood cell transfusion
E. Intravenous crystalloid bolus

36. An 85-year-old woman is admitted to the ICU with chest pain, new onset of atrial fibrillation, and an exacerbation of her chronic congestive heart failure (CHF). After several days, she starts to improve. Heparin was initiated at admission, and she has recently started transitioning to warfarin. Starting on the fifth hospital day, her platelets decrease to 100,000/μL from 220,000/μL on admission. She is now noted to have new right lower extremity pain and edema.

In addition to discontinuing heparin, which of the following is the next best step?
A. Await results of lower extremity ultrasound
B. Initiate argatroban
C. Initiate low-molecular-weight heparin
D. Continue transition to warfarin
E. Await results of platelet factor 4 (PF4) antibody

37. An 85-year-old woman is admitted to the ICU after having a stroke. She is intubated for altered mental status and inability to protect her airway.

Which of the following interventions could increase her risk of ventilator-associated pneumonia?
A. Elevation of the head of the bed to 30 degrees
B. Oropharyngeal decontamination
C. Gastrointestinal decontamination
D. Continuous drainage of subglottic secretions
E. Stress ulcer prophylaxis

38. A 52-year-old man with coronary artery disease is admitted with hematemesis. He is intubated, and an esophagogastroduodenoscopy (EGD) demonstrates a bleeding gastric ulcer. Over the next 48 hours his condition stabilizes, and a repeat EGD demonstrates no further bleeding. His ICU course is complicated by delirium and pneumonia presumed to be due to aspiration. His hemoglobin stabilizes at 7.5 g/dL.

Which of the following is the most accurate statement about the role of red blood cell transfusion?
A. Transfusion is indicated due to concomitant coronary artery disease.
B. Transfusion is indicated due to his recent gastrointestinal bleed.
C. Transfusion is associated with fewer ventilator-dependent days.
D. Transfusion may be associated with an increase in mortality.
E. Transfusion may result in hypokalemia.

39. A 75-year-old man is admitted for pneumonia and sepsis. He requires vasopressors and is intubated for respiratory failure. He is placed on midazolam and fentanyl. He is treated with ceftriaxone and azithromycin for severe community-acquired pneumonia and continued on his outpatient aspirin, atorvastatin, and sertraline. Over the course of the next 18 hours, he is weaned off of vasopressors, and his white blood cell count improves; however, he is noted to become increasingly agitated. Additional midazolam and fentanyl are given, and he also receives haloperidol for presumed delirium. His vital signs are notable for a new fever to 103°F, heart rate 120 beats per minute, and blood pressure 100/60 mm Hg. His examination is notable for dry mucous membranes, increased muscle tone, and tremor and hyperreflexia with clonus, particularly in his lower extremities. His pupils are dilated with oscillatory eye movements.

Which of the following is the next best step?
A. Discontinue sertraline
B. Discontinue sertraline and fentanyl
C. Initiate propofol
D. Discontinue haloperidol
E. Add vancomycin

40. A 45-year-old man has a witnessed cardiac arrest in a shopping mall. Bystander cardiopulmonary resuscitation is initiated. An automated external defibrillator is applied. It advises a shock, which is delivered, but there is no return of spontaneous circulation. Paramedics arrive, and after two doses of epinephrine and additional shocks are given according to advanced cardiac life support (ACLS) protocol, the patient regains a pulse. When he arrives in the emergency department, he is tachycardic but normotensive. He withdraws to painful stimuli but is otherwise unresponsive. Laboratory data are notable for a white blood cell count of 18,000/μL, lactate 8 mEq/L, potassium 5.8 mEq/L, bicarbonate 18 mEq/L, and creatinine 1.5 mg/dL.

Which of the following is the most accurate statement about therapeutic hypothermia in this setting?
A. Therapeutic hypothermia is contraindicated due to risk of infection.

B. Therapeutic hypothermia is contraindicated due to hyperkalemia.
C. Therapeutic hypothermia results in increased frequency of malignant arrhythmias.
D. Therapeutic hypothermia should be initiated after reassessment of neurologic status at 12 hours.
E. Therapeutic hypothermia should be continued for 24 hours.

41. A 45-year-old man is intubated for a severe asthma exacerbation. His chest x-ray demonstrates only hyperinflation. His initial ventilator settings are volume-targeted, assist-control mode ventilation; tidal volume 450 mL (7 mL/kg of ideal body weight); set rate 28 breaths per minute; PEEP 5 cm H_2O; and Fio_2 0.5. The patient is not triggering additional breaths and appears synchronous with the ventilator, and he has a measured end-expiratory pressure of 15 cm H_2O with a peak inspiratory pressure of 45 cm H_2O. His blood pressure is 89/55 mm Hg. His arterial blood gases reveal the following: pH 7.38, Pco_2 40 mm Hg, and Po_2 120 mm Hg.

Which of the following ventilator changes would you recommend?
A. No change
B. Increase PEEP
C. Decrease respiratory rate
D. Increase respiratory rate
E. Increase inspiratory-to-expiratory time (I:E) ratio

42. An 84-year-old man is intubated for aspiration pneumonia.

Which of the following interventions is most likely to be associated with an increased duration of mechanical ventilation?
A. Daily interruption of sedation
B. Daily spontaneous breathing trials
C. Use of midazolam instead of propofol
D. Use of dexmedetomidine instead of midazolam
E. Avoidance of routine sedative medication

43. A 55-year-old man is admitted with altered mental status. He has a history of heavy alcohol abuse. In the emergency department, his vital signs are notable for tachycardia to 110 beats per minute but are otherwise normal. Laboratory values include the following: serum sodium 145 mEq/L, potassium 4 mEq/L, chloride 105 mEq/L, bicarbonate 15 mEq/L, BUN 25 mg/dL, glucose 150 mg/dL, and creatinine 1.5 mg/dL. Urinalysis demonstrates no ketones but is noted to have needle-shaped crystals. His serum alcohol level is 10 mg/dL, and his serum osmolarity is 325 mOsm/kg.

Which of the following is the most appropriate next step in his treatment?
A. Ethanol
B. Benzodiazepines
C. Fomepizole
D. Hemodialysis
E. Bicarbonate

44. A 65-year-old man is admitted with several days of progressive weakness, dyspnea, and cough. His temperature is 99°F, blood pressure is 82/58 mm Hg, heart rate is 105 beats per minute, and respiratory rate is 22 breaths per minute. His oxygen saturation is 93% on supplemental oxygen at 2 L/min delivered by nasal cannulae. Laboratory values demonstrate an elevated white blood cell count; asymmetric bilateral lower lobe opacities are demonstrated on his chest x-ray. He is given intravenous fluids and antibiotics for pneumonia. Over the course of the next several hours, his hypotension worsens. Blood lactate is elevated, and his extremities are cool. A central venous catheter is placed for initiation of vasopressors. His central venous pressure is 14 cm H_2O, and a blood gas drawn from this catheter reveals an oxygen saturation of 40%.

Which of the following is the best interpretation of his hemodynamics?
A. Distributive shock due to sepsis
B. Distributive shock due to underlying liver disease
C. Hypovolemic shock due to sepsis
D. Hemorrhagic shock
E. Cardiogenic shock

45. A 55-year-old man is scheduled to undergo an esophagogastroduodenoscopy for Barrett esophagus. His vital signs, including oxygen saturation, are normal. He receives topical anesthesia with benzocaine, and conscious sedation is achieved using midazolam and fentanyl. Shortly after the procedure begins, his oxygen saturation drops to the mid-80% range. Other vital signs have not changed. He is placed on supplemental oxygen, but his oxygen saturation does not improve. Chest examination demonstrates clear lung fields.

Which of the following is the next best diagnostic step?
A. Chest x-ray
B. Chest CT angiography
C. Arterial blood gas with cooximetry
D. Arterial blood gas
E. Electrocardiogram

46. A 75-year-old man with severe chronic obstructive pulmonary disease is intubated for an exacerbation of his lung disease. His initial ventilator settings are volume-cycled ventilation in assist-control mode, tidal volume 500 mL (8 mL/kg), PEEP 5 cm H_2O, and Fio_2 0.5. His initial peak inspiratory pressures are 18 cm H_2O. Several hours after intubation, his ventilator alarms indicate increased peak inflation pressures. His new peak inspiratory pressure is 35 cm H_2O. His plateau pressure is 15 cm H_2O.

Which of the following is the next best step in management?
A. Obtain a chest x-ray
B. Needle decompression
C. Endotracheal suctioning
D. Chest tube placement
E. Diuresis

47. A 27-year-old woman with epilepsy and a history of poor adherence to therapy is admitted to the hospital after a tonic-clonic seizure. Shortly after admission, she has two more seizures. She is given lorazepam and intubated. She is afebrile and normotensive; head CT scan and serum chemistries, including blood glucose, are all within normal limits.

Which of the following statements about her management is most accurate?

A. Infusion with phenytoin should be the initial treatment.
B. Fosphenytoin is preferred over phenytoin because of a decreased risk of hypotension.
C. Diazepam has a slower onset of action than lorazepam.
D. Lorazepam infusion followed by fosphenytoin is a reasonable treatment.
E. Propofol is ineffective for this condition.

48. A 67-year-old patient with COPD and coronary disease is admitted to the hospital for pneumonia. During the evening of his admission, his tachypnea worsens, and he is placed on increased supplemental oxygen. Several hours later, he becomes hypotensive and more lethargic. He is found soon thereafter without a pulse. The cardiac arrest team is called.

Which of the following statements about his resuscitation is most accurate?

A. Inadequate bag-and-mask ventilation is a common cause of failure to recover from an arrest not due to ventricular tachycardia or ventricular fibrillation.
B. A rapid response team would not have reduced the likelihood of cardiac arrest.
C. A pulse check should be performed immediately after administration of medications.
D. A pulse check should be performed immediately after defibrillation.
E. End-tidal CO_2 detection may help determine the quality of cardiopulmonary resuscitation (CPR) and return of spontaneous circulation.

49. A 75-year-old man is admitted with right lower lobe opacities and septic shock. He is treated with broad-spectrum antibiotics. His condition worsens over the first 24 hours. His initial infiltrate progresses to become bilateral, and he requires intubation. His shock worsens to the point of requiring two vasopressors despite adequate fluid resuscitation.

Which of the following is the most accurate statement about administration of corticosteroids in this patient?

A. Corticosteroids improve mortality in patients who have a low response to adrenocorticotropic hormone (ACTH) stimulation.
B. Corticosteroids improve mortality in patients who have inappropriately normal serum cortisol.
C. Corticosteroids will likely improve his response to vasopressors.
D. Corticosteroids, if initiated for his ARDS, will be of greater benefit if initiated after 14 days.
E. High-dose corticosteroids demonstrate mortality benefit in sepsis but have an unacceptable rate of complications.

50. An 85-year-old man with hypertension, coronary artery disease, and chronic kidney disease is admitted after an overdose of verapamil. His initial blood pressure is 130/80 mm Hg with a pulse of 75 beats per minute. His mental status is normal, and his serum chemistries and complete blood count are unchanged from baseline. His electrocardiogram shows a prolonged PR interval. He is given activated charcoal and intravenous calcium and is admitted to the ICU. Over the next several hours, he develops bradycardia and hypotension. He is given additional calcium, atropine, and glucagon with some transient improvement. However, his bradycardia and hypotension continue to worsen, and he requires intubation and escalating doses of vasopressors.

Which of the following therapies should be initiated?

A. Hemodialysis
B. Bicarbonate infusion
C. Physostigmine
D. Intravenous corticosteroids
E. High-dose insulin therapy

Chapter 4 Answers

1. ANSWER: D. Respiratory failure and death

In the Salmeterol Multicenter Asthma Research Trial (SMART), approximately 26,000 patients were randomly assigned to receive either inhaled salmeterol or placebo for 6 months, added to their "usual care." Study outcomes included deaths and near-deaths (respiratory failure requiring admission to an intensive care unit) resulting from asthma. Although these events were rare, they occurred more commonly in the group randomized to receive salmeterol than in a placebo group. Episodes of respiratory failure occurred 37 times in the salmeterol-treated group versus 22 times in the placebo-treated group; deaths resulting from asthma occurred 13 times in the salmeterol-treated group versus 3 times in the placebo-treated group (both differences were statistically significant). The explanation for these adverse outcomes remains uncertain. The possibility that this effect would be eliminated if all patients used an inhaled corticosteroid at the same time that they received a long-acting beta-agonist bronchodilator or placebo is currently being investigated. The SMART study of adverse outcomes related to salmeterol revealed no increase in serious atrial or ventricular arrhythmias (Answers

A and B), cardiovascular events (heart attacks or strokes) (Answer C), or drug-induced allergic events (angioedema or anaphylaxis) (Answer E). Of note, the increased mortality found with use of long-acting beta agonists alone has not been found in studies comparing long-acting beta agonist/inhaled steroid combination inhalers with inhaled steroids alone.

Nelson HS, Weiss ST, Bleecker ER, et al. The Salmeterol Multicenter Asthma Research Trial: a comparison of usual pharmacotherapy for asthma or usual pharmacotherapy plus salmeterol. [Published erratum appears in *Chest.* 2006;129(5):1393.] *Chest.* 2006;129(1):15–26.

Stempel DA, Raphiou IH, Kral KM, et al. Serious asthma events with fluticasone plus salmeterol versus fluticasone alone. *N Engl J Med.* 2016;374(19):1822–1830.

2. **ANSWER: A. FEV_1 2.0 L (66% of predicted), FVC 4.0 L (100% of predicted), FEV_1/FVC 0.5 (66% of predicted)**

Let us offer a simple strategy for interpreting spirometry results. After you have checked to see if the test has been properly performed, with a smooth graphic display (volume–time plot) and at least 6 seconds of forced expiratory time, look at the FEV_1/FVC ratio. If this ratio is reduced (as in example A), there is an obstructive pattern. A reduced ratio is typically defined as a value below the 95% confidence interval (not given in these examples). The Global Initiative for Chronic Obstructive Lung Disease (GOLD) guidelines attempt to simplify this definition by using a cutoff for a reduced ratio of <0.7. This cutoff is generally accurate except for all but the oldest of patients, in whom an FEV_1/FVC ratio <0.7 may still be normal. (The FEV_1/FVC ratio declines with age because of loss of lung elastic recoil during the normal aging process.) If the FEV_1/FVC ratio is normal or increased, there is no obstruction.

Having established the presence of airflow obstruction based on a reduced FEV_1/FVC ratio, one can judge the severity of the obstruction by looking at the FEV_1 expressed as a percentage of normal. By widely accepted convention, in this context, an FEV_1 80%–99% of normal indicates mild obstruction; 50%–79% of normal indicates moderate obstruction; 35%–49% of normal indicates severe obstruction; and <35% of normal indicates very severe obstruction. The patient in example A has moderate airflow obstruction. The degree to which the FEV_1 is reduced (in the absence of an acute exacerbation) correlates directly with disease morbidity and mortality in chronic obstructive pulmonary disease (COPD).

The pattern in Answer B suggests severe restriction; Answer C shows normal spirometry; and in Answer D, the results suggest a pattern of moderate restriction. Restriction is confirmed with full measurement of lung volumes, including total lung capacity, functional residual capacity, and residual volume, as measured by the helium dilution technique or plethysmography. Obstructive lung disease would be expected in a patient with a long smoking history and evidence of airflow obstruction on examination.

Vestbo J, Hurd SS, Agustí AG, et al. Global strategy for the diagnosis, management, and prevention of chronic obstructive pulmonary disease: GOLD executive summary. *Am J Respir Crit Care Med.* 2013;187(4):347–365.

3. **ANSWER: A. The diagnosis is established by a blood test.**

The presence of widespread (panlobular) emphysema in a nonsmoker should raise the possibility of alpha-1 antitrypsin deficiency; other suggestive findings include COPD that develops in a cigarette smoker at an unusually young age (e.g., before age 50) or a strong family history of emphysema. However, many patients with homozygous alpha-1 antitrypsin deficiency do not have these "classic" characteristics, and some experts recommend widespread testing for alpha-1 antitrypsin deficiency among patients with COPD. Testing for alpha-1 antitrypsin begins with measurement of serum alpha-1 antitrypsin level, a routine blood test done in the chemistry laboratory. Patients who are homozygous for alpha-1 antitrypsin deficiency will have a very low blood level of the protein, on the order of 15% of normal. This finding reflects the fact that most patients with alpha-1 antitrypsin deficiency make an alpha-1 antitrypsin protein that is transported ineffectively out of the liver, rather than making no alpha-1 antitrypsin protein (the homozygous null/null genotype is rare). Further testing of the patient with a very low serum alpha-1 antitrypsin level can be performed by protein electrophoresis or genetic analysis to determine the specific genetic abnormality.

Patients with heterozygous alpha-1 antitrypsin abnormality will have low serum alpha-1 antitrypsin levels (often on the order of approximately 50% of normal). There is controversy regarding whether heterozygous persons are at a modest increased risk for developing COPD. In any case, a blood level less than the lower limits of normal does not establish homozygous deficiency (Answer B). It is estimated that as many as 30% of nonsmoking persons with alpha-1 antitrypsin deficiency will never develop obstructive lung disease (Answer C). The percentage of adult patients with alpha-1 antitrypsin deficiency who develop clinical evidence of liver disease (specifically those with ZZ phenotype and other forms in which abnormal protein accumulates in the liver) is estimated to be approximately 20% and varies with age (Answer D). Emphysema due to alpha-1 antitrypsin deficiency, such as emphysema due to smoking in persons with a normal alpha-1 antitrypsin level, is associated with a reduced diffusing capacity of the lung for carbon monoxide due to impaired transfer of carbon monoxide across decreased alveolar-capillary membrane surface area (Answer E).

Stoller JK, Aboussouan LS. A review of α1-antitrypsin deficiency. *Am J Respir Crit Care Med.* 2012;185(3):246–259.

4. ANSWER: D. "Given your history, a leukotriene modifier such as montelukast, zafirlukast, or zileuton might be particularly helpful as treatment for your asthma."

Aspirin-sensitive asthma (also called *aspirin-intolerant asthma* and, most recently, *aspirin-exacerbated respiratory disease*) occurs in approximately 3%–5% of adults with asthma. It is exceedingly rare in children and does not have a familial predisposition. Although the precise biochemical abnormality leading to asthmatic exacerbations after aspirin ingestion is unknown, it involves some aspect of the cyclooxygenase pathway, and specifically cyclooxygenase-1. Thus any cyclooxygenase-1 inhibitor, including ibuprofen, naproxen, and other nonsteroidal antiinflammatory drugs (NSAIDs), can precipitate an attack and need to be avoided (Answer B). Acetaminophen and specific cyclooxygenase-2 inhibitors (e.g., celecoxib) have weak cyclooxygenase-1 inhibition and are safe to use in most patients. The dose of aspirin that triggers an asthmatic reaction varies among aspirin-sensitive asthmatics, but some patients will respond to 81 mg or less (Answer A).

A feature of patients with aspirin-sensitive asthma is that they synthesize more than the normal amount of cysteinyl leukotrienes at baseline and markedly excess amounts after ingestion of aspirin or other cyclooxygenase-1 inhibitors. As a result, it is logical to try antileukotriene therapy (either a leukotriene receptor antagonist or lipoxygenase inhibitor) to treat their asthma (but not to make aspirin or other NSAID ingestion safe) (Answer D). The reaction to aspirin/NSAIDs is not IgE mediated and is not associated with IgE-mediated allergic reactions, such as food allergy to nuts (Answer C). Aspirin sensitivity is not associated with an increased risk of adverse reactions to beta-agonist bronchodilators (Answer E).

5. ANSWER: B. Stage 1C

The latest GOLD classification of COPD uses severity of FEV_1 impairment, number of exacerbations, and dyspnea scores to classify patients.

Group A: Mild (GOLD 1, FEV_1 >80% predicted) to moderate (GOLD 2, FEV_1 50%–80% predicted) airflow limitation, 0 to 1 exacerbation per year, and low scores on dyspnea scales (either CAT or mMRC scales).

Group B: Mild or moderate airflow limitation, 0 to 1 exacerbation per year, but higher scores on dyspnea scales.

Group C: Severe (GOLD 3, FEV_1 <50% predicted) or very severe (GOLD 4, <30% predicted) airflow limitation or >2 exacerbations per year or one hospitalization, with low dyspnea scale scores.

Group D: Severe or very severe airflow limitation, >2 exacerbations per year or one hospitalization, plus high dyspnea scale scores.

Based on his exacerbation history, this patient would fall into GOLD stage 1C.

Vestbo J, Hurd SS, Agustí AG, et al. Global strategy for the diagnosis, management, and prevention of chronic obstructive pulmonary disease: GOLD executive summary. *Am J Respir Crit Care Med.* 2013;187(4):347–365.

6. ANSWER: B. Chest tube drainage of pleural space, with thoracoscopic lysis of pleural adhesions if necessary

The clinical scenario of fever, productive cough, chest pain, and leukocytosis is consistent with an acute pneumonia and parapneumonic effusion. The effusion is moderate to large and appears to be loculated, based on difficulty aspirating more than 60 mL of fluid during thoracentesis. The pleural fluid is serous without frank pus or bacteria in the pleural space; that is, there is no evidence of an empyema. In this context, the pleural fluid pH is helpful. The "normal" pleural fluid pH is >7.4. A value of 7.2 or less indicates a "complicated" parapneumonic effusion, one that is likely to behave like an empyema, with formation of adhesions and difficulty clearing the infection without drainage of the pleural space. Together with the rest of the clinical picture, the need for chest tube drainage of the pleural space and possibly surgical lysis of adhesions and decortication of the pleura are indicated. It is thought that in this setting the low pleural fluid pH is caused by anaerobic metabolism of glucose by infection (not found in the sampled fluid) and inflammation in the pleural space, leading to generation of carbon dioxide and lactate.

Like managing an empyema, antibiotics alone without pleural drainage will have a low likelihood of success (Answer A). Pleural biopsy might be considered if malignancy or tuberculosis were high in the differential diagnosis, which they are not (Answer C). A history of recurrent vomiting or recent upper endoscopy with severe retrosternal or upper abdominal pain might suggest esophageal rupture with spillage of gastric fluid into the pleural space. A high pleural fluid amylase is typical of this syndrome (Answer D). A low pleural fluid pH may be seen in pleural effusions due to collagen vascular disease, especially in rheumatoid effusions, but the clinical history does not support this diagnosis (Answer E).

7. ANSWER: A. Lymphangioleiomyomatosis (LAM)

Chylothorax is typically milky in appearance (white to beige in color) and (in the absence of cirrhosis) has a high triglyceride concentration (>110 mg/dL). The diagnosis of chylothorax can be confirmed by identification of chylomicrons in the pleural fluid on lipoprotein electrophoresis. Chylothorax results from disruption of the flow of chyle from the small intestines through the thoracic duct into the left brachiocephalic vein. Causes of thoracic duct obstruction or rupture include the proliferation of tumor-like smooth muscle cells in LAM; malignancy such as lymphoma; radiation fibrosis; and direct surgical trauma. The other choices above—parapneumonic effusion (Answer B), malignant effusion

(Answer C), pulmonary infarction (Answer D), and sarcoidosis (Answer E)—typically cause an exudative pleural effusion with low lipid content.

8. **ANSWER: C. Idiopathic pulmonary fibrosis**

This patient presents with a typical history for chronic interstitial lung disease. He has progressive dyspnea, a nonproductive cough, crackles on chest examination, and restriction on pulmonary function testing. His chest x-ray is confirmatory, with bilateral linear and nodular opacities, the radiographic correlate of an interstitial process. The chest CT scan shows a pattern that is suggestive of the pathologic process called *usual interstitial pneumonitis* (UIP). In particular, there are dense bands of opacity suggesting fibrosis with associated traction bronchiectasis (bronchial walls pulled apart by the retraction of scar formation) and honeycombing (dilated alveolar spaces, likewise enlarged by the retractive forces from surrounding scar formation). The peripheral and basilar predominance are consistent with UIP.

Potential causes of this pathologic process include collagen vascular diseases, pneumoconioses, and medications such as bleomycin and nitrofurantoin. In the absence of an identifiable cause or association, the diagnosis is idiopathic pulmonary fibrosis (IPF). Of note, clubbing is found in as many as 50% of patients with IPF. In this case example, bronchoscopy was performed to exclude a potential infectious etiology, with results that were nonspecific, consistent with but not diagnostic of UIP.

Neither the radiographic findings nor the transbronchial lung biopsy results were suggestive of alternative diagnoses. Sarcoidosis (Answer A) is typically bronchocentric in location, generally with an upper lobe predominance, and often associated with hilar and mediastinal lymphadenopathy. Transbronchial lung biopsy will often reveal noncaseating granulomas. Like IPF, nonspecific interstitial pneumonia (Answer B) is an idiopathic chronic inflammatory lung disease. It usually presents with areas of ground-class opacities on a chest CT scan (Fig. 4.10), and transbronchial lung biopsy findings are often nonspecific, as in this case.

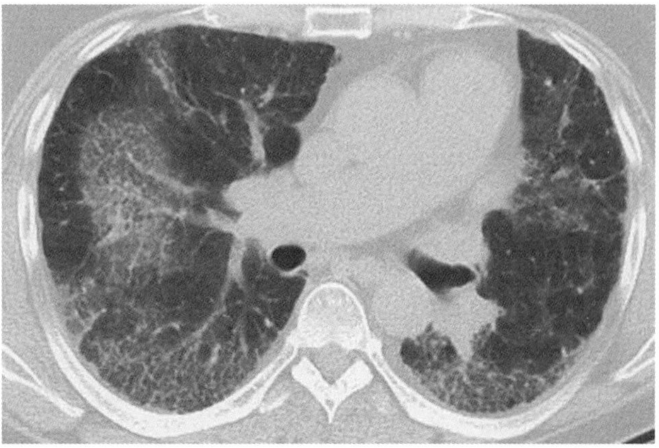

• **Fig. 4.10** Ground-class opacities on chest CT scan (Answer 8).

Cryptogenic organizing pneumonia (Answer D), also referred to as *bronchiolitis obliterans organizing pneumonia* (BOOP), mimics infectious pneumonia, with areas of consolidation on chest imaging. Transbronchial lung biopsy may identify areas of organizing pneumonia and occasionally the endobronchiolar polypoid tissue of bronchiolitis obliterans. Finally, Langerhans cell histiocytosis (Answer E) presents with cystic lung disease and associated small lung nodules; on immunohistochemical staining of bronchoalveolar lavage fluid, one may be able to identify the characteristic Langerhans cells.

9. **ANSWER: A. Normal oxygen saturation at rest that falls to 82% with exertion**

Characteristic of the interstitial lung diseases is oxygen desaturation with exercise. The alveolar-to-arterial gradient for oxygen widens with exertion for two reasons. In part, there is likely worsened ventilation/perfusion mismatching when minute ventilation and cardiac output increase. In part, diffusion impairment is made manifest when cardiac output increases, circulation time decreases, and the transit time for red blood cells in alveolar capillaries shortens, limiting the amount of oxygen that can diffuse across thickened alveolar-capillary membranes. In the patient with idiopathic pulmonary fibrosis or asbestosis, as described in this case, one might find a normal oxygen saturation at rest, but oxygen saturation characteristically decreases with exertion (Answer A). In IPF and other diffuse interstitial lung diseases, the diffusion capacity of the lung for carbon monoxide (DLCO) is decreased; lungs are stiffer than normal and so exhibit reduced lung compliance (a measure of the change in lung volume for any change in transpulmonary pressure); and lung volumes are reduced, characteristic of restrictive pulmonary processes

10. **ANSWER: E. Pirfenidone**

Recent studies suggest that both pirfenidone, an antifibrotic agent, and nintedanib, a tyrosine kinase inhibitor, may slow disease progression in IPF. Supplemental oxygen should be given to chronically hypoxemic patients, and some patients may be eligible for lung transplant.

High-dose steroids (Answer A) are often used as a "therapeutic trial" to treat chronic idiopathic inflammatory lung disease when the diagnosis is uncertain. However, there is no role for high-dose systemic steroids when the diagnosis of idiopathic pulmonary fibrosis has been established. A randomized, controlled clinical trial of high-dose steroids, azathioprine, and *N*-acetylcysteine (Answer B) versus placebo in patients with idiopathic pulmonary fibrosis, referred to as the PANTHER-IPF trial, was terminated early when it was found that mortality was greater in the group randomized to receive steroids, azathioprine, and *N*-acetylcysteine than in the placebo group. Rituximab (Answer C), a monoclonal antibody directed at the CD20 protein found on the surface of B cells, is used to treat granulomatosis with polyangiitis (Wegener granulomatosis) and may be effective in interstitial lung disease associated with rheumatoid arthritis; it is not known to be effective in the treatment of idiopathic pulmonary fibrosis. Hydroxychloroquine (Answer D) is used to treat collagen vascular disease, especially rheumatoid arthritis, but it is not a therapy for chronic inflammatory lung disease.

Idiopathic Pulmonary Fibrosis Clinical Research Network. Prednisone, azathioprine, and N-acetylcysteine for pulmonary fibrosis. *N Engl J Med.* 2012;366(21):1968–1977.

King Jr TE, Bradford WZ, Castro-Bernardini S, et al. A phase 3 trial of pirfenidone in patients with idiopathic pulmonary fibrosis. [Published erratum appears in *N Engl J Med.* 2014; 371(12):1172.] *N Engl J Med.* 2014;370(22):2083–2092.

Richeldi L, du Bois RM, Raghu G, et al. Efficacy and safety of nintedanib in idiopathic pulmonary fibrosis. [Published erratum appears in *N Engl J Med.* 2015;373(8):782.] *N Engl J Med.* 2014;370(22):2071–2082.

11. ANSWER: A. Retrognathia

Persons with a narrowed posterior pharyngeal opening are at increased risk for critical narrowing and occlusion of the upper airway during sleep. The posterior pharynx may be narrowed due to a large tongue, posteriorly extending soft palate, large tonsils, or posteriorly positioned jaw and tongue (retrognathia). A large neck circumference (>16 inches in women and >17 inches in men) correlates with excess fatty deposition in the upper airway (Answer B). Nasal obstruction, such as with large nasal polyps (Answer C), can aggravate preexisting obstructive sleep apnea, but it is not a risk factor for the presence of obstructive sleep apnea. Short stature in the absence of obesity is not a risk factor for sleep-disordered breathing (Answer D). Insomnia (Answer E) may be a manifestation of obstructive sleep apnea syndrome, but it is nonspecific and not closely associated with the presence of obstructive sleep apnea.

12. ANSWER: D. Motor vehicle accidents

Persons with obstructive sleep apnea (OSA) have a sevenfold increased risk of being involved in a motor vehicle accident as a consequence of their associated daytime hypersomnolence. Strong epidemiologic evidence indicates that OSA is also an independent risk factor for adverse cardiovascular events. These include heart attacks and strokes as well as heart failure. In addition, OSA is a cause of hypertension, likely as a result of repetitive sympathetic stimulation associated with episodic hypoxemia and sudden awakenings, and evidence indicates that treatment of OSA results in a meaningful lowering of blood pressure. OSA does not increase the risk of aspiration (Answer A), laryngospasm (Answer B), diabetic ketoacidosis (Answer C), or hypoxemic respiratory failure (Answer E).

Gottlieb DJ, Yenokyan G, Newman AB, et al. Prospective study of obstructive sleep apnea and incident coronary heart disease and heart failure: the sleep heart health study. *Circulation.* 2010;122(4):352–360.

Somers VK, White DP, Amin R, et al. Sleep apnea and cardiovascular disease: an American Heart Association/American College of Cardiology Foundation Scientific Statement from the American Heart Association Council for High Blood Pressure Research Professional Education Committee, Council on Clinical Cardiology, Stroke Council, and Council on Cardiovascular Nursing. *J Am Coll Cardiol.* 2008;52(8):686–717.

Tregear S, Reston J, Schoelles K, Phillips B. Obstructive sleep apnea and risk of motor vehicle crash: systematic review and meta-analysis. *J Clin Sleep Med.* 2009;5(6):573–581.

13. ANSWER: C. Relapsing polychondritis

Relapsing polychondritis, the rarest of the collagen vascular diseases listed, is associated with airway disease, including tracheomalacia and subglottic stenosis, but not with diffuse interstitial lung disease. The other choices are all associated with interstitial lung disease. In addition, scleroderma is associated with pulmonary hypertension and with esophageal and sometimes oropharyngeal dysfunction with an increased risk of aspiration pneumonia. Systemic lupus erythematosus can cause pleural effusions, diffuse alveolar hemorrhage, and "shrinking lung syndrome," possibly due to diaphragmatic weakness. Mixed connective tissue disease may also cause pulmonary hypertension.

14. ANSWER: C. Central apneas

The case history is a classic description of obesity hypoventilation syndrome (OHS), previously referred to as *pickwickian syndrome*, defined as the combination of morbid obesity (BMI >30 kg/m^2), P_{CO_2} >45 mm Hg, and sleep-disordered breathing in the absence of other causes of alveolar hypoventilation. This morbidly obese young man has evidence of chronic hypoxemia causing secondary polycythemia, pulmonary hypertension, and cor pulmonale. He also has daytime hypercapnia, which, in the absence of known lung disease, is likely due to central hypoventilation. In some cases of OHS, prolonged obstructive apneas (with associated acute hypercapnia) without adequate compensatory hyperventilation following these apneas can lead to daytime hypercapnia. Continuous positive airway pressure (CPAP) may successfully treat OHS in these instances. In other patients, central apneas persist despite CPAP therapy, reflecting a primary abnormality of ventilatory drive (Answer A).

Orthodeoxia (Answer B) refers to a decrease in arterial oxygenation in the upright position that improves when lying supine; it is the objective manifestation of the symptom of platypnea (dyspnea in the upright position that lessens when supine). Intracardiac right-to-left shunts and intrapulmonary arteriovenous shunts at the lung bases may cause orthodeoxia. Morbid obesity is more likely to cause the opposite positional effects, that is, orthopnea and worsened hypoxemia when supine. Nothing in the history suggests the presence of restless legs syndrome (Answer D), characterized by repetitive readjustment of the positioning of the legs while awake and jerking movements of the legs while asleep. A shortened (rather than prolonged) sleep latency period (Answer E) is a nonspecific marker of sleepiness and is found in many sleep-related disorders, including narcolepsy.

Chau EH, Lam D, Wong J, et al. Obesity hypoventilation syndrome: a review of epidemiology, pathophysiology, and perioperative considerations. *Anesthesiology.* 2012;117(1):188–205.

15. ANSWER: B. Blood gas on room air

Obesity hypoventilation syndrome is marked by daytime hypoventilation and is often associated with nocturnal sleep apnea. The daytime hypoxemia in an obese patient without significant evidence of intrinsic lung disease suggests obesity hypoventilation, which is diagnosed with a room air blood gas showing hypercapnia. A chest x-ray or chest CT might be done, but with a normal pulmonary exam and only mild restriction on pulmonary function tests (likely from body habitus), the yield will be lower. A CBC might show an elevated hemoglobin resulting from chronic hypoxemia, but it cannot confirm the diagnosis. A 6-minute walk test would demonstrate the degree of desaturation with exercise but would again not be diagnostic.

Bilevel positive airway pressure with a mandatory backup respiratory rate applied during sleep in patients with obesity hypoventilation syndrome that fails to improve with CPAP can correct or ameliorate sleep-related hypercapnia and improve daytime gas exchange as well. The latter "spillover" effect may be due to a reduction in the renal compensation for hypercapnia with less blunting of the ventilatory drive by metabolic alkalosis. Daytime hypersomnolence will also improve. Supplemental oxygen will address the hypoxemia and its consequences, but it may worsen the patient's hypoventilation and does not address the underlying disease pathophysiology.

16. Answer: E. Fig. 4.6 Flow–volume loop

The flow–volume loop displays the results of the same maximal forced expiratory maneuver used to generate the spirogram. Instead of displaying the results as a plot of volume versus time as in spirometry, it displays flow (vertical axis) versus volume (horizontal axis). It also typically adds display of flow versus volume during completion of a maximal inspiration performed immediately after maximal exhalation. The expiratory limb of the flow–volume curve is displayed above the horizontal "zero flow" line; the inspiratory limb is displayed below the "zero flow" line; and together they form the flow–volume loop.

Characteristic of the flow–volume curves in asthma and COPD is the scooped, concave appearance of the expiratory curve (Answers C and D), reflecting diffuse intrathoracic airway narrowing. This appearance is seen in all diffuse obstructive lung diseases and is not diagnostic of any specific disease. On the other hand, a large tracheal tumor causing upper airway narrowing results in flow at a single, fixed rate throughout a large portion of exhalation and again during inhalation. The resulting appearance on the flow–volume loop is distinctive: a horizontal portion (referred to as a "plateau" pattern) of the expiratory and inspiratory curves. Although not true of Answer E, often the rate of flow is similar on expiration and inspiration at the midportion of the curves (50% of the vital capacity), unlike in diffuse intrathoracic airflow obstruction, in which inspiratory flow at 50% of the vital capacity typically exceeds expiratory flow (e.g., Fig. 4.11). Normal flow–volume curves (Answer A) or flow–volume curves with a pattern suggesting restriction (Answer B) would not be expected in the presence of a large tracheal tumor.

17. ANSWER: B. Serum immunoglobulin G

Many cases of bronchiectasis are "idiopathic," presumably the result of a prior necrotizing infection that caused irreversible damage to the airway walls. In other instances, however, an underlying predisposition can be identified. Among the potential conditions that may predispose to the development of bronchiectasis are hypogammaglobulinemia and primary ciliary dyskinesia (also called *immotile cilia syndrome*). The former is typically treated with intravenous gamma-globulin replacement therapy, which would be expected to slow the progression of the disease. The latter (primary ciliary dyskinesia), which is diagnosed by electron microscopic examination of nasal or bronchial epithelial tissue and associated ciliary ultrastructure (Answer D), does not have therapeutic options that would alter treatment of flares at this time. Pulmonary vasculitides, such as granulomatosis with polyangiitis

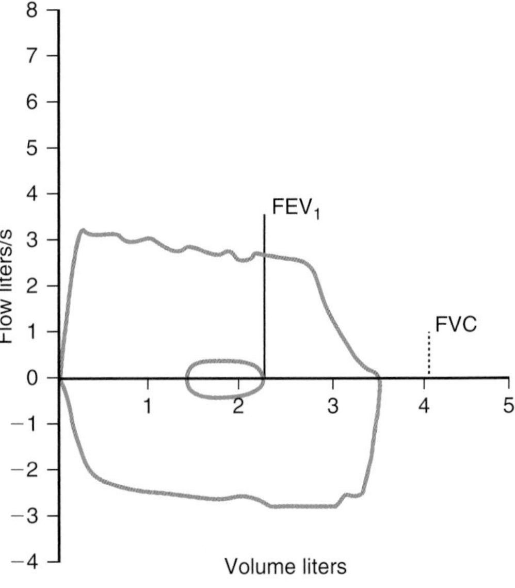

• **Fig. 4.11** Diffuse intrathoracic airflow obstruction (Answer 16).

(Wegener syndrome) or eosinophilic granulomatosis with polyangiitis (Churg-Strauss syndrome), do not typically cause bronchiectasis, making assay for antinuclear cytoplasmic antibodies (ANCA) associated with vasculitis unhelpful (Answer A). Celiac disease (Answer C) is associated with idiopathic pulmonary hemosiderosis (called *Lane-Hamilton disease)* but not bronchiectasis. The etiology of bronchiectasis cannot be discerned by detailed characterization of its physiologic consequences on pulmonary function testing (Answer E).

Knowles MR, Daniels LA, Davis SD, et al. Primary ciliary dyskinesia. Recent advances in diagnostics, genetics, and characterization of clinical disease. *Am J Respir Crit Care Med.* 2013;188(8):913–922.

McShane PJ, Naureckas ET, Tino G, Strek ME. Non-cystic fibrosis bronchiectasis. *Am J Respir Crit Care Med.* 2013;188(6): 647–656.

18. ANSWER: D. Tree-in-bud nodules

The CT image displayed in Question 18 has the following abnormality: small lung nodules (2–3 mm in diameter) grouped around peripheral blood vessels in the lung periphery. The image is suggestive of some trees in early spring, with their buds (the "nodules") sprouting along the distal branches before leaves appear (Fig. 4.12).

Pathologically, the nodules on CT imaging correspond to an inflammatory reaction, often granulomatous, around bronchioles (which run in parallel to peripheral vessels). The nodules are the pathologic correlate of a bronchiolitis or peribronchiolitis, such as may be seen in sarcoidosis, mycobacterial infection, aspiration, and other conditions.

Examples of ground-glass opacity (Answer A) (Fig. 4.13), consolidation with air bronchograms (Answer B) (Fig. 4.14), honeycombing (Answer C) (Fig. 4.15), and atelectasis (Answer E) (Fig. 4.16) are shown, each with a distinctive and very different appearance than "tree-in-bud" nodules.

Eisenhuber E. The tree-in-bud sign. *Radiology.* 2002;222(3): 771–772.

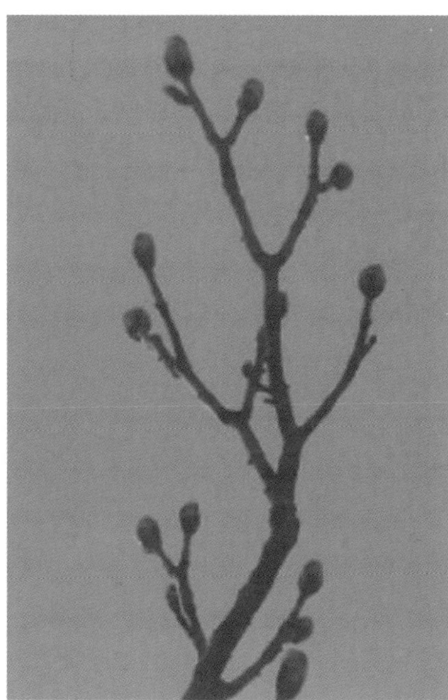

• **Fig. 4.12** Tree-in-bud nodules (Answer 18).

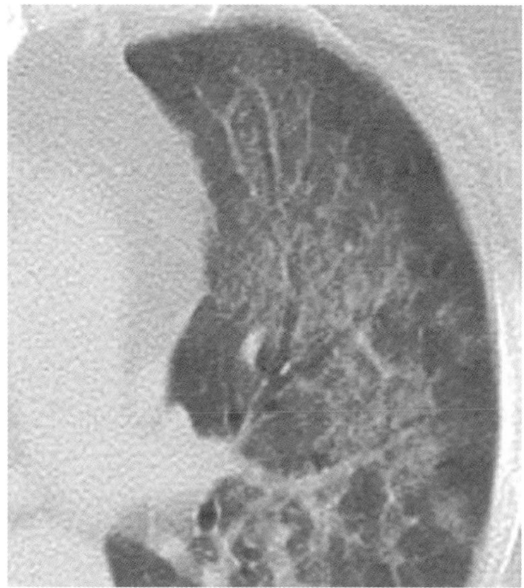

• **Fig. 4.13** Ground-glass opacity (Answer 18).

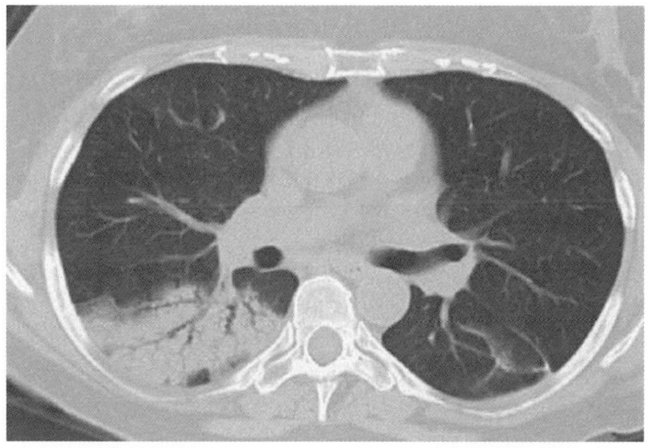

• **Fig. 4.14** Consolidation with air bronchograms (Answer 18).

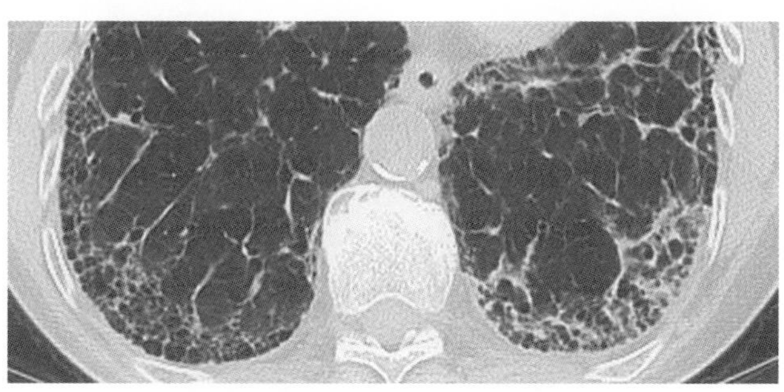

• **Fig. 4.15** Honeycombing (Answer 18).

19. ANSWER: A. Alpha-1 antitrypsin deficiency

The radiographic appearance of alpha-1 antitrypsin deficiency is that of emphysema, with hyperinflation (as demonstrated by large lung volumes and flattened diaphragms) and hyperlucency (due to a decrease in the normal vascular markings) of the lung fields. In some cases of emphysema due to alpha-1 antitrypsin deficiency, a distinctive finding is predominance of emphysema in the lower lung fields (rather than the typical predisposition for the upper lobes). In the chest x-ray shown in Question 19, one can see blood vessels in the upper halves of the lungs bilaterally but few in the lower halves. The cause of the basilar predominance of emphysema in some patients with alpha-1 antitrypsin deficiency is unknown.

The chest x-ray does not have the bilateral upper lobe opacities consistent with ankylosing spondylitis (Answer B); upper lobe-predominant linear markings in the orientation of bronchi, with oval cystic spaces and hyperinflation, suggestive of cystic fibrosis (Answer C); multiple lung nodules, potentially some with cavitation, as may be seen in granulomatosis with polyangiitis (Wegener granulomatosis) (Answer D); or hyperinflation with diffuse, thin-walled cystic spaces typical of lymphangioleiomyomatosis.

20. ANSWER: D. Surgical resection of the lung nodule

A new (over the course of 1 year), PET-positive lung nodule in a middle-aged cigarette smoker is highly suspicious for lung cancer. Benign etiologies are possible, including benign tumors, infections, and inflammatory reactions, but the risk of lung cancer is high, especially given the relatively large size of the nodule (>1 cm in diameter). The evaluation described in the case history serves to exclude obvious evidence for metastatic disease (based on the absence of other areas of increased uptake on the PET scan) and contraindications to surgical resection (adequate ventilatory reserve based on his spirometry results and low risk for myocardial infarction based on his negative cardiac stress test). The next step in his management should be referral to a thoracic surgeon for surgical excision of the lung nodule. Surgical resection not only provides definitive diagnosis but also, if this nodule is indeed a lung cancer, offers the best chance for cure.

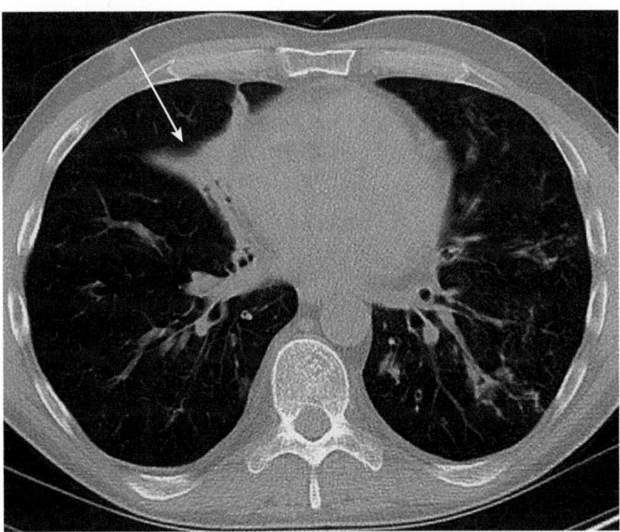

• **Fig. 4.16** Atelectasis (Answer 18).

The argument against attempting to establish a preoperative diagnosis with fiberoptic bronchoscopy and transbronchial lung biopsy (Answer B) or transthoracic needle aspirate/biopsy (Answer C) is the following. If a diagnosis of lung cancer is confirmed, the patient will then be referred for surgical resection of the nodule. If the sample returns with nonspecific findings ("no malignant cells seen"), there remains an unacceptably high chance (10% or greater) of a false-negative result. The likelihood of the sample providing a specific diagnosis of a benign lesion, such as a histoplasmoma, is small, estimated at 5% or less.

In the absence of suggestive symptoms or a known extrathoracic primary malignancy, the likelihood that this nodule represents a solitary pulmonary metastasis is low, especially with the PET scan indicating no abnormal areas of increased glucose uptake outside the chest. Workup for an alternative primary malignancy from which this nodule might be a solitary pulmonary metastasis (Answer A) is unnecessary beyond the results of the PET scan. Monitoring for growth of the nodule before proceeding with surgical excision (Answer E) may be appropriate for small or PET-negative nodules, but in this example, the probability of lung cancer is sufficiently high that delay in excision poses an unnecessary risk of growth and spread of malignancy.

Gelbman BD, Cham MD, Kim W, et al. Radiographic and clinical characterization of false negative results from CT-guided needle biopsies of lung nodules. *J Thorac Oncol.* 2012;7(5):815–820.

21. ANSWER: B. Fluticasone

A common side effect of inhaled corticosteroids is hoarse voice or dysphonia (a change in voice quality). The precise pathophysiology is uncertain, but it likely is the consequence of deposition of corticosteroid onto the larynx, with consequent irritative effect, mucosal thinning, or muscular atrophy. The dysphonia tends to be intermittent and fully reversible with cessation of medication. It cannot be prevented by rinsing the posterior pharynx or hypopharynx after each use of the medication. Sometimes this unpleasant side effect can be ameliorated by addition of a valved holding chamber ("spacer") to the metered-dose inhaler being used to deliver the inhaled steroid or changing the delivery system (e.g., from a dry-powder inhaler to a metered-dose inhaler with spacer). The inhaled steroid ciclesonide is released as a prodrug that is activated by esterases along the bronchial mucosa. It is said to have fewer oropharyngeal (and possibly laryngeal) side effects as a result of this unique mechanism of activation.

Although any inhaled medication can potentially cause occasional hoarseness, none of the other choices (salmeterol, tiotropium, albuterol, or ipratropium) commonly cause this problem.

22. ANSWER: C. She has ulcerative colitis.

Bronchiolitis obliterans is a potential cause of severe obstructive lung disease and should be considered in a patient without other common causes of chronic airflow obstruction, such as asthma, cigarette smoking, or genetic predisposition to emphysema (alpha-1 antitrypsin deficiency). Physical findings may include evidence for pulmonary hyperinflation and sometimes an inspiratory squeak. Findings on chest CT scan may be few, sometimes with areas of mosaic oligemia or tree-in-bud nodularity. Airflow obstruction is often poorly reversible to bronchodilators or corticosteroids.

Bronchiolitis obliterans may be immune mediated, as a pulmonary manifestation of ulcerative colitis, rheumatoid arthritis, or graft-versus-host disease following bone marrow transplant or rejection following lung transplant. A poorly ventilated office building is not a cause of bronchiolitis obliterans (Answer A). Chronic exposure to parrots (Answer B) may cause hypersensitivity pneumonitis, a restrictive lung disease. Mixed connective tissue disease (Answer D) can cause interstitial lung disease with fibrosis, likewise a cause of restriction on pulmonary function testing. The peripheral lung scarring that results from radiation therapy for localized breast cancer (Answer E) typically has no impact on pulmonary function.

23. ANSWER: D. Start antibiotics because the patient has a change in sputum quantity and character.

The bacterial pathogens causing exacerbations of COPD are most often *Streptococcus pneumoniae, Haemophilus influenzae,* and *Moraxella catarrhalis,* bacteria that can be treated with a variety of antibiotics chosen empirically (including macrolides, cephalosporins, amoxicillin/clavulanate, trimethoprim-sulfamethoxazole, doxycycline, and quinolones). Empiric treatment of exacerbations of COPD without need for sputum Gram stain and culture has proven effective in numerous clinical trials. Although many flares of COPD are triggered by events other than bacterial infection, omission of antibiotics when there is evidence for increased cough, sputum purulence, and/or fever results in less frequent resolution and more frequent deterioration than treatment with a short course of antibiotics. Oral steroids given for 2 weeks result in identical outcomes (in terms of resolution of the exacerbation and risk of recurrence) to 8 weeks (Answer A), and recent evidence suggests that 5 days of therapy may suffice in many cases. Oral steroids are equally effective compared with intravenous steroids in the treatment of COPD exacerbations with no greater incidence of gastrointestinal side effects (Answer B). Noninvasive mechanical ventilation, such as with bilevel positive airway pressure, can reduce the need for intubation with mechanical ventilation in severe exacerbations of COPD (Answer C).

de Jong YP, Uil SM, Grotjohan HP, et al. Oral or IV prednisolone in the treatment of COPD exacerbations: a randomized, controlled, double-blind study. *Chest.* 2007;132(6):1741–1747.

Leuppi JD, Schuetz P, Bingisser R, et al. Short-term vs conventional glucocorticoid therapy in acute exacerbations of chronic obstructive pulmonary disease: the REDUCE randomized clinical trial. *JAMA.* 2013;309(21):2223–2231.

Niewoehner DE, Erbland ML, Deupree RH, et al. Effect of systemic glucocorticoids on exacerbations of chronic obstructive pulmonary disease. *N Engl J Med.* 1999;340(25):1941–1947.

Quon BS, Gan WQ, Sin DD. Contemporary management of acute exacerbations of COPD: a systematic review and metaanalysis. *Chest.* 2008;133(3):756–766.

24. ANSWER: E. No therapy

This case history strongly points to a diagnosis of stage 1 pulmonary sarcoidosis. The patient has a mild, dry cough but is otherwise asymptomatic. No treatment is necessary. The rate of spontaneous remission of his disease over the next 2 years is approximately 80%. Treatment with systemic steroids (Answers A and B) may hasten resolution, but at an unacceptably high cost of medication side effects. Importantly, there is no evidence to suggest that early treatment of sarcoidosis prevents long-term progression or sequelae of the disease. Consequently, there is no justification for treating an asymptomatic or minimally symptomatic patient, whose disease has a high rate of spontaneous remission, with a medication that entails frequent short-term and long-term adverse side effects.

Hydroxychloroquine (Answer C) has been used to treat cutaneous sarcoidosis, including erythema nodosum, but it is not effective in most cases of pulmonary sarcoidosis. Methotrexate (Answer D) is a potential steroid-sparing agent in the treatment of severe pulmonary sarcoidosis.

Baughman RP, Lower EE. Treatment of sarcoidosis. *Clin Rev Allergy Immunol.* 2015;49(1):79–92.

25. ANSWER: B. Acute metabolic alkalemia due to "unmasking" of compensatory chronic metabolic alkalosis

In patients with chronic hypercapnia, such as from COPD with severe airflow obstruction, the sudden reversal of hypercapnia with mechanical ventilation leads to a rapid change in extracellular pH (from acidemic to alkalemic). The resulting electrolyte shifts across myocardial cell membranes can result in serious, potentially life-threatening cardiac arrhythmias. By a similar mechanism, seizures may develop. The target arterial P_{CO_2} during mechanical ventilation for exacerbations of COPD in patients with acute-on-chronic hypercapnia should be values close to baseline hypercapnia rather than a normal arterial P_{CO_2}. If lowering the arterial Pco_2 to this goal involves excessively high peak inflation pressures or auto-PEEP, one may choose to accept persistently higher arterial Pco_2 values until lung function improves, the ventilatory strategy referred to as *permissive hypercapnia.*

Reversing chronic hypoxemia with high inspired oxygen concentrations (Answer A) may lead to worsened hypercapnia in the spontaneously breathing patient with chronic hypercapnia, but it will have no adverse consequences in a patient receiving mechanical ventilation. Inadequate time for exhalation during mechanical ventilation of patients with severe expiratory airflow obstruction may lead to the development of high airway and transpulmonary pressures at the end of exhalation (auto-PEEP) (Answer C). Auto-PEEP can cause hypotension and increased risk of barotrauma, but cardiac arrhythmias would not be expected in the absence of hypotension. This patient does not have respiratory acidosis (Answer D); his $Paco_2$ is 36 mm Hg, and his arterial pH is 7.56. One cannot exclude a chronic metabolic alkalosis (Answer E) based on the blood gas results. However, corticosteroids and inhaled beta-agonist bronchodilators are not likely to cause a metabolic alkalosis of this severity, and chronic metabolic alkalosis does not precipitate ventricular arrhythmias.

26. ANSWER: B. Dopamine is more likely to cause cardiac arrhythmias.

In a double-blind, randomized, controlled trial of initial treatment of shock, treatment with dopamine versus norepinephrine demonstrated a significant increase in arrhythmias with dopamine. No statistically significant difference in overall mortality was seen, but a subgroup analysis demonstrated increased mortality in patients with cardiogenic shock treated with dopamine (Answer D). The trend in other subgroups did not favor dopamine, and norepinephrine was not associated with more adverse effects (Answer C). Dopamine has been studied for its renal protective effects; this trial did not show improvement in renal function, and previous trials in early renal dysfunction also demonstrated no benefit of dopamine (Answer A). Based on data from this trial and others, the Surviving Sepsis guidelines recommend norepinephrine as the first-line vasopressor in septic shock.

De Backer D, Biston P, Devriendt J. Comparison of dopamine and norepinephrine in the treatment of shock. *N Engl J Med.* 2010;362(9):779–789.

Dellinger RP, Levy MM, Rhodes A, et al. Surviving Sepsis Campaign: international guidelines for management of severe sepsis and septic shock, 2012. *Intensive Care Med.* 2013;39(2):165–228.

27. ANSWER: B. A reduction in mortality

Neuromuscular blockade in severe acute respiratory distress syndrome (ARDS) has traditionally been used for refractory cases and with great caution due to concerns for complications, in particular neuromuscular weakness related to critical illness (neuropathy, myopathy, or polyneuromyopathy). However, patient respiratory efforts and ventilator dyssynchrony may result in lung injury that may be mitigated by paralysis (Answer C). A recent randomized controlled trial demonstrated a reduction in organ failure (Answer E) and an overall mortality benefit for 48 hours of paralysis in relatively severe ARDS (Pao_2/Fio_2 ratio <150 with at least 5 cm H_2O of PEEP). Despite the concern for weakness, there was no increase in weakness noted at 28 days or ICU discharge compared with placebo (Answer A). Neuromuscular blockade requires deep sedation to avoid anesthesia awareness and would not be expected to decrease sedation requirements. Indeed, sedation was similar in the two groups in this trial (Answer D).

Papazian L, Forel JM, Gacouin A, et al. Neuromuscular blockers in early acute respiratory distress syndrome. *N Engl J Med.* 2010;363(12):1107–1116.

28. ANSWER: D. Volume targeted, tidal volume 410 mL

This patient has acute respiratory distress syndrome (ARDS). His Pao_2/Fio_2 ratio is <100, which meets criteria for severe ARDS. Low tidal volume ventilation results in decreased mortality and is the standard of care for ARDS. The goal tidal volume of 6 mL/kg is calculated based on the ideal rather than actual body weight. For a male of 5 feet 8 inches, the ideal body weight is 68.4 kg; thus 6 mL/kg would equal 410 mL. The protocol used in the ARDSNet trial started at 8 mL/kg, or 550 mL; thus tidal volumes of 650 mL, 700 mL, and 800 mL (Answers A, B, and C) are too large. Mechanical ventilation breaths can be delivered either by setting a volume or by setting a pressure, and plateau pressures are of importance in ARDS. Thus pressure-targeted assist-control mode (pressure control) is a reasonable ventilator mode for ARDS. However, without knowing the respiratory mechanics and tidal volume achieved by this setting, it is impossible to know whether this ventilator setting is more—or even potentially less—injurious (Answer E).

Acute Respiratory Distress Syndrome Network. Ventilation with lower tidal volumes as compared with traditional tidal volumes for acute lung injury and the acute respiratory distress syndrome. *N Engl J Med.* 2000;342(18):1301–1308.

29. ANSWER: E. Hyperkalemia

Succinylcholine is a neuromuscular blocking agent that is frequently used for intubation due to its rapid onset, brief duration, and predictable response. Succinylcholine acts as a depolarizing agent and thus can result in hyperkalemia. In the setting of preexisting hyperkalemia, particularly if severe, this side effect can be life threatening. Succinylcholine is also contraindicated in patients with a history of malignant hyperthermia and in cases where acetylcholine receptors are expected to be upregulated (e.g., denervation from stroke, inherited myopathies). Neuroleptic malignant syndrome is not related to malignant hyperthermia and is not a contraindication to succinylcholine or propofol (Answer A). Propofol may cause hypotension, and thus hypertension is not a contraindication (Answer D). Hypernatremia and corticosteroid use are not contraindications to sedatives and neuromuscular blockers in general (Answer B and C). Etomidate is an alternative sedative commonly used at the time of intubation because of its general lack of hemodynamic side effects; it can be associated with adrenal suppression.

30. ANSWER: D. Measurement of bladder pressure

This patient is at high risk for abdominal compartment syndrome. Initially recognized in surgical conditions (e.g., trauma, abdominal surgery), this syndrome is increasingly being recognized in medical settings, particularly in the context of large-volume resuscitation and intraabdominal pathology. Among the consequences of increased intraabdominal pressure are a decrease in venous return with associated hypotension and extrinsic compression of the lung, resulting in increased atelectasis and dead space. The normal intraabdominal pressure in a nonobese, critically ill patient, traditionally measured by transducing bladder pressure, is <7 mm Hg. Intraabdominal hypertension is defined as a sustained intraabdominal pressure >12 mm Hg. Abdominal compartment syndrome is defined as organ dysfunction with intraabdominal hypertension and is common with intraabdominal pressures >20 mm Hg.

Conservative treatment includes bowel decompression and patient positioning; surgical decompression may be required for severe cases. Although imaging may be helpful in identifying an alternative etiology for his abdominal distention, it would diagnose abdominal compartment syndrome. Thus abdominal ultrasound and portable radiographs are not the best choice (Answers C and E). Given his instability, transportation to a CT scanner may be risky (Answer A). Empiric antibiotics may be considered in severe pancreatitis with necrosis or if the etiology of his worsening is due to sepsis, but these processes are less likely than intraabdominal hypertension (Answer B).

31. ANSWER: D. *N*-acetylcysteine

Acetaminophen poisoning remains a major cause of acute liver failure in the United States. Treatment with *N*-acetylcysteine is the standard of care and should begin as soon as possible, ideally within 8 hours after ingestion. The suspicion for overdose is high, and one should not wait for the results of toxicology screening (Answer A). Administration of activated charcoal can be helpful, but it is most effective if given within 4 hours (preferably within 1 hour) of ingestion, and the time of this patient's ingestion is unknown (Answer C). Gastric lavage and induced vomiting are not recommended (Answer E). Sodium bicarbonate is a therapy for other ingestions (e.g., tricyclic and salicylate poisoning). Whereas it may be helpful for cases of severe acidosis, in this case acidosis is not mentioned (Answer B).

32. ANSWER: C. Noninvasive ventilation

The arterial blood gases are consistent with acute-on-chronic respiratory acidosis. In the setting of a COPD exacerbation with hypercapnia (P_{CO_2} >45 mm Hg), several studies have demonstrated that noninvasive positive pressure ventilation decreases mortality and need for intubation. Her oxygen saturation is adequate, and increasing supplemental oxygen is unlikely to result in significant improvement in her dyspnea and may worsen hypercapnia (Answer A). Conversely, decreasing supplemental oxygen is likely to result in suboptimal oxygen saturation and is unlikely to result in improvement in the patient's dyspnea (Answer D). Intubation may eventually be needed. However, this patient is not in severe distress and does not have any clear contraindications to noninvasive ventilation (e.g., impaired consciousness, high aspiration risk, or severe respiratory failure). Therefore noninvasive ventilation should be attempted first (Answer B).

Plant PK, Owen JL, Elliott MW. Early use of non-invasive ventilation for acute exacerbations of chronic obstructive pulmonary disease on general respiratory wards: a multicentre randomised controlled trial. *Lancet.* 2000;355(9219):1931–1935.

33. ANSWER: B. Spontaneous breathing trial

Increased duration of mechanical ventilation is associated with an increased risk of complications, especially ventilator-associated pneumonia. Patients should be assessed daily for their readiness for discontinuation of mechanical ventilation. In most patients who are not requiring high levels of support, a spontaneous breathing trial is a reasonable next step. A spontaneous breathing trial has the patient breathe on minimal to no support for at least 30 minutes. Many ICUs also include a rapid shallow breathing index (RSBI) prior to, or as a part of, the spontaneous breathing trial. The RSBI is performed with the patient breathing spontaneously without pressure support or PEEP and is the ratio of respiratory rate divided by tidal volume (in liters). An RSBI <105 identifies patients more likely to be ready to be extubated. However, the decision to extubate should not be based solely on the RSBI. The RSBI has only moderate specificity to predict readiness to extubate; can be artificially low in the setting of sedation; and does not take into account mental status, airway secretions, and other factors (Answer A). In several ventilator "weaning" trials, a substantial number of patients were able to be extubated immediately after a successful spontaneous breathing trial. Thus the decision to proceed with decreasing amounts of pressure support should ideally be initiated only after the results of the spontaneous breathing trial are known and the decision regarding immediate extubation is made (Answer C). Weaning via SIMV results in a longer duration of mechanical ventilation than daily spontaneous breathing trials or pressure support (Answer E). Decreasing PEEP and FiO_2 to levels required to adequately support oxygenation is reasonable if the patient is unable to be extubated, but it is not the most appropriate next step in this patient's care (Answer D).

Brochard L, Rauss A, Benito S, et al. Comparison of three methods of gradual withdrawal from ventilatory support during weaning from mechanical ventilation. *Am J Respir Crit Care Med.* 1994;150(4):896–903.

Esteban A, Frutos F, Tobin MJ, A comparison of four methods of weaning patients from mechanical ventilation. *N Engl J Med.* 1995;332(6):345–350.

34. ANSWER: A. Continuous renal replacement therapy (CRRT) does not have a mortality benefit compared with intermittent hemodialysis (IHD).

Acute renal failure in the setting of septic shock is a frequent and morbid problem. Although only a minority of patients go on to require renal replacement therapy, the appropriate modality has been controversial. CRRT and IHD have been compared in several studies; overall, the evidence is most consistent with CRRT being equivalent to IHD (Answer A). Although CRRT may be easier to tolerate in the setting of vasopressors (or mechanical ventilation), a study by Vinsonneau and colleagues did not demonstrate any mortality benefit in a population where the vast majority required both vasopressor and mechanical ventilator support (Answers C and D). In this study, despite the use of vasopressors, most patients were able to be treated with IHD (Answer E). The available data on dialysis intensity suggest that this factor may be important. However, study results have been conflicting. Harm may be associated with low-intensity therapy, and whereas some studies have demonstrated improved mortality with high-intensity renal replacement, several others have not demonstrated a benefit over standard-intensity dialysis (Answer B).

Vinsonneau C, Camus C, Combes A, et al. Continuous venovenous haemodiafiltration versus intermittent haemodialysis for acute renal failure in patients with multiple-organ dysfunction syndrome: a multicentre randomised trial. *Lancet.* 2006;368(9533):379–385.

RENAL Replacement Therapy Study Investigators. Intensity of continuous renal-replacement therapy in critically ill patients. *N Engl J Med.* 2009;361(17):1627–1638.

35. ANSWER: E. Intravenous crystalloid bolus

Adequate fluid resuscitation is a mainstay of hemodynamic support in septic shock. A randomized controlled trial of early goal-directed therapy (EGDT) demonstrated improved mortality with early and aggressive resuscitation in septic shock. Adequate resuscitation in this trial was demonstrated by a CVP from 8 to 12 cm H_2O. This specific numeric target has been controversial because a static measurement of CVP is poorly predictive of fluid responsiveness. Nonetheless, the 2.5 L of fluid that this patient received is a relatively low amount, particularly in someone who is obese, and other indicators, such as respiratory variation in CVP, may also serve as indicators of volume responsiveness. Debate persists about which aspect of the Rivers protocol may have led to improved outcomes. A more recent trial comparing protocolized care in the emergency room versus usual care (which now include early antibiotic therapy) did not show a decrease in mortality, but patients in the control arm received 2.3 L in the first 6 hours, reflecting a change in general practice toward earlier resuscitation.

Adequate resuscitation is preferred over increasing vasopressors (Answer A). Fluid should be given as a bolus and not as a continuous infusion, both to treat hypotension quickly and to be able to gauge responsiveness (Answer B). Although colloid is likely safe in this setting, there is no clear justification for its added expense (Answer C). Although the patient is anemic, a baseline hematocrit is not given, and in the absence of active cardiac ischemia or ongoing blood loss, a transfusion would not be worth the risks (e.g., transfusion reaction or increased susceptibility to ARDS) (Answer D).

ProCESS Investigators. A randomized trial of protocol-based care for early septic shock. *N Engl J Med.* 2014;370(18):1683–1693.

Rivers E, Nguyen B, Havstad S, et al. Early goal-directed therapy in the treatment of severe sepsis and septic shock. *N Engl J Med.* 2001;345(19):1368–1377.

36. ANSWER: B. Initiate argatroban

This patient has a high likelihood of having heparin-induced thrombocytopenia with thrombosis (HITT). The pretest probability of HITT is often given as the "4 Ts": thrombocytopenia, timing, thrombosis, and exclusion of other causes of thrombocytopenia. Her thrombocytopenia has no other clear etiology; the timing is within 5–10 days after exposure; her platelet count has fallen by over 50%; and she has evidence suggesting a new deep venous thrombosis (DVT) of her right leg. Treatment is indicated for most patients with HIT, and certainly for patients with HITT. Additional testing should be done, but therapy should not be delayed (Answers A and E). Of the available agents, only argatroban is indicated (alternatives may include fondaparinux or bivalirudin). Low-molecular-weight heparin is also associated with a risk of HIT, albeit lower than unfractionated heparin, and therefore is still contraindicated in HIT (Answer C). Warfarin rapidly lowers protein C levels and thus is associated with increased risk of thrombosis during initiation (Answer D). Transition to warfarin should be considered when the patient's platelet count has improved and she has been stably anticoagulated.

Greinacher A. Heparin-induced thrombocytopenia. *N Engl J Med.* 2015;373(3):252–261.

37. ANSWER: E. Stress ulcer prophylaxis

Ventilator-associated pneumonias (VAP) (or more broadly, ventilator-associated complications) are an important cause of morbidity and mortality in the ICU. Several practices have been shown to reduce the incidence of VAP. Many of these therapies have been included in ventilator "bundles" (grouped practices to reduce complications in mechanically ventilated patients). These therapies include elevation of the head of the hospital bed, oropharyngeal decontamination, and daily assessment of readiness to extubate (to reduce the duration of mechanical ventilation) (Answers A and B). Continuous drainage of subglottic secretions has been shown in several studies to decrease VAP. However, this approach requires specially designed endotracheal or tracheostomy tubes (Answer D). Selective decontamination of the gastrointestinal tract has also been shown to decrease VAP, though use has been limited in part due to concerns about promotion of antibiotic resistance (Answer C). Whereas stress ulcer prophylaxis is usually included as part of a ventilator "bundle," acid suppression actually results in an increased, not decreased, risk of VAP. The mechanism is thought to be bacterial overgrowth in the stomach in the absence of suppressive gastric acid, with risk of reflux and aspiration of these bacterial pathogens.

Dodek P, Keenan S, Cook D, et al. Evidence-based clinical practice guideline for the prevention of ventilator-associated pneumonia. *Ann Intern Med.* 2004;141(4):305–313.

Koeman M, van der Ven AJ, Hak E, et al. Oral decontamination with chlorhexidine reduces the incidence of ventilator-associated pneumonia. *Am J Respir Crit Care Med.* 2006;173(12):1348–1355.

38. ANSWER: D. Transfusion may be associated with an increase in mortality.

Anemia results in decreased oxygen delivery. However, correction of anemia via transfusion of packed red blood cells is associated with risks, including hemolytic transfusion reactions, immunosuppression, transfusion-associated circulatory overload (TACO), and transfusion-related acute lung injury (TRALI). In the Transfusion Requirements in Critical Care trial, over 800 critically ill patients were randomized to a restrictive or liberal transfusion strategy. There was no benefit to the liberal transfusion group. In a subgroup analysis of patients less acutely ill and those <55 years of age, a restrictive strategy (transfusion of hemoglobin <7 g/dL) was associated with decreased mortality. Although patients with a primary cardiac diagnosis appeared less likely to be enrolled in this trial, analysis of patients with coronary disease demonstrated no increased risk of complications in the restrictive transfusion group (Answer A) and no benefit from transfusions in terms of duration of mechanical ventilation in the liberal transfusion group (Answer C). The patient's gastrointestinal bleed has stabilized. Particularly in the absence of active blood loss, there is no compelling reason to transfuse, and a randomized trial has demonstrated a benefit for a restrictive (hemoglobin <7 g/dL) transfusion strategy for most patients with upper gastrointestinal bleeding (Answer B). Transfusions are associated with several electrolyte abnormalities, including hypocalcemia and hyperkalemia, but not hypokalemia (Answer E).

Hébert PC, Wells G, Blajchman MA, et al. A multicenter, randomized, controlled clinical trial of transfusion requirements in critical care. [Published erratum appears in *N Engl J Med.* 1999;340(13):1056.] *N Engl J Med.* 1999;340(6):409–417.

Villanueva C, Colomo A, Bosch A, et al. Transfusion strategies for acute upper gastrointestinal bleeding. [Published erratum appears in *N Engl J Med.* 2013;368(24):2341.] *N Engl J Med.* 2013;368(1):11–21.

39. ANSWER: B. Discontinue sertraline and fentanyl

The differential diagnosis for fever in the ICU is broad. Although infectious etiologies are the most common causes, certain toxidromes are important to recognize. The serotonin syndrome is a life-threatening condition associated with increased serotonergic activity and is characterized by mental status changes, autonomic hyperactivity, and neuromuscular changes. In addition to agents traditionally associated with serotonin reuptake, many other medications can increase serotonin, such as metoclopramide, carbidopa-levodopa, meperidine, and fentanyl. The serotonin syndrome shares many features with neuroleptic malignant syndrome (NMS), including fever, mental status change, and increased muscle tone. However, in contrast to NMS (Answer D), serotonin syndrome is characterized by hyperreflexia, not bradyreflexia, and clonus, which can be inducible, spontaneous, and ocular. In addition, this patient's agitation began before administration of haloperidol; the onset of serotonin syndrome usually occurs within 24 hours of initiation of medication and is dose related, whereas the onset of NMS begins within days to weeks. Management of serotonin syndrome consists of discontinuation of all serotonergic agents (thus Answer A is incorrect), sedation with benzodiazepines, and consideration of cyproheptadine, a serotonergic antagonist. Propofol would not treat serotonin syndrome (Answer C). Whereas haloperidol should probably not be continued because of anticholinergic effects, its discontinuation would not address the life-threatening serotoninergic effects of the sertraline and fentanyl (Answer D). There is no evidence for an infectious etiology for this patient's fever, so vancomycin is not appropriate (Answer E).

40. ANSWER: E. Therapeutic hypothermia should be continued for 24 hours.

In patients who survive an out-of-hospital cardiac arrest, anoxic-ischemic encephalopathy is a major cause of morbidity and mortality. The benefit of induced hypothermia in ventricular fibrillation and pulseless ventricular tachycardia was demonstrated in two randomized controlled trials, which both demonstrated a significant improvement in favorable neurologic outcomes. Although the data are less robust, recommendations for therapeutic hypothermia have been extended to include all causes of cardiac arrest. Risks of therapeutic hypothermia include increased risk of infection, coagulopathy, hypokalemia (not hyperkalemia, Answer B), and bradycardia. Although these risks must be weighed against the benefits of hypothermia, there was no statistically significant increase in sepsis or lethal arrhythmias in these two trials (Answer C). In the larger of the two trials, development of infection was not associated with increased mortality (Answer C). Based on results from these trials and other observational data, hypothermia should be initiated early (that is, within 4–6 hours) and not delayed for reassessment of neurologic status (Answer D), and it should be continued for 12–24 hours. Of note, in a more recent trial, targeted temperature management with a goal of 36°C led to outcomes equivalent to a target of 33°C, suggesting that it may be active temperature management and possibly prevention of fever, rather than hypothermia per se, that leads to improved outcomes after cardiac arrest.

Bernard SA, Gray TW, Buist MD, et al. Treatment of comatose survivors of out-of-hospital cardiac arrest with induced hypothermia. *N Engl J Med.* 2002;346(8):557–563.

Hypothermia after Cardiac Arrest Study Group. Mild therapeutic hypothermia to improve the neurologic outcome after cardiac arrest. *N Engl J Med.* 2002;346(8):549–556.

Nielsen N, Wetterslev J, Cronberg T, et al. Targeted temperature management at 33°C versus 36°C after cardiac arrest. *N Engl J Med.* 2013;369(23):2197–2206.

41. ANSWER: C. Decrease respiratory rate

Ventilator support for obstructive lung disease should allow for longer exhalation times to avoid hyperinflation and barotrauma (i.e., pneumothorax and pneumomediastinum). In this case, the measured end-expiratory pressure is above the set PEEP (i.e., auto-PEEP is present), and the patient's blood pressure is borderline low. Thus decreasing the respiratory rate and allowing adequate exhalation time should reduce auto-PEEP and, as a result of decreased intrathoracic pressure, improve hemodynamics. Without any change in ventilator settings, the patient will continue with relative hypotension and risk of barotrauma from high inflation pressures (Answer A). Increasing the respiratory rate or increasing the I:E ratio would worsen hyperinflation (Answers C and E). Increasing PEEP in the setting of obstructive lung disease with auto-PEEP could improve triggering and patient-ventilator dyssynchrony, but these are not problems in this case (Answer B).

42. ANSWER: C. Use of midazolam instead of propofol

Providing appropriate control of discomfort during mechanical ventilation is an important goal in the intensive care unit. Although keeping patients heavily sedated may appear to be most appropriate, excessive sedation is associated with prolonged mechanical ventilation and other adverse outcomes, such as greater likelihood of delirium. Randomized trials have demonstrated more rapid extubation with daily interruption of sedation (Answer B), daily spontaneous breathing trials (Answer B), and a combination of daily interruption of sedation with spontaneous breathing trials. The type of sedation used may also be important. Trials have demonstrated decreased duration of mechanical ventilation with propofol versus midazolam (thus Answer C is associated with an increased duration of mechanical ventilation), as well as dexmedetomidine, an alpha-2 agonist with analgesic and sedative properties, versus midazolam (Answer D). Avoidance of routine sedatives altogether can be achieved in many intubated patients, and this approach has also been associated with decreased duration of mechanical ventilation (Answer E).

Brochard L, Rauss A, Benito S, et al. Comparison of three methods of gradual withdrawal from ventilatory support during weaning from mechanical ventilation. *Am J Respir Crit Care Med.* 1994;150(4):896–903.

Girard TD, Kress JP, Fuchs BD, et al. Efficacy and safety of a paired sedation and ventilator weaning protocol for mechanically ventilated patients in intensive care (Awakening and Breathing Controlled trial): a randomised controlled trial. *Lancet.* 2008;371(9607):126–134.

Kress JP, Pohlman AS, O'Connor MF, Hall JB. Daily interruption of sedative infusions in critically ill patients undergoing mechanical ventilation. *N Engl J Med.* 2000;342(20):1471–1477.

43. ANSWER: C. Fomepizole

This patient's presentation is highly suspicious for ethylene glycol intoxication. His osmolar gap is 15 if one includes ethanol in the calculation of the expected serum osmolarity: expected osmolarity = 2 × (sodium in mEq/L) + (glucose in mg/dL)/18 + (BUN in mg/dL)/2.8 + (ethanol in mg/dL)/3.7. Ingestion of a toxic alcohol should be considered when the osmolar gap is >10. However, it is important to note that this gap reflects the presence only of the parent alcohols and may be normal in late presentations. The combination of an osmolar gap and anion-gap metabolic acidosis should raise concern for ethylene glycol toxicity. The presence of crystals in the urine is consistent with calcium oxalate, which is a consequence of ethylene glycol metabolism. The treatment for ethylene glycol ingestion is fomepizole (Answer C). Fomepizole is an inhibitor of alcohol dehydrogenase and thereby inhibits the metabolism of ethylene glycol to its toxic compounds. Administration of ethanol would also help prevent ethylene glycol metabolism, but it is associated with additional side effects (Answer A). Alcohol withdrawal is a concern in this patient, for which benzodiazepines would be appropriate, but this intervention would not treat ethylene glycol poisoning (Answer B). Bicarbonate would be more appropriate therapy for a non–anion gap acidosis (Answer E). Hemodialysis is indicated for severe ingestions with refractory acidosis, renal failure, deterioration in vital signs, or a markedly elevated level of ethylene glycol (Answer D).

44. ANSWER: E. Cardiogenic shock

The central venous pressure is elevated, inconsistent with hemorrhagic or hypovolemic shock (Answers C and D). The central venous oxygen saturation reflects oxygen extraction for blood returning via the superior vena cava and approximates the mixed venous oxygen saturation. In septic shock following adequate fluid resuscitation, this value is typically elevated, reflecting impaired tissue oxygen extraction. A low value indicates elevated tissue extraction and is consistent with impaired cardiac output. Impaired cardiac output can be due to inadequate filling (e.g., hypovolemia), obstruction of blood flow (e.g., massive pulmonary embolus), or intrinsic cardiac causes (e.g., systolic dysfunction). In this case, the low venous oxygen saturation and elevated central venous pressure, together with his physical examination (cool extremities), are more consistent with cardiogenic shock. Although myocardial dysfunction is not uncommon in the setting of severe sepsis, it is also possible that his bilateral radiographic opacities reflect pulmonary edema. Although central venous oxygen saturation is typically high in the setting of sepsis, it can at times be low, particularly in settings of inadequate fluid resuscitation or concomitant impaired cardiac output (Answer A). A high central venous oxygen saturation can also be seen in end-stage liver disease, although shock is usually due to superimposed infection or bleeding (Answer B).

45. ANSWER: C. Arterial blood gas with cooximetry

The most common causes of hypoxemia are ventilation–perfusion mismatch and shunt; these abnormalities can be due to a variety of parenchymal and vascular causes, such as atelectasis, aspiration, pulmonary edema, and pulmonary embolism. Hypoventilation is another important cause of hypoxemia, particularly in the setting of sedation. In this situation, another important cause of hypoxemia to consider is methemoglobinemia. Methemoglobin is formed when the ferrous (Fe^{2+}) iron in heme is oxidized to the ferric (Fe^{3+}) state; the ferric state is unable to bind oxygen. Increases in methemoglobin can be due to genetic conditions resulting in deficiencies of cytochrome b5 reductase or globin mutations, but they are more commonly due to medications. The list of medications potentially causing methemoglobinemia includes nitrates; dapsone; metoclopramide; and topical anesthetics, particularly benzocaine.

Standard pulse oximeters use photodetectors to identify oxyhemoglobin and deoxyhemoglobin; methemoglobin cannot be specifically detected and instead causes an artifactual change (usually decrease) in oxygen saturation with increasing concentrations of methemoglobin, generally to around 85%–87%. An arterial blood gas with cooximetry can quantify the degree of methemoglobinemia, if present. In severe cases, methemoglobinemia is treated with methylene blue. An arterial blood gas alone can provide the actual oxygen saturation, but without cooximetry, it cannot diagnosis methemoglobinemia (Answer D). A chest x-ray and electrocardiogram are reasonable initial tests for this patient, but they would not be diagnostic of this patient's condition (Answers A and E). Pulmonary embolism can certainly cause a sudden reduction in oxygen saturation, but chest CT angiography would not be the first test of choice (Answer B).

46. ANSWER: C. Endotracheal suctioning

The pressure required to deliver a breath to a mechanically ventilated patient can be simplified into two components: airway resistance and lung compliance (or conversely, lung elastance). Problems with airway resistance and lung compliance can increase peak inspiratory pressures, but only problems affecting lung compliance will increase the plateau pressure. The plateau pressure is calculated by performing a breath-hold at end-inspiration and subtracting PEEP from the measured pressure. Because this pressure is calculated at zero flow, it reflects the pressure required to distend the lung parenchyma by the given tidal volume, independent of airway resistance. In this case, although the plateau pressure before the event is not given, it is not likely to be significantly increased, because the plateau pressure must be lower than the peak pressure and because in COPD, one anticipates a low peak pressure due to high lung compliance. Thus these findings (a high peak inspiratory pressure with a low plateau pressure) are consistent with an airway problem. Increases in ventilator pressures due to airway resistance can be due to mucous plugging, obstructed or kinked endotracheal tubes, or bronchospasm. Thus endotracheal suctioning is a reasonable first step. A chest x-ray may be helpful, but it should not delay a potentially beneficial intervention (Answer A). Needle decompression and chest tube placement would treat a pneumothorax or pleural effusion (Answers B and D), and diuresis would treat pulmonary edema (Answer E), all of which typically would be expected to increase the plateau pressures.

47. ANSWER: D. Lorazepam infusion followed by fosphenytoin is a reasonable treatment.

Status epilepticus is defined as seizures that persist or recur frequently enough so that recovery between attacks does not occur. Management of status epilepticus includes assessment of the underlying etiology and supportive care of respiratory and circulatory status, which may include intubation. Initial management is generally through administration of benzodiazepines, most often lorazepam, although others can be used. In a randomized controlled trial comparing several treatments, lorazepam alone was found to be superior to phenytoin alone (Answer A). Fosphenytoin is preferred over phenytoin because it is water soluble, may be infused more rapidly, and results in less local irritation. Although the absence of the propylene glycol carrier in fosphenytoin should in theory lead to fewer cardiovascular side effects, several studies suggest that the risk of hypotension does not differ between the two drugs (Answer B). Diazepam has higher lipid solubility and likely faster, not slower, onset of action than lorazepam (Answer C). For some cases of status epilepticus, treatment with lorazepam alone is sufficient. However, in many cases, addition of phenytoin or fosphenytoin can help provide a prolonged antiseizure effect and thus represents a reasonable treatment in this case. Although propofol has not been as well studied as benzodiazepines or phenytoin, it has been used successfully to treat status epilepticus in several small trials (Answer E).

Rossetti AO, Reichhart MD, Schaller MD, et al. Propofol treatment of refractory status epilepticus: a study of 31 episodes. *Epilepsia.* 2004 Jul;45(7):757–763.

Treiman DM, Meyers PD, Walton NY, et al. A comparison of four treatments for generalized convulsive status epilepticus. *N Engl J Med.* 1998;339(12):792–798.

48. ANSWER: E. End-tidal CO_2 detection may help determine the quality of cardiopulmonary resuscitation (CPR) and return of spontaneous circulation.

Carbon dioxide is detected in exhaled breath in the presence of circulation. Thus end-tidal carbon dioxide detection has been advocated as a method both to assess for adequacy of CPR and to detect the return of spontaneous circulation. Over the past several years, advanced cardiac life support (ACLS) guidelines have been updated to reflect studies highlighting the detrimental effects of inadequate and interrupted chest compressions, which result in decreased cardiac and cerebral perfusion. They have also discouraged emphasis on establishing an advanced airway with assisted ventilation, which not only interrupts chest compressions but also may lead to overventilation, increased intrathoracic pressure, and decreased venous return.

Although hypoxemia and hypercapnia can cause cardiac arrest, inadequate bag-and-mask ventilation is usually not the cause of failure to recover from an arrest (Answer A). In this case, overventilation is a particular concern, given the patient's COPD. ACLS guidelines have recognized a detrimental effect on effective CPR from frequent interruptions for pulse checks and consequently recommend immediately resuming compressions for 2 minutes after administration of drugs (such as epinephrine) or a defibrillation attempt (Answers C and D). Rapid response teams have not convincingly been shown to decrease mortality, but several studies have demonstrated that they can reduce the incidence of in-hospital cardiac arrest (Answer B).

Chan PS, Jain R, Nallmothu BK, et al. Rapid response teams: a systematic review and meta-analysis. *Arch Intern Med.* 2010;170(1):18–26.

49. ANSWER: C. Corticosteroids will likely improve his response to vasopressors.

Despite decades of study, the use of corticosteroids in sepsis and septic shock remains controversial. Older studies using high-dose steroids found no beneficial effect and a possible increase in mortality (Answer E). A study of moderate-dose corticosteroids (200 mg of hydrocortisone) appeared to demonstrate benefit, limited to those who were deemed to have inadequate adrenal reserve after an ACTH stimulation test. However, this favorable finding was not confirmed in a subsequent trial (Answer A). Experts continue to recommend moderate-dose steroids for septic shock with continued need for vasopressors, based on a consistent improvement in hemodynamics and response to vasopressors.

The use of corticosteroids in ARDS, as in septic shock, is controversial. More data are available for the use of steroids late in the course of ARDS. In an ARDSNet trial of late rescue (after 7 days), use of steroids was associated with fewer days in shock and shorter duration of mechanical ventilation but a higher rate of reintubation. Mortality was increased in the subgroup that received therapy after 14 days (Answer D). Assessment of adrenal insufficiency in critically ill patients is challenging, owing to wide variations in serum cortisol levels and in free versus bound cortisol. However, in the absence of true adrenal insufficiency, neither the absolute serum cortisol level nor the response to ACTH appears reliably to identify patients who will benefit from corticosteroids (Answer B).

Annane D, Bellissant E, Bollaert PE, et al. Corticosteroids in the treatment of severe sepsis and septic shock in adults: a systematic review. *JAMA.* 2009;301(22):2362–2375.

Sprung CL, Annane D, Keh D, et al. Hydrocortisone therapy for patients with septic shock. *N Engl J Med.* 2008;358(2): 111–124.

Steinberg KP, Hudson LD, Goodman RB, et al. Efficacy and safety of corticosteroids for persistent acute respiratory distress syndrome. *N Engl J Med.* 2006;354(16):1671–1684.

50. ANSWER: E. High-dose insulin therapy

Calcium channel blocker overdose is associated with substantial morbidity and mortality. The effects of overdose depend on the type and dose of calcium channel blocker. In addition to vasodilation and decreased inotropy, diltiazem and verapamil, but not the dihydropyridines, typically result in bradycardia. Recognition of the overdose is important because hemodynamic deterioration can be delayed by hours after the ingestion. In addition to supportive and symptomatic care, treatment usually includes intravenous calcium and glucagon. Whole-bowel irrigation may be appropriate for ingestion of extended-release preparations. Temporary pacemaker support may be indicated for persistent bradycardia. High-dose insulin therapy has been increasingly advocated for cases of calcium channel blocker (and beta-blocker) overdose. The mechanisms of action are unclear, but calcium channel blockers may cause insulin resistance in the myocardium that is overcome by high doses of insulin. Although this therapy is usually instituted with a concomitant glucose infusion, calcium channel blocker overdose itself can cause impaired glucose metabolism, and patients are often hyperglycemic and may not require additional glucose. Recently, another treatment, intravenous lipid emulsion, has been advocated for use in several types of severe overdoses, including calcium channel blocker overdose. Although this therapy has not been well studied, results from animal studies and case reports of severe toxicity in humans have demonstrated evidence of benefit. The mechanism of action is unclear, but it may work by acting as a "lipid sink" for the toxic medication.

Hemodialysis is not effective for removing verapamil, because verapamil is highly protein bound (Answer A). Bicarbonate infusion may be indicated in the setting of severe acidemia or a widened QRS complex due to sodium channel blockade, as in tricyclic overdose (Answer B). Physostigmine is a therapy for anticholinergic overdose (Answer D). Intravenous corticosteroids are not helpful in calcium channel blocker overdose (Answer E).

Greene SL, Gawarammana I, Wood DM, et al. Relative safety of hyperinsulinaemia/euglycaemia therapy in the management of calcium channel blocker overdose: a prospective observational study. *Intensive Care Med.* 2007;33(11):2019–2024.

Doepker B, Healy W, Cortez E, Adkins EJ. High-dose insulin and intravenous lipid emulsion therapy for cardiogenic shock induced by intentional calcium-channel blocker and beta-blocker overdose: a case series. *J Emerg Med.* 2014;45(4):486–490.

Acknowledgment

The authors and editors gratefully acknowledge the contributions of the previous authors, Christopher Fanta and Michael Cho.

5 Endocrinology

OLE-PETTER R. HAMNVIK

1. An 89-year-old Caucasian woman is seen at your clinic for a routine physical examination. She is known to have prediabetes for many years, and you have recently diagnosed her with new-onset type 2 diabetes. She is asymptomatic, but her fasting blood glucose was 145 mg/dL, and her recent hemoglobin A_{1c} (HbA_{1c}) was 7.5%. Her past medical history is significant for hypertension, hypercholesterolemia, and coronary artery disease with ischemic cardiomyopathy (ejection fraction 40%). Medications include amlodipine, aspirin, atorvastatin, and metoprolol. On physical exam, she weighs 39 kg; her blood is pressure 99/64 mm Hg; and her heart rate is 67 beats per minute. Her jugular venous pulse is estimated at 5 cm. She has normal heart sounds with no added sounds or murmurs. Her lungs are clear to auscultation with no wheeze or crackles. She has normal pedal pulses and no edema. Her abdominal and neurologic exams were normal. Serum creatinine was measured at 1.3 mg/dL. You refer the patient for diabetes education and to a dietitian for nutritional counseling. She wishes to start metformin because her husband has been taking this for diabetes for the past 15 years with good glycemic control.

   How would you advise her regarding metformin therapy?

   A. An extended-release formulation of metformin should be started at 2000 mg once daily.
   B. Metformin should be started at 500 mg once daily and slowly increased to a target daily dose of 2000 mg per day.
   C. Metformin should be started at 500 mg twice daily with no further dose escalation.
   D. Metformin therapy is contraindicated on the basis of renal dysfunction.
   E. Metformin therapy is contraindicated due to her history of congestive heart failure.

2. A 60-year-old woman is found to have mild primary hyperparathyroidism on routine chemistry screening with serum calcium 10.9 mg/dL (normal 8.6–10.4), albumin 4.0 g/dL, and intact parathyroid hormone (PTH) 76 pg/mL (normal 10–65). Vitamin D levels are normal. Screening bone density shows osteoporosis at the femoral neck. She generally feels well and denies any history of kidney stones. She refuses to consider parathyroid surgery at this time.

   What do you recommend for her?

   A. 24-hour urine to measure calcium excretion
   B. Alendronate 70 mg orally weekly
   C. Annual calcium, creatinine, and bone mineral density testing
   D. Cinacalcet 30 mg orally twice daily
   E. Neck ultrasound and sestamibi scanning

3. A 20-year-old woman presents to the clinic because of oligomenorrhea. She went through menarche and adrenarche at the same age as her peers. She is currently obese and has struggled with her weight since her teens. She is concerned about several years of hair thinning, male pattern balding, and facial and chest terminal hair growth. She has minimal acne. She has the following laboratory test results: total testosterone 42.4 ng/dL (mildly elevated), sex hormone–binding globulin (SHBG) 12 nmol/L, prolactin 9.6 ng/mL, follicle-stimulating hormone (FSH) 5.2 mIU/mL, luteinizing hormone (LH) 11.8 mU/mL, and HbA_{1c} 5.2%. She also has a normal dexamethasone suppression test result and normal 17-hydroxyprogesterone. You diagnose her with polycystic ovarian syndrome (PCOS). She is not currently interested in pregnancy, and you start treatment with an estrogen-progestin contraceptive. After 6 months her hirsutism persists, and she is very concerned about this.

   In addition to continuing the oral contraceptive pill, what is the next best treatment strategy for her hirsutism?

   A. Encourage weight loss.
   B. Reassure her that her hirsutism will improve with prolonged treatment.
   C. Start letrozole.
   D. Start metformin.
   E. Start spironolactone.

4. A 48-year-old man had a history of hypertension for the past 7 years. His treatment included lisinopril, amlodipine, and hydrochlorothiazide. Despite taking these three medications, his blood pressure remained at 170/100 mm Hg. On a routine physical examination, his serum potassium was found to be 2.7 mEq/L. Previously, while on hydrochlorothiazide, his potassium had been between 3.3 and 3.7 mEq/L. He was given potassium chloride supplementation, but his serum potassium remained less than 3.5 mEq/L. To further address his hypokalemia, his hydrochlorothiazide was stopped, and instead he was treated with spironolactone. With the addition of spironolactone for 4 weeks, his blood pressure improved to 140/80 mm Hg, and his potassium stabilized at 3.7 mEq/L. At that time, a biochemical workup for hyperaldosteronism revealed a serum aldosterone of 42 ng/dL and a plasma renin activity of 4.2 ng/mL/h.

What is the best interpretation of these laboratory results?

A. Essential hypertension
B. Insufficient information to confirm a diagnosis
C. Primary hyperaldosteronism
D. Renal tubular acidosis
E. Secondary hyperaldosteronism

5. A 39-year-old man is admitted to the intensive care unit (ICU) for severe community-acquired pneumonia requiring intubation. He is otherwise healthy except for obesity, and he is not known to have diabetes. Random blood glucose levels obtained during the first day in the ICU are 183, 195, and 182 mg/dL. HbA_{1c} was 5.5%.

What would be your next step in glucose management of this patient?

A. Initiation of intravenous insulin with glucose target of 140–180 mg/dL
B. Initiation of sliding-scale insulin, with a rapid-acting insulin every 4 hours for fingerstick glucose values above 180 mg/dL
C. Initiation of subcutaneous agonist of the glucagon-like peptide 1 receptor with a target glucose of 80–180 mg/dL
D. Initiation of subcutaneous long-acting basal insulin and titration of dose until glucose values are 80–110 mg/dL
E. Monitoring of fingerstick glucose values every 4 hours only

6. A 55-year-old woman is admitted with a severe headache. She also complains of double vision. On physical exam, her blood pressure is 89/48 mm Hg; her heart rate is 99 beats per minute; and she is afebrile. She is slightly drowsy, and she has partial palsy of left cranial nerves III, IV, and VI. A CT scan of the head shows a large pituitary mass with extension into the left cavernous sinus and with an area of likely hemorrhage. Blood test results have not yet been returned.

What is the best initial treatment for this patient?

A. Bromocriptine 2.5 mg daily
B. Hydrocortisone 50 mg IV every 8 hours
C. Levothyroxine 100 µg orally once daily
D. Urgent surgical resection of the mass
E. Vitamin K 10 mg daily

7. A 31-year-old woman presents with a 5-week history of weight loss and symptomatic palpitations. Laboratory tests demonstrate thyrotoxicosis. She is diagnosed with Graves disease on the basis of clinical findings, including goitrous enlargement of her thyroid, mild proptosis, and periorbital swelling. She is effectively treated with methimazole for 12 months, and then treatment is held to see if she may have entered a state of remission. Laboratory tests checked 2 months after stopping methimazole show thyroid-stimulating hormone (TSH) <0.001 mU/L, free thyroxine (T4) 1.9 ng/dL, T4 12.1 µg/dL, and triiodothyronine (T3) 243 ng/dL. After options for further management are reviewed, the patient elects to proceed with radioactive iodine treatment.

What should you tell her?

A. She should wait until she is 6 months out from treatment before trying to conceive.
B. She will need to be strictly isolated from family members for 2 weeks.
C. She will not have to take any more medication after treatment.
D. The treatment may improve her thyroid eye disease.
E. The treatment should work immediately.

8. A 50-year-old woman with multiple sclerosis was treated for over 1 year with high-dose prednisone. Her prednisone dose was as high as 60 mg daily, and over the course of the last year, as her neurologic symptoms improved, her prednisone dose was decreased gradually and ultimately stopped. Two weeks after her last prednisone dose, she was scheduled for an elective orthopedic surgical procedure.

What empiric hormone treatment should be administered perioperatively?

A. Cosyntropin
B. Dehydroepiandrosterone (DHEA)
C. Epinephrine
D. Fludrocortisone
E. Hydrocortisone

9. A 50-year-old obese woman with a history of gestational diabetes and a family history of diabetes and coronary artery disease was diagnosed with type 2 diabetes during a visit with her primary care physician, at which time she was found to have an HbA_{1c} level of 8.7% on routine screening blood tests. Despite implementing dietary changes under the supervision of a dietitian, engaging in moderate exercise several times

weekly, and complying with treatment with metformin 1000 mg twice daily, her HbA_{1c} remains above target at 7.7%. You wish to add a second medication to intensify her treatment, but she is resistant due to concern for hypoglycemia. You learn that her brother-in-law died after a motor vehicle accident thought to be caused by insulin-induced hypoglycemia.

Which of the following would be the best option for this patient, given the above considerations?

A. Add glipizide
B. Add insulin degludec
C. Add nateglinide
D. Add pioglitazone
E. No change in treatment

10. A 75-year-old man with a remote history of papillary thyroid cancer is diagnosed with metastatic prostate cancer. He undergoes prostate surgery, local radiation, and androgen deprivation therapy. He also receives 4 mg of zoledronic acid intravenously to prevent bone loss. Five days later, he presents to the emergency room with severe paresthesias and muscle cramping. On examination, he has positive Chvostek and Trousseau signs and a well-healed neck scar. Laboratory data include TSH 0.54 μIU/mL (normal), alkaline phosphatase 120 U/L (normal), 25-hydroxyvitamin D 25 ng/mL, serum calcium 6.5 mg/dL (normal 8.6–10.4), albumin 4.0 g/L, and phosphate 6.0 mg/dL.

What is the most likely etiology of the hypocalcemia?

A. Hungry bone syndrome
B. Hypomagnesemia
C. Hypoparathyroidism
D. Osteoblastic bone metastases
E. Vitamin D deficiency

11. A 65-year-old Caucasian woman is noted to have osteopenia on bone mineral density screening. When you calculate her FRAX score, you find that she has a 22% chance of sustaining a major osteoporotic fracture over the next 10 years. According to the National Osteoporosis Foundation, antiresorptive therapy should be considered when the 10-year absolute risk of a major osteoporotic fracture is above what level?

A. 5%
B. 10%
C. 15%
D. 20%
E. 25%

12. A 48-year-old man with a history of obesity and type 2 diabetes mellitus presents with low serum total testosterone. He notes decreased libido and erectile dysfunction. An afternoon total testosterone was 200 ng/dL (normal range 220–1000 ng/dL). On examination, he has a BMI of 34 kg/m^2 but is normally virilized with testicular size of 15 mL bilaterally.

What is the next best step?

A. Karyotyping
B. Measure a morning total testosterone and sex hormone–binding globulin.
C. Pituitary MRI
D. Testicular ultrasound
E. Start testosterone replacement therapy.

13. A 46-year-old previously healthy woman is admitted to the hospital after presenting with lethargy, polyuria, polydipsia, and 2-kg weight loss. On physical examination, her vital signs showed a respiratory rate of 32 breaths per minute, heart rate of 132 beats per minute, blood pressure of 92/50 mm Hg, and temperature of 37.0°C. She is noted to be obese with a BMI of 34 kg/m^2. Her cardiac exam is notable for tachycardia but no murmurs. Her lungs are clear to auscultation bilaterally. Her neurologic exam is normal. Her skin exam shows acanthosis nigricans of the neck and axillae.

Her laboratory tests confirmed diabetic ketoacidosis with glucose 623 mg/dL, bicarbonate 10 mmol/L, and an anion gap of 24 mmol/L. The patient is treated with intravenous normal saline, potassium, and insulin and transitioned to a subcutaneous basal-bolus regimen (NPH insulin 10 U twice daily and insulin lispro 5 U with each meal). The test for GAD65 antibodies was negative.

She returns 4 weeks later to her primary care physician for follow-up. She reports that she has a strong family history of type 2 diabetes in two sisters and both her parents. She has been compliant with the insulin that she was prescribed on discharge, but she has had increasing problems with hypoglycemia, now occurring almost every day. She is frustrated with the frequent injections and also upset that she has gained 2.5 kg since before her admission.

What is the next best step in the treatment of this patient's hyperglycemia?

A. Advise her that she can likely stop insulin therapy; initiate metformin and reduce insulin doses to help achieve this.
B. Advise her that she does not need antidiabetic therapy; stop insulin now and monitor her fingerstick glucose values three times per day.
C. Advise her that she will need lifelong insulin treatment; switch her basal insulin to insulin degludec to reduce hypoglycemic episodes.
D. Advise her that she will need to remain on insulin for the rest of her life and reduce the doses to prevent the frequent hypoglycemic episodes.

14. A 48-year-old woman presents for follow-up of her type 2 diabetes mellitus. She was diagnosed 1 year ago and has been taking metformin, her only medication, since then. She checks fingerstick glucose values at home before breakfast and always has values above 230 mg/dL. She has checked her glucose later in the day only twice over the past month, and her glucose values were 289 mg/dL and 300 mg/dL. A recent HbA_{1c} was 6.5%, and a recent glucose value sent as part of a basic metabolic panel was 274 mg/dL. The remainder of her menstrual history is notable for menorrhagia, a hemithyroidectomy for a benign nodule, and overweight (BMI 28.9 kg/m^2).

What is the best intervention for this patient?

A. Evaluate for mutations of the *HBB* gene.
B. Provide her with a new glucose meter.
C. Provide the patient with a continuous glucose monitor.
D. Reassure her that her HbA_{1c} is at her goal of <7%.
E. Send for a complete blood count.

15. A 55-year-old woman is noted to be tachycardic with a resting pulse of 104 beats per minute during a routine physical examination. Laboratory tests checked to evaluate this show TSH 0.002 mU/L with follow-up laboratory tests showing free T4 2.3 ng/dL, T4 14.7 µg/dL, and T3 289 ng/dL. She denies any history of anterior neck discomfort, weight loss, palpitations, anxiety, tremor, heat intolerance, or insomnia. Physical examination reveals tachycardia with a regular rhythm, a slightly enlarged thyroid without any discrete nodularity, and no evidence of proptosis or ocular irritation. A radioiodine uptake scan shows diffuse uptake consistent with Graves disease. She is started on methimazole with normalization of her thyroid function within 2 months; she is currently taking it at a dose of 5 mg per day without any adverse effects. Eighteen months later, she asks you if she can stop the methimazole because she is concerned about side effects. Her last TSH was 4.1 mU/L.

What do you recommend as the next step?

A. Continue methimazole indefinitely.
B. Measure erythrocyte sedimentation rate (ESR).
C. Refer for radioiodine ablation.
D. Refer to a thyroid surgeon for a thyroidectomy.
E. Stop methimazole.

16. A 22-year-old man presents with headache and peripheral vision loss. Brain imaging reveals a large sellar mass with both solid and cystic components that is compressing the optic chiasm. Humphrey visual field testing demonstrates bitemporal hemianopsia. He has no previous medical history, his BMI is 20 kg/m^2, and he is taking no medications. His initial pituitary functional evaluation revealed central hypogonadism and central hypothyroidism. His adrenal function was normal. MRI characteristics suggested the mass was a craniopharyngioma. He was taken to surgery to remove the pituitary mass in an attempt to decompress the optic chiasm and restore his vision. He did well in the immediate postoperative period, but within 24 hours, he began to develop polyuria. His urine output increased to 400 mL/h with a urine specific gravity <1.001. He complained of extreme thirst. His serum sodium increased to 148 mEq/L, and his fasting glucose was elevated at 106 mg/dL.

What diagnosis are you suspecting in this patient?

A. Central diabetes insipidus
B. Nephrogenic diabetes insipidus
C. Psychogenic polydipsia
D. Syndrome of inappropriate antidiuretic secretion (SIADH)
E. Type 2 diabetes mellitus

17. A 25-year-old woman with hypothyroidism presented to the emergency room complaining of weakness. She was feeling dizzy and lightheaded while out on a hot summer day. In the preceding weeks, her friends had noticed that she had lost weight and was increasingly fatigued during the day. In the emergency room, the patient appeared lethargic and weak. Her sodium was 133 mEq/L, and her potassium was 5.7 mEq/L. At 2:00 p.m., her plasma adrenocorticotropic hormone (ACTH) level was 550 pg/mL (10–60) and serum cortisol was 2.4 µg/dL (2.3–19.4). The patient was given 250 µg of ACTH for a stimulation test, and 60 minutes later her cortisol was 4.1 µg/dL.

What is the most likely diagnosis?

A. Primary adrenal insufficiency
B. Secondary adrenal insufficiency
C. Ectopic ACTH syndrome
D. Cushing disease
E. Cushing syndrome

18. A 56-year-old woman presents complaining of genital discomfort manifesting as daily itching and stinging, with more severe symptoms upon attempted intercourse, including dyspareunia and slight bleeding. Her last menstrual period was 3 years prior. She has hot flashes once or twice per week. A pelvic exam reveals pale vaginal mucosa. The cervix appears normal and a Pap smear was negative for cytologic changes suggestive of cervical cancer. The patient otherwise has a history of atypical hyperplasia of the breast, and her mother had breast cancer.

What is the best management of this patient's climacteric symptoms?

A. Bazedoxifene with conjugated equine estrogens 1 tablet daily
B. Estradiol 10-µg vaginal pill
C. Gabapentin 600 mg PO at bedtime
D. Lubricant with intercourse
E. Weekly estradiol patch with daily medroxyprogesterone acetate

19. A 56-year-old woman presented to the emergency room with right lower quadrant abdominal pain. An abdominal CT scan was performed to evaluate for appendicitis. No abnormal bowel findings or other abnormalities to account for the pain were identified. However, a 1.2-cm adrenal mass was incidentally detected in the medial limb of the left adrenal gland. The mass was described as homogeneous, round, with smooth borders and a lipid-rich density (6 Hounsfield units). She denied any episodic adrenergic symptoms, weight gain, or muscle weakness. She had no history of hypertension, impaired glucose handling, or low bone density.

Which of the following would you advise?

A. Corticotropin stimulation test
B. Dexamethasone suppression test
C. MRI of the adrenal gland
D. No further testing needed
E. Serum catecholamines

20. A 44-year-old man is referred to your clinic for diabetes management. Following a routine screening 6 months ago, he was found to have a fasting glucose level of 129 mg/dL and HbA_{1c} of 6.8%. He was started on metformin 1000 mg twice daily, which was effective for several months in controlling his blood sugar. For the last month, the patient's fasting blood glucose levels have been elevated again at 150–180 mg/dL. After meals, most of his readings are in the 200–300 mg/dL range, and his most recent HbA_{1c} was 8.6%. The patient has no other medical conditions. Blood pressure is 125/76 mm Hg, and body mass index is 23.4 kg/m^2. The rest of the physical examination is unremarkable, with no acanthosis nigricans or skin tag and no other physical exam features of endocrinopathies. Blood tests were significant for HDL cholesterol of 46 mg/dL and fasting triglycerides of 132 mg/dL. The patient has no other family members with diabetes.

How would you further evaluate this patient?

A. Obtain a 24-hour urine collection for cortisol levels.
B. Obtain a serum insulin-like growth factor-1 level.
C. Obtain MRI of the pancreas.
D. Test for maturity-onset diabetes of youth (MODY) mutations.
E. Test for the presence of antiglutamic acid decarboxylase (GAD) antibodies.

21. A 55-year-old Caucasian woman has recently been diagnosed with type 2 diabetes mellitus. Her only past medical history is gastritis treated with *Helicobacter pylori* eradication therapy 3 years ago. Her current medications are metformin and a multivitamin. Her family history is notable for a myocardial infarction in her father at age 83. Physical examination is significant for a body mass index of 27.1 kg/m^2 and blood pressure of 132/84 mm Hg. Her laboratory tests show fasting blood glucose 118 mg/dL, HbA_{1c} 6.3%, total cholesterol 205 mg/dL, low-density lipoprotein (LDL) cholesterol 127 mg/dL, high-density lipoprotein (HDL) cholesterol 46 mg/dL, and triglycerides 165 mg/dL. Although the patient denies chest pain or shortness of breath, she is concerned about her risk of cardiovascular disease and asks you how she can reduce this risk.

Based on the guidelines from the American Diabetes Association, what is the best strategy for cardiovascular risk reduction in this patient?

A. Initiate aspirin 81 mg daily.
B. Initiate rosuvastatin 20 mg daily.
C. Initiate chlorthalidone 25 mg daily.
D. Initiate insulin glargine 10 U at night.
E. Obtain a coronary artery calcium score.

22. A 33-year-old man is noted to have palpable enlargement of the right side of his thyroid on a routine physical examination. A thyroid ultrasound reveals a solitary 3.1-cm right-sided nodule with smooth borders. Laboratory tests show TSH 0.1 mU/L and T4 11.5 μg/dL. He reports a history of occasional symptomatic palpitations and weight loss of 5 lb over the course of 3 months despite an increase in his appetite. He is not taking any medications and has not noted any problems with dysphagia or dysphonia.

What should you do next?

A. Administer a 15 mCi dose of ^{131}I.
B. Obtain a thyroid scan.
C. Perform a fine-needle aspiration biopsy of the right-sided nodule.
D. Refer the patient to a thyroid surgeon.
E. Start methimazole at a dose of 5 mg daily.

23. A 47-year-old woman has a long history of having difficulty losing weight. She has multiple members in her extended family who are overweight but states that her parents and siblings are all of normal weight. She states that she has always struggled to maintain her weight, but in the last 2 years she has gained 20 kg despite exercising daily and watching her caloric intake. She has recently been diagnosed with both type 2 diabetes mellitus and hypertension. Last year, she fell while riding her bicycle, broke her elbow, and was found to have osteoporosis. She reports menarche at age 12 with regular menses until the last year, when they have become increasingly unpredictable. She has been distressed by her weight gain and recently started taking an antidepressant. On physical examination, she is found to be obese with a BMI of 35 kg/m^2, blood pressure of 160/100 mm Hg, and heart rate of 72 beats per minute. She has a very round face with fine, thin hair on her lateral cheeks. She has supraclavicular fat accumulation and multiple pigmented striae on her abdomen. She has several bruises on her lower extremities. You are concerned that she may have Cushing syndrome.

Which of these is an appropriate first-line screening test for hypercortisolism?

A. 8:00 a.m. ACTH level
B. 8:00 a.m. serum cortisol level
C. Overnight 8-mg dexamethasone suppression test
D. Cosyntropin stimulation test
E. Late-night salivary cortisol test

24. A 53-year-old man with a history of acromegaly presented to establish routine care with a primary care provider. He underwent surgical resection of a pituitary macroadenoma 6 years prior to your visit and has been lost to endocrine follow-up.

He has a history of diabetes mellitus, hypertension, and obstructive sleep apnea. He has been feeling poorly the last few months and presents with fatigue, diffuse joint pain, and excessive sweating. He feels his hands and feet have been swollen. He denies headaches or visual changes. His medications include metformin and lisinopril. On examination, he has the classic coarse facial features of acromegaly: enlarged tongue and spaces between his teeth. His blood pressure is 152/80 mm Hg, and his heart rate is 64 beats per minute. His visual fields are normal on confrontation testing. He has multiple skin tags, and his hands are very large and sweaty. The remainder of his examination is unremarkable. Laboratory testing of his pituitary reveals normal thyroid, adrenal, and gonadal function. However, his insulin-like growth factor-1 (IGF-1) and growth hormone (GH) levels are elevated at twice the upper limit of normal. Suspecting recurrence of his acromegaly, you obtain a pituitary MRI, which does not show obvious significant tumor burden. An oral glucose tolerance test performed to assess GH suppression confirms that his acromegaly is not in biochemical remission.

Which of the following is the initial treatment of choice for this patient?

A. Medical therapy with a dopamine agonist
B. Medical therapy with a somatostatin analogue
C. Observation only
D. Radiation therapy to the pituitary
E. Repeat transsphenoidal pituitary tumor resection

25. A 76-year-old woman presenting with a 1-week history of a cough, fever, and audible stridor is diagnosed with community-acquired pneumonia. A chest x-ray does not show evidence of an infiltrate, but it does reveal marked rightward tracheal deviation with a visible mediastinal soft tissue mass. A noncontrast chest CT scan reveals multiple bilateral thyroid nodules with an 8.5-cm left lower pole nodule extending below the clavicle and sternum with compression and narrowing of the trachea. Laboratory tests show TSH <0.001 mU/L, free T4 2.8 ng/dL, T4 12.9 µg/dL, and T3 245 ng/dL. A thyroid uptake and scan reveals 24-hour uptake of 37% with tracer accumulation localized to two right-sided thyroid nodules and the substernal left-sided thyroid nodule.

What is the next appropriate step in management?

A. Administer a 30-mCi dose of ^{131}I.
B. Check pulmonary function tests with flow–volume loops.
C. Refer the patient to a thyroid surgeon.
D. Start levothyroxine at a dose of 137 µg daily.
E. Start methimazole at a dose of 10 mg daily.

26. A 55-year-old man presents to your office as a new patient to establish care after he recently moved to the area. His past medical history is significant for hypertension, which is well controlled with hydrochlorothiazide 25 mg once daily, as well as dyslipidemia treated with atorvastatin 80 mg once daily. He also has a history of type 2 diabetes diagnosed at age 36, which was initially poorly controlled due to difficulty with affording his medications, although his HbA_{1c} has been at goal of 6.5%–7.0% for the past 5 years on metformin 1000 mg twice daily and exenatide once weekly. He also takes aspirin 81 mg daily. He reports that a recent eye exam showed background diabetic retinopathy. He is allergic to lisinopril, which caused a cough; the remainder of his history was unremarkable. His physical exam is notable for blood pressure of 120/70 mm Hg and heart rate 72 beats per minute. He has intact sensation to monofilament and normal ankle jerk reflexes; the remainder of the physical examination is normal. Laboratory data reveal normal electrolytes, serum creatinine 0.8 mg/dL, fasting glucose 140 mg/dL, normal liver function tests, total cholesterol 170 mg/dL, HDL 45 mg/dL, triglycerides 135 mg/dL, LDL 90 mg/dL, and HbA_{1c} 7.2%. A urine test shows a ratio of urine albumin to creatinine of 89 mg/g (normal <30 mg/g). These results are all similar to blood test results obtained by his prior physician 5 months earlier.

What is the best intervention to reduce this patient's risk of developing complications of his diabetes?

A. Initiate therapy with labetalol.
B. Prescribe niacin.
C. Refer for intravitreal injection of bevacizumab.
D. Replace metformin with insulin glargine.
E. Start therapy with telmisartan.

27. A 38-year-old woman is evaluated for progressive shortness of breath, decreased exercise tolerance, and extreme fatigue. Heart and lung examination results are negative, but chest x-ray shows bilateral hilar lymphadenopathy with reticular opacities in the lower lung zones. Routine serum chemistries show serum calcium 11.8 mg/dL, albumin 4.0 g/dL, and intact PTH <10 pg/mL.

Which test is most likely to explain her hypercalcemia?

A. 1,25-dihydroxyvitamin D
B. 24-hour urinary calcium excretion
C. 25-hydroxyvitamin D
D. Parathyroid hormone–related peptide (PTHrP)
E. Technetium-99m bone scan

28. A 19-year-old man with an unremarkable medical history presents because of delayed puberty. His height is 171.5 cm, arm span is 178 cm, and weight is 92 kg. On physical examination, he has Tanner stage 1 pubic hair, gynecomastia, and small testes. Sense of smell is intact. He has no history of testicular injury or mumps orchitis. Laboratory evaluation shows total testosterone 88 ng/dL (normal 220–1000; confirmed by repeat testing), LH 30 mU/mL (normal 1.7–8.6), FSH 32 mIU/mL (normal 1.5–12.4), normal prolactin, and HbA_{1c} 6.6%.

What other testing would be warranted?

A. Echocardiogram
B. Ferritin, iron/total iron-binding capacity
C. Karyotyping
D. Pituitary MRI
E. Renal ultrasound

29. A 35-year-old Asian American man with history of advanced melanoma was diagnosed with panhypopituitarism secondary to ipilimumab-related hypophysitis. His biochemical testing included an undetectable total testosterone level and very low LH and FSH levels. You start him on testosterone replacement therapy with a daily topical gel. Three months later, he returns for follow-up and feels greatly improved.

What tests are recommended?

A. Hematocrit
B. LH
C. Liver function tests
D. Prolactin
E. Prostate-specific antigen (PSA)

30. A 45-year-old woman presents to the clinic for her annual examination. She is doing well overall but reports new-onset fatigue, constipation, and a 3-kg weight gain over the last year. She attributes these to work-related stress. On further questioning, she reports oligomenorrhea. Her mother went through menopause at the age of 50, and the patient believes she may be perimenopausal. Laboratory results show the following: sodium 130 mEq/L, potassium 3.5 mEq/L, creatinine 0.80 mg/dL, glucose 90 mg/dL, FSH 5.7 IU/L, TSH 60 (mIU/L), prolactin 35 ng/mL, total cholesterol 276 mg/dL, HDL 47 mg/dL, and LDL 169 mg/dL.

What is the best treatment option for this patient?

A. 1 liter fluid restriction
B. Treatment with a statin
C. Treatment with cabergoline
D. Treatment with levothyroxine
E. Treatment with menopausal hormone replacement therapy

31. A 44-year-old man is referred to your clinic for the management of type 2 diabetes. This was diagnosed 3 years prior and has been treated with metformin and nutrition referral. The patient lost 4 kg by dieting with the help of a smartphone app; despite this, his HbA_{1c} values have remained in the 7.2%–8.1% range; the most recent value was 7.6%, and his recent fasting fingerstick glucose values have been in the range of 130–150 mg/dL. Past medical history is significant for obesity (body mass index 31.2 kg/m^2) and asthma; he has no complications of his diabetes. He is not taking any medications other than metformin, with which he is compliant. Liver and kidney function are normal. He wishes to improve his glucose control, but it is important for him that he does not regain any of the weight that he lost.

What would be the next best step in the management of this patient's hyperglycemia?

A. Initiate glipizide 5 mg twice daily.
B. Initiate insulin glargine 10 U at bedtime.
C. Initiate linagliptin 5 mg daily.
D. Initiate pioglitazone 30 mg daily.
E. Initiate repaglinide 0.5 mg before each meal.

32. A 54-year-old man who was previously healthy is being worked up for weakness and generalized body aches, progressively worsening over 10 months. He denies any change in food intake or bowel habits. Other than acetaminophen, he has not taken any medications. He does not smoke or consume alcohol. Physical examination was remarkable for bony tenderness throughout. A plain x-ray of a particularly painful right humerus showed severe osteopenia and metaphysial changes consistent with osteomalacia. Laboratory testing found phosphorus of 0.9 mg/dL (reference range 3.5–5.0 mg/dL), alkaline phosphatase 234 IU/L, 25-hydroxyvitamin D 35 ng/mL, and normal basic metabolic panel and complete blood count.

Which of the following laboratory tests is most likely to be elevated?

A. 1,25-dihydroxyvitamin D
B. 24-hour urine calcium
C. Calcitonin
D. Fibroblast growth factor 23 (FGF23)
E. Intact PTH

33. A 28-year-old woman presents to clinic with new-onset amenorrhea of 6 months' duration. She had menarche at the age of 13. She has had normal 28-day menstrual cycles for the majority of her life until approximately 6 months ago. She specifically denies acne, hirsutism, galactorrhea, headaches, visual changes, and heat or cold intolerance. She does, however, report that she has recently started running competitively and is currently training for her third marathon. She reports that after experiencing a stress fracture during training for her second marathon, she was disappointed by her marathon results. She is now following a calorie-restricted diet and training 6 days per week to improve her results at an upcoming marathon.

What is the most likely etiology of this patient's secondary amenorrhea?

A. Cushing disease
B. Hyperprolactinemia
C. Hypothalamic amenorrhea
D. PCOS
E. Pregnancy

34. A 74-year-old man with metastatic prostate cancer developed weakness of his legs and incontinence. Imaging studies revealed metastatic foci of cancer in his spine with evidence of spinal cord compression. He was started on dexamethasone 2 mg every 6 hours to reduce spinal cord edema, and radiation therapy was initiated. The following day, he experienced transient tachycardia and lightheadedness with mild orthostatic hypotension. A morning cortisol level was 0.5 μg/dL.

What is the best interpretation of this cortisol value?

A. Primary adrenal insufficiency
B. Secondary adrenal insufficiency due to metastatic lesion to the pituitary
C. Secondary adrenal insufficiency due to radiation therapy
D. This cortisol value cannot be adequately interpreted.

35. A 62-year-old man with a history of poorly controlled type 2 diabetes is hospitalized for treatment of acute pyelonephritis after presenting with a 5-day history of fever, dysuria, and left-sided flank pain. Blood cultures obtained on admission grow *Escherichia coli.* Laboratory tests checked on intake reveal TSH 0.22 mU/L, T4 3.1 μg/dL, and T3 64 ng/dL. He is treated with broad-spectrum intravenous antibiotics with minimal improvement. An abdominal CT scan checked 6 days after admission reveals findings consistent with a left-sided perinephric abscess that requires management with percutaneous drainage. The patient is discharged to a rehabilitation facility 23 days after admission and has laboratory tests checked on intake that show TSH 16.4 mU/L. His current weight is 218 lb. What would you recommend?

A. Obtain a pituitary MRI scan.
B. Obtain a thyroid uptake and scan.
C. Start levothyroxine 50 μg daily.
D. Start liothyronine 5 μg twice daily.
E. Wait 6 weeks and recheck a full profile of thyroid hormone levels.

36. A 61-year-old man who has a history of a nonfunctioning pituitary macroadenoma presents for routine follow-up. He underwent surgical resection a number of years ago for a large tumor and has had no evidence of recurrence. He has hypopituitarism and is on hormone replacement therapy for hypothyroidism, adrenal insufficiency, and hypogonadism. He takes levothyroxine, hydrocortisone, and a topical testosterone gel. He returns for routine follow-up. He denies headaches or visual changes. He complains of fatigue and inability to lose weight. He has noted very dry skin but attributes it to the weather. He denies tremor, palpitations, insomnia, or change in bowel movements, although he tends toward constipation. He denies sexual dysfunction. On physical examination, he has gained 2.5 kg since his last visit. His blood pressure is 126/82 mm Hg, and his pulse is 76 beats per minute. He does not have lid lag, and his visual fields by confrontation are normal. His neurologic examination is otherwise normal. No tremor is noted. He does not look cushingoid. His thyroid function tests show the following: TSH 0.1 mIU/L (normal 0.5–5 mIU/L) and free T4 0.6 ng/dL (normal 0.9–1.7 ng/dL).

What adjustments should be made to his levothyroxine dose?

A. Decrease levothyroxine dose.
B. Discontinue levothyroxine completely.
C. Increase levothyroxine dose.
D. No change; continue current levothyroxine dose.

37. A 78-year-old woman is seen for type 2 diabetes diagnosed over 25 years ago. She also has hypertension and had an anterior wall myocardial infarction diagnosed 2 years ago. A recent eye examination is significant for a mild nonproliferative diabetic retinopathy, which has been stable for many years. She has no evidence of any other diabetes-related complications. For the last 5 years, her HbA_{1c} has been consistently around 6.5%. She is treated with metformin, liraglutide, and 22 U of insulin glargine once daily. Following her repeated episodes of asymptomatic hypoglycemia as low as 39 mg/dL, you have decreased her insulin dose to 18 U. She has come today to review her blood glucose readings. Morning glucose levels are between 90 and 125 mg/dL, and before lunch and dinner, her glucose levels range between 125 and 165 mg/dL. She has had no hypoglycemic events since the adjustment of the insulin dose. However, her HbA_{1c} has increased to 7.4%. The patient is concerned about the recent increase in HbA_{1c}, and she would like to optimize her regimen to meet treatment goals.

What is the best next step in management of this patient's diabetes?

A. Add glyburide.
B. Discontinue liraglutide and start insulin aspart with her meals.
C. Increase insulin glargine.
D. No further adjustment of her regimen.
E. Provide the patient with a continuous glucose-monitoring device.

38. A 45-year-old man with a history of dyslipidemia was recently found to have an HbA_{1c} of 6.3% on routine screening blood tests. He has no known history of heart disease but has a strong family history of premature coronary artery disease. His only medications are aspirin 81 mg daily and atorvastatin 80 mg daily. The patient states that he tries to eat a healthy diet but admits to eating large portion sizes. His wife feels that there is certainly much room for improvement as far as the patient's diet. He exercises on a treadmill for 20–30 minutes twice weekly. He is overweight and reports that his weight has been stable for many years.

The patient feels well overall and has no specific complaints today.

On examination, his blood pressure was 126/78 mm Hg, heart rate was 70 beats per minute, and BMI was 27 kg/m^2. His physical examination was otherwise unremarkable. You obtain screening laboratory tests; the results show a fasting blood glucose level of 110 mg/dL, and a repeat HbA_{1c} is 6.2%. In addition, you receive copies of his old medical records, which indicate that his HbA_{1c} was 6% about 1 year ago.

What would you recommend as the first step in the treatment of this patient's dysglycemia?

A. Dietary/lifestyle interventions
B. Start metformin.
C. Start insulin therapy.
D. Start a dipeptidyl peptidase-4 (DPP-4) inhibitor.

39. A 50-year-old man presents with a wrist fracture after a minor fall. He is generally in good health other than a history of irritable bowel syndrome and some weight loss. He takes 1200 mg calcium and 800 IU vitamin D_3 daily because his mother had osteoporosis. Bone mineral density measurement shows a T-score of −2.5 at the hip and −3.0 at the 1/3 distal radius of the nonfractured wrist. On examination, he has a scaly skin rash on his arms and trunk. Laboratory test results reveal serum calcium 8.7 mg/dL, 25-hydroxyvitamin D 24 ng/dL, intact PTH 120 pg/mL, and 24-hour urine calcium excretion of 38 mg with creatinine 1000 mg.

What intervention is most likely to improve his skeletal health?

A. Doubling his calcium intake to 2400 mg daily
B. Doubling his vitamin D intake to 1600 IU daily
C. Oral alendronate 70 mg weekly
D. Parathyroidectomy
E. Starting a gluten-free diet

40. A 28-year-old man presents for evaluation of infertility. His serum LH, FSH, and testosterone levels are all normal. Semen analysis reveals azoospermia.

Which of the following gene mutations is most likely related to the above findings?

A. *CFTR* gene
B. *FGFR1* gene
C. *KAL1* gene
D. *KISS1* gene
E. *TAC3* gene

41. A 40-year-old woman presents to the clinic for new-onset amenorrhea of 12 months' duration. She has two children and had previously had regular 28-day menstrual cycles for her reproductive life. Her mother went through menopause at the age of 50, and she is concerned that she is now going through early menopause. On further questioning, she reports a 10-kg weight gain over the last year. She also reports new-onset fatigue and has found it difficult to keep up with her children. She had no previous history of headaches, but over the last 6 months, she has noted several episodes of headaches. On examination, her BMI is 31 kg/m^2, and she has a round, plethoric face with supraclavicular fullness. She has evidence of abdominal striae. She has no expressible galactorrhea.

Which laboratory test would most likely help determine the cause of this woman's secondary amenorrhea?

A. 24-hour urine free cortisol
B. HbA_{1c}
C. LH-to-FSH ratio
D. Serum prolactin
E. TSH, FT4

42. A 45-year-old woman had a 5-year history of hypertension and anxiety. She was treated with lisinopril and venlafaxine. She reports a new increase in anxiety along with palpitations in the preceding 5 weeks, and her blood pressure has been trending higher than usual at approximately 145/80 mm Hg (typically 135–140/80 mm Hg). She has been under a lot of pressure at work, which has heightened her anxiety. She denies any illicit drug use. Plasma metanephrines were ordered and revealed plasma metanephrines <0.20 nmol/L (0–0.49) and plasma normetanephrines 1.6 nmol/L (0–0.89).

What is the most likely cause of the elevated normetanephrine levels in this patient?

A. Extraadrenal paraganglioma
B. Lisinopril use
C. Methamphetamine use
D. Pheochromocytoma
E. Venlafaxine use

43. A 55-year-old man with type 2 diabetes mellitus, coronary artery disease, hypertension, dyslipidemia, and obesity returns for follow-up after a recent hospitalization for an acute myocardial infarction. He was diagnosed with diabetes 5 years ago and was treated initially with metformin alone and subsequently a combination of metformin 1000 mg twice daily and glipizide 10 mg twice daily. Although he reports compliance with his medications, his HbA_{1c} at the time of his hospital admission was 9.1%. He was discharged to home on a regimen of insulin glargine 40 U once daily, insulin aspart 10 U before each meal, and metformin 1000 mg twice daily. He has been monitoring his glucose levels at home and has worked with a pharmacist in your clinic to optimize his insulin dose; he is currently taking insulin glargine 80 U twice daily and aspart 30 U with each meal using insulin pens. His fingerstick glucose values at home are in the 200s at all times, and his HbA_{1c} has decreased to 8.6%.

What is the most appropriate treatment of his hyperglycemia at this point?

A. Add a DPP-4 inhibitor such as sitagliptin.
B. Add quick-release bromocriptine.
C. Increase the dose of insulin glargine and insulin aspart by 15%.
D. Switch from glargine to NPH insulin.
E. Switch to regular insulin, U-500.

44. A 74-year-old woman is complaining of left hip pain for the past year, which has been progressively worsening. She denies early morning stiffness, fevers, chills, weight loss, or trauma. On physical examination, her left hip has intact range of motion with no pain on active or passive range of motion. Routine laboratory work reveals an elevated alkaline phosphatase of 205 IU/L and a 25-hydroxyvitamin D level of 32 ng/mL; the remainder of her laboratory panel was normal, including calcium, phosphate, creatinine, γ-glutamyltransferase, and aminotransferases. A plain x-ray of the hip and pelvis shows patchy areas of osteolysis with multifocal sclerotic patches of the left hemipelvis, including near the hip joint. A bone scan shows uptake of radiotracer in the pelvic lesion.

Which of the following is the best management strategy at this time?
A. Monitor alkaline phosphatase levels with no treatment unless it exceeds 400 IU/L.
B. Prescribe alendronate 70 mg by mouth once weekly.
C. Prescribe salmon calcitonin, 50 units subcutaneously once daily.
D. Refer for zoledronic acid infusion 5 mg intravenously.

45. A 68-year-old woman presents for follow-up after her first bone mineral density (BMD) scan showed osteoporosis, with T-scores of –2.6 at the lumbar spine and –2.4 at the femoral neck. She has had no fractures and no other relevant past medical history. She underwent menarche at age 11 and menopause at age 49, with normal menstrual cycles throughout her life except during her two pregnancies. Her physical examination was normal with no features of endocrinopathies, no kyphosis or spinal tenderness, and normal dentition.

Which of the following laboratory tests is indicated at this time?
A. 24-hour urine free cortisol
B. Complete blood count
C. Insulin-like growth factor-1 (IGF-1)
D. Serum protein electrophoresis
E. Tryptase

46. A 55-year-old man had an abdominal CT scan to evaluate the source of abdominal pain. No acute abnormalities to explain his abdominal pain were found, and his pain spontaneously resolved. However, a 3-cm adrenal mass was noted in his left adrenal gland. The mass was described as round, without calcifications, and with a very lipid-rich density (–50 Hounsfield units). He had a normal blood pressure and denied any episodic adrenergic symptoms, weight gain, muscle weakness, alopecia, or abnormal hair growth. He denied melena or blood in his stools, and he had recently had a normal colonoscopy and prostate-specific antigen test. He had smoked one pack of cigarettes per day for more than 25 years, but he denied cough, bloody sputum, shortness of breath, or fever.

What is the most likely diagnosis?
A. Adrenal adenoma
B. Adrenal carcinoma
C. Adrenal myelolipoma
D. Adrenal pheochromocytoma
E. Lung cancer metastases to the adrenal gland

47. A 74-year-old man with a history of hypertension and hypercholesterolemia is hospitalized after presenting with a 3-month history of progressive fatigue and dyspnea on exertion. His weight on admission is 74 kg; his pulse is 44 beats per minute; and laboratory tests show creatine phosphokinase (CPK) 528 U/L, TSH 65 mU/L, free T4 0.2 ng/dL, and T4 2.3 μg/dL. A pharmacologic nuclear stress test reveals findings consistent with diffuse ischemia. Subsequent coronary angiography reveals diffuse three-vessel disease that is not amenable to percutaneous stenting. A consulting cardiologist has recommended that he undergo coronary artery bypass surgery.

What would you recommend?
A. Administer 70 μg of levothyroxine intravenously once daily.
B. Check antithyroid peroxidase and antithyroglobulin antibodies.
C. Defer further evaluation and treatment until after he has undergone revascularization.
D. Start levothyroxine at a dose of 25 μg daily.
E. Start liothyronine 5 μg three times daily.

48. A 27-year-old woman presents with a 3-month history of amenorrhea. She reports menarche at age 12 and regular menses. She states she is healthy and denies other medical problems; she takes no medications. She denies galactorrhea. She is not currently talking any medications except a birth control pill. She noted a 10-pound weight gain over the last 6 months and occasionally feels cold. She attributes the weight gain to dietary changes and lack of exercise. Her examination is unremarkable, except that she had expressible galactorrhea on breast examination. A prolactin level is ordered and comes back elevated at 52 ng/dL (normal <22 ng/dL); her TSH level was normal at 3.1 mU/L.

In addition to repeating the prolactin test, what is the next test that should be ordered in this patient?
A. Humphrey visual field testing
B. Pelvic ultrasound
C. Pituitary MRI
D. Serum dopamine level
E. Urine pregnancy test

49. A 28-year-old woman with a 6-year history of hypothyroidism due to Hashimoto thyroiditis is treated with levothyroxine at a dose of 125 μg daily; her last TSH was 1.6 mIU/L. She is currently planning pregnancy and is asking for your advice about management of her hypothyroidism in this setting.

How do you advise her?

A. Increase the dose of levothyroxine to 137 μg while attempting pregnancy.
B. Increase the dose of levothyroxine to nine pills per week once she is pregnant.
C. Obtain monthly TSH levels until she is pregnant.
D. Recommend fetal thyroid ultrasound.
E. Switch from levothyroxine to a preparation of combined T4 and T3.

50. A 35-year-old woman with a history of regular menses presents with complaints of bilateral galactorrhea. She notes that her menses have been more irregular over the last year and that her last menstrual period was approximately 6 weeks ago. She reports occasional headaches but otherwise feels well. She does not take any medications or herbal supplements. Laboratory testing reveals a negative pregnancy test, TSH 2.2 mIU/L, and prolactin of 360 ng/mL. You suspect a prolactinoma and order a pituitary MRI, which reveals a 10-mm × 12-mm pituitary lesion. There is no cavernous sinus invasion or compression of the optic nerves by the pituitary tumor.

What is the initial treatment of choice?

A. Medical therapy with a dopamine agonist
B. Medical therapy with a somatostatin analogue
C. Observation only
D. Radiation therapy to the pituitary
E. Transsphenoidal pituitary tumor resection

Chapter 5 Answers

1. ANSWER: D. Metformin therapy is contraindicated on the basis of renal dysfunction.

Learning objective: Determine suitability of metformin therapy in a patient on the basis of comorbidities.

The first-line treatment for most patients with type 2 diabetes is metformin. However, there is a concern of using metformin in patients with decreased glomerular filtration rate (GFR) due to the potential for lactic acidosis. The Food and Drug Administration (FDA) recently changed the label information for metformin-containing products. Prior recommendations considered metformin contraindicated in men and women with serum creatinine concentrations ≥1.5 and ≥1.4 mg/dL, respectively. The new recommendation suggests that metformin use is safe in patients with an estimated GFR as low as 30 mL/min/1.73 m^2. However, the FDA recommends against initiating metformin in patients whose estimated GFR is below 45 mL/min/1.73 m^2. This recommendation is also endorsed by the American Diabetes Association (ADA) and the European Association for the Study of Diabetes. In this elderly woman, the estimated GFR ranges from 17 to 41 mL/min/1.73 m^2, depending on the calculation used. It is therefore not appropriate to start metformin in this patient at any dose. Her heart failure appears stable, with no evidence of decompensation, and therefore it is not a contraindication. In this patient, lifestyle interventions alone are appropriate because recent diabetes guidelines suggest that less-stringent HbA_{1c} goals (such as <8%) may be appropriate for patients with a limited life expectancy.

Lipska KJ, Bailey CJ, Inzucchi SE. Use of metformin in the setting of mild-to-moderate renal insufficiency. *Diabetes Care.* 2011;34(6):1431–1437.

2. ANSWER: B. Alendronate 70 mg orally weekly

Learning objective: Choose appropriate therapies to improve bone strength in a patient with primary hyperparathyroidism who is refusing parathyroidectomy.

This patient has osteoporosis and therefore meets criteria for parathyroid surgery. However, because she refuses surgery, there is no reason to proceed with imaging procedures to localize an adenoma. Similarly, a 24-hour urine test will not change management if she refuses surgery. Cinacalcet will reduce both serum calcium and PTH levels but does not improve bone mineral density (BMD) in patients with primary hyperparathyroidism. Annual monitoring would be appropriate in the absence of already established osteoporosis. Given that primary hyperparathyroidism is associated with bone loss and increased fracture risk, the best answer is to treat the patient with an antiresorptive agent for osteoporosis, such as alendronate. She should, however, be advised that recent data show much better results with surgical management of primary hyperparathyroidism compared with treatment with antiresorptive agents.

Marcocci C, Bollerslev J, Khan AA, Shoback DM. Medical management of primary hyperparathyroidism: Proceedings of the fourth international workshop on the management of asymptomatic primary hyperparathyroidism. *J Clin Endocrinol Metab.* 2014;99(10):3607–3618.

3. ANSWER: E. Start spironolactone.

Learning objective: Select appropriate treatment for hirsutism in PCOS.

Although there are several different treatment strategies for PCOS, the best treatment strategy should be tailored to the patient's presenting symptoms and goals. This patient is not interested in pregnancy and is most concerned about symptoms of hirsutism. Although metformin and weight loss may eventually help ameliorate her symptoms, they are unlikely to help in the short term. After 6 months of treatment on an oral contraceptive, it is unlikely that continued treatment would provide further improvement. Spironolactone, an antiandrogenic agent, has been shown to help with hirsutism. However, it has teratogenic effects and should be used in conjunction with an oral contraceptive in young women of reproductive age.

Legro RS, Arslanian SA, Ehrmann DA, et al. Diagnosis and treatment of polycystic ovary syndrome: an Endocrine Society clinical practice guideline. *J Clin Endocrinol Metab.* 2013;98(12):4565–4592.

4. ANSWER: B. Insufficient information to confirm a diagnosis

Learning objective: Identify medications that interfere with testing for primary hyperaldosteronism.

This patient's progressive and resistant hypertension and newly worsening hypokalemia both likely suggest that he has underlying primary hyperaldosteronism. However, there is insufficient information at this time to confirm that diagnosis. The initial screening test for hyperaldosteronism involves obtaining a serum aldosterone level and plasma renin activity together. These should be considered in the following settings: moderate to severe or resistant hypertension, spontaneous or diuretic-induced hypokalemia in hypertensive individuals, and when there is hypertension in the setting of an incidentally discovered adrenal mass. An aldosterone-to-renin ratio (ARR) that is greater than at least 20–30 should be considered as a positive screen for primary hyperaldosteronism that requires further confirmatory testing (for example, a salt/saline suppression test). It is expected that in addition to a high ARR, the plasma renin activity will also be very low or suppressed in primary hyperaldosteronism as the expected physiologic response to the volume retention induced by the high aldosterone levels.

Many antihypertensive medications alter the function of the renin-angiotensin-aldosterone system; therefore, the patient's medications must be carefully considered before interpreting the ARR. Spironolactone, a mineralocorticoid inhibitor, functions to inhibit the negative feedback of aldosterone on renin release and therefore will cause a rise in plasma renin activity. This patient has an ARR <20 and unsuppressed plasma renin activity, both of which are more consistent with secondary hyperaldosteronism and likely reflect the effect of spironolactone. Therefore, to obtain a reliable screening ARR to diagnose primary hyperaldosteronism, spironolactone should be stopped and substituted for another medication to control blood pressure that does not interfere with the ARR (such as an alpha-antagonist), and measurement of ARR should be repeated after several weeks.

Funder JW, Carey RM, Fardella C, et al. Case detection, diagnosis, and treatment of patients with primary aldosteronism: an Endocrine Society clinical practice guideline. *J Clin Endocrinol Metab.* 2008;93(9):3266–3281.

5. ANSWER: A. Initiation of intravenous insulin with glucose target of 140–180 mg/dL

Learning objective: Determine appropriate targets and management strategies for hyperglycemia in inpatients.

The current standards of care and guidelines, including the American Diabetes Association guidelines published in 2012 for the medical care of patients with diabetes, recommend that in critically ill patients in the hospital, insulin therapy be initiated for the treatment of persistent hyperglycemia starting at a threshold of no greater than 180 mg/dL, and once insulin therapy is started, a glucose range of 140–180 mg/dL is recommended for the majority of these patients. The optimal target range is a topic that has been debated. Van den Berghe et al. conducted the first prospective randomized trial comparing tight blood glucose control (target 80–110 mg/dL) with intensive insulin therapy with conventional blood glucose control (180–200 mg/dL) in critically ill surgical patients. In this study, which included over 1500 patients, 63% of whom had undergone cardiac surgery before ICU admission, researchers found that tight blood glucose control resulted in a significant reduction in mortality (10.6% with intensive treatment vs. 20.2% with conventional treatment, $p = .005$) in patients who required ≥5 days of ICU care with multiorgan failure and sepsis. In addition, cardiac surgical mortality was reduced in those patients requiring ≥5 days of ICU care with other conditions. After this study, for a while, it was widely accepted that tight blood glucose control (80–110 mg/dL) is better than conventional control in surgery or in the ICU. However, since then, several randomized trials have failed to show a benefit of tight blood glucose control with intensive insulin therapy, and authors of a meta-analysis of 29 randomized studies focusing on the benefits and risks of tight glucose control (very tight ≤110 mg/dL or moderately tight <150 mg/dL) in critically ill adult patients concluded that tight glucose control was not associated with significantly reduced hospital mortality but was associated with an increased risk of hypoglycemia. In addition, a recent large prospective randomized multicenter trial (the NICE-SUGAR study) demonstrated that intensive blood glucose control with a target of 81–108 mg/dL increased mortality among adults in the ICU compared with conventional blood glucose control with a target of ≤180 mg/dL. Therefore, although stricter glycemic control (110–140 mg/dL) may be appropriate in selected patients if it can be achieved without significant hypoglycemia, on the basis of currently available evidence and guidelines, maintaining a blood glucose target between 140 and

180 mg/dL would be the appropriate/recommended target for this patient. The patient will need to be transitioned to a subcutaneous insulin regimen before the intravenous insulin infusion is discontinued, but he may be discharged on no antidiabetic agents or on an oral regimen only.

Subcutaneous insulin regimens are not recommended in critically ill patients, owing to the many variables that impact blood glucose levels, including hypermetabolic neurohormonal stress responses in the setting of critical illness/surgery, the patient's nutritional status (e.g., taking nothing or very little by mouth), potential requirement for pressors, and so forth. In this setting, a continuous intravenous infusion of insulin yields better blood glucose control and is the optimum and recommended method for management of hyperglycemia. Glucagon-like peptide 1 receptor agonists are not recommended in critically ill patients.

NICE-SUGAR Investigators. Intensive versus conventional glucose control in critically ill patients. *N Engl J Med.* 2009;360(13):1283–1297.

6. ANSWER: B: Hydrocortisone 50 mg IV every 8 hours

Learning objective: Recognize and treat pituitary apoplexy.

This patient has pituitary apoplexy: ischemia and/or hemorrhage into the pituitary gland. It may occur in a normal gland, but often it occurs in a gland that is abnormal due to a preexisting adenoma or diffuse enlargement such as that seen in pregnancy. She is at high risk for central adrenal insufficiency, and she is hypotensive. She should therefore be given a glucocorticoid such as hydrocortisone as soon as possible (ideally after blood has been drawn for cortisol and adrenocorticotropic hormone [ACTH]). Bromocriptine is appropriate management for a prolactinoma but is not indicated in the emergent management of pituitary apoplexy. The patient may have central hypothyroidism, but this does not manifest for several days, owing to the long half-life of thyroxine, and therefore treatment with levothyroxine is not indicated at this point. The patient may require surgical resection, but empiric treatment for adrenal insufficiency is more important at this point. Although the patient had hemorrhage into the pituitary gland, there is no indication that she is coagulopathic and therefore no indication for vitamin K administration.

Rajasekaran S, Vanderpump M, Baldeweg S, et al. UK guidelines for the management of pituitary apoplexy. *Clin Endocrinol (Oxf).* 2011;74(1):9–20.

7. ANSWER: A. She should wait until she is 6 months out from treatment before trying to conceive.

Learning objective: Counsel a patient on the risks and benefits of radioactive iodine treatment for Graves disease.

Pregnancy should be delayed until at least 6 months after radioactive iodine treatment to minimize the risk of fetal exposure. Patients treated with radioactive iodine need to take some precautions to avoid exposing family members to excreted ^{131}I for the first 2–4 days after treatment, but strict, prolonged isolation is not necessary. Radioactive iodine treatment may exacerbate thyroid eye disease. Pretreatment with glucocorticoids may help minimize this risk in patients with moderate to severe changes. Most patients with Graves disease who are treated with radioactive iodine will progress to develop postablative hypothyroidism that will require treatment with levothyroxine replacement. It may take up to 2–6 months to see the full effects of treatment after administration of a dose of radioactive iodine.

American Thyroid Association Taskforce on Radioiodine Safety. Radiation safety in the treatment of patients with thyroid diseases by radioiodine ^{131}I: practice recommendations of the American Thyroid Association. *Thyroid.* 2011;21(4):335–346.

8. ANSWER: E. Hydrocortisone

Learning objective: Implement empiric steroid treatment in a patient at high risk of adrenal insufficiency.

The patient has recently ceased use of chronic glucocorticoids. She likely still has an element of chronic secondary adrenal insufficiency. Exogenous glucocorticoids suppress pituitary ACTH release and thereby cause a decline in adrenal cortisol production. With chronic glucocorticoid therapy and chronic ACTH inhibition, endogenous ACTH and cortisol production may require many days, weeks, or even months to normalize following the cessation of glucocorticoid therapy. It is for this reason that glucocorticoids are typically tapered gradually after prolonged use. Although exogenous prednisone use in this patient likely resulted in ACTH suppression and thereby cortisol deficiency, the stimulation and production of endogenous adrenal mineralocorticoids remain intact secondary to stimulation by the renin-angiotensin system and potassium. Therefore, this patient should receive empiric hydrocortisone therapy to prevent precipitating an adrenal crisis in the setting of the physiologic stress of surgery. She does not need treatment for mineralocorticoid deficiency (with agents such as fludrocortisone), androgen deficiency (with DHEA), or catecholamine deficiency (epinephrine). A preoperative assessment of the patient's adrenal function with a baseline morning cortisol level followed by a stimulation test with synthetic ACTH (cosyntropin) would also be reasonable, but these should be done several days in advance of the surgery and not perioperatively.

Oelkers W. Adrenal insufficiency. *N Engl J Med.* 1996;335(16):1206–1212.

9. ANSWER: D. Add pioglitazone

Learning objective: Select appropriate antidiabetic treatment to avoid hypoglycemia when metformin monotherapy has failed.

This patient's HbA_{1c} of 7.7% is still higher than goal (<7%) despite her maximum efforts with lifestyle interventions and metformin, and therefore adding a second agent would be indicated. Of the choices provided, given this patient's concerns for hypoglycemia, pioglitazone (a thiazolidinedione) would be the best option because all the other agents can cause hypoglycemia. Glipizide, a sulfonylurea, and nateglinide, a meglitinide, both act on the beta-cells of the pancreas to stimulate insulin release, whereas insulin degludec is a long-acting insulin.

Inzucchi SE, Bergenstal RM, Buse JB, et al. Management of hyperglycemia in type 2 diabetes, 2015: a patient-centered approach: update to a position statement of the American Diabetes Association and the European Association for the Study of Diabetes. *Diabetes Care.* 2015;38(1):140–149.

10. ANSWER: C. Hypoparathyroidism

Learning objective: Distinguish between causes of hypocalcemia on the basis of other laboratory findings.

Osteoblastic bone metastases from prostate cancer can lead to hypocalcemia from deposition of calcium in the bone metastases, particularly in patients with widespread disease along with calcium and vitamin D deficiencies. This patient has a normal alkaline phosphatase and no evidence of widely metastatic disease. His vitamin D, though on the low end, should not result in this degree of hypocalcemia. Hungry bone syndrome generally presents after surgical cure of hyperparathyroidism and would result in both hypocalcemia and hypophosphatemia because both electrolytes are rapidly deposited into previously unmineralized bone. Hypomagnesemia can lead to functional hypoparathyroidism, but there is nothing in the history to suggest that this patient would be at risk for low magnesium. The most likely etiology is hypoparathyroidism resulting from previous thyroid cancer surgery. Patients with decreased parathyroid reserve may manifest overt hypocalcemia when given a potent antiresorptive agent such as zoledronic acid or denosumab for osteoporosis or cancer. In this situation, the sudden loss of calcium resorption from bone and inadequate PTH response can lead to profound hypocalcemia and hyperphosphatemia, as seen in this case.

Shoback D. Hypoparathyroidism. *N Engl J Med.* 2008;359 (4):391–403.

11. ANSWER: D. 20%

Learning objective: Initiate antiresorptive therapy in patients with osteopenia based on current guidelines.

Though the risk of a major osteoporotic fracture (spine, forearm, hip, or shoulder fractures) is highest in those with osteoporosis by bone mineral density criteria (T-score below −2.5), most fractures occur in patients with osteopenia because the prevalence of osteopenia in the population is much higher. As a result, several clinical prediction rules have been developed to identify those patients with osteopenia at highest risk of fractures, who would presumably benefit the most from therapy. The most validated risk prediction tool is the FRAX calculator, which gives the 10-year absolute risk of major osteoporotic fractures and of hip fractures. The current recommendation in the United States is to initiate therapy in osteopenic individuals when the risk of a major osteoporotic fracture exceeds 20% or when the risk of a hip fracture exceeds 3%.

Cosman F, de Beur SJ, LeBoff MS, et al. Clinician's guide to prevention and treatment of osteoporosis. *Osteoporos Int.* 2014;25(10):2359–2381.

12. ANSWER: B. Measure a morning total testosterone and sex hormone–binding globulin.

Learning objective: Choose diagnostic tests for male hypogonadism.

The diagnosis of male hypogonadism requires measurement of early-morning serum total testosterone levels. A low value should be confirmed by repeating the measurement along with a serum sex hormone–binding globulin (SHBG) level. Men with obesity and type 2 diabetes mellitus often have low SHBG, resulting in low total testosterone but normal "free" ("biologically active") testosterone levels. Because the reliability of "free testosterone" assays varies greatly, it is best to measure total testosterone plus SHBG and then calculate the free testosterone level using a widely available calculation tool. Prior to confirmation of hypogonadism, it is too early to perform other tests or to begin treatment.

Bhasin S, Cunningham GR, Hayes FJ, et al. Testosterone therapy in men with androgen deficiency syndromes: an Endocrine Society clinical practice guideline. *J Clin Endocrinol Metab.* 2010;95(6):2536–2559.

13. ANSWER: A. Advise her that she can likely stop insulin therapy; initiate metformin and reduce insulin doses to help achieve this.

Learning objective: Recognize ketosis-prone diabetes and initiate appropriate therapy.

This patient presented with diabetic ketoacidosis but has several features of type 2 diabetes: family history of type 2 diabetes, obesity and acanthosis nigricans on physical exam, and negative anti-GAD65 antibodies. She therefore is unlikely to have type 1 diabetes (which would require lifelong insulin therapy); she is more likely to have type 2 diabetes. Certain individuals with type 2 diabetes present with diabetic ketoacidosis, thought to be secondary to acute insulin deficiency due to toxic effects of hyperglycemia on beta-cells leading to reduced insulin secretion. Upon correction of the hyperglycemia, beta-cell function often recovers, and patients can be managed with standard therapies for type 2 diabetes. Therefore, this patient who is experiencing weight gain and hypoglycemia as a result of her insulin regimen should be started on metformin as the standard first-line therapy for diabetes, and her total daily dose of insulin should be reduced with a goal of stopping it completely if she does well on metformin alone.

Balasubramanyam A, Nalini R, Hampe CS, Maldonado M. Syndromes of ketosis-prone diabetes mellitus. *Endocr Rev.* 2008;29(3):292–302.

14. ANSWER: E. Send for a complete blood count.

Learning objective: Indicate appropriate workup of a discrepant HbA_{1c} value.

This patient has an HbA_{1c} value that is discrepant from her glucose measurements; the first step in management should be to identify the etiology of the discrepancy. Common causes of inaccurate HbA_{1c} values include conditions that change erythrocyte survival (the shortened survival in patients with blood loss or hemolytic anemias will falsely lower HbA_{1c} values; patients with B_{12}/folate anemias can have falsely elevated HbA_{1c} values). In addition, certain hemoglobin variants can interfere with the HbA_{1c} measurement.

In this patient, the most likely cause of a falsely low HbA_{1c} is a blood loss anemia related to her menorrhagia, and a complete blood count will diagnose this. Her HbA_{1c} is not accurate, and the patient should therefore not be reassured. Although glucometer errors could also cause discrepancies, her glucose value as measured in the laboratory corroborates the values from her glucometer. Mutations in the *HBB* gene could cause hemoglobinopathies such as sickle cell disease, but this could also be diagnosed on the basis of the complete blood count, so genetic testing is not yet indicated. A continuous glucose monitor will just show the same findings as her fingerstick glucose values, namely persistent hyperglycemia, and it is therefore not the next best intervention.

Saudek CD, Derr RL, Kalyani RR. Assessing glycemia in diabetes using self-monitoring blood glucose and hemoglobin A1c. *JAMA.* 2006;295(14):1688–1697.

15. ANSWER: E. Stop methimazole

Learning objective: Develop a long-term management strategy for Graves disease.

This patient with Graves disease appears to be in remission on the basis of a normal TSH while taking only a low dose of methimazole. At this point, it is reasonable to stop her methimazole and monitor her TSH for any evidence of recurrence of hyperthyroidism. Should she have recurrence, radioiodine ablation or thyroidectomy may be reasonable options. Long-term therapy with methimazole is also an option, but often it is not the preferred option, owing to concerns for agranulocytosis and liver abnormalities. An ESR is not helpful in the determination of management of Graves disease.

Bahn RS, Burch HB, Cooper DS, et al. Hyperthyroidism and other causes of thyrotoxicosis: management guidelines of the American Thyroid Association and American Association of Clinical Endocrinologists. *Endocr Pract.* 2011;17(3):456–520.

16. ANSWER: A. Central diabetes insipidus

Learning objective: Diagnose disorders of water balance after pituitary surgery.

The symptoms and presentation in this case are most concerning for the development of postoperative central diabetes insipidus. Diabetes insipidus is a syndrome of hypotonic polyuria and is due to either a deficiency of arginine vasopressin, also known as antidiuretic hormone (ADH), or an inadequate renal response to ADH. Patients with diabetes insipidus often complain of extreme thirst and will excrete large amounts of very dilute urine. Without this hormone, individuals cannot adequately concentrate their urine and, if not allowed access to liquids, may develop severe, life-threatening hypernatremia. Central diabetes insipidus is due to deficiency, either partial or complete, of ADH. Central diabetes insipidus can occur after any pituitary surgery. It can be transient or permanent and is seen more frequently in patients with larger tumors or those that tend to invade the pituitary stalk, such as craniopharyngiomas. Given the clinical presentation of a pituitary lesion, this patient's diabetes insipidus would be much more likely to be central than nephrogenic. Psychogenic polydipsia, a primary disorder of increased water intake, is associated with polyuria and dilute urine, but it would be associated with a low or low-normal serum sodium level, not hypernatremia as seen in this patient. The diagnosis is not likely SIADH, because this condition is typically associated with hyponatremia. Type 2 diabetes mellitus would also not be a likely cause of this patient's acute severe polyuria and polydipsia, because the fasting glucose is only mildly elevated.

Lamas C, del Pozo C, Villabona C; Neuroendocrinology Group of the SEEN. Clinical guidelines for management of diabetes insipidus and syndrome of inappropriate antidiuretic hormone secretion after pituitary surgery. *Endocrinol Nutr.* 2014;61(4):e15–e24.

17. ANSWER: A. Primary adrenal insufficiency

Learning objective: Interpret hormone levels in the patient with adrenal insufficiency.

This patient has primary adrenal insufficiency (Addison disease) that is most likely secondary to an autoimmune process, given her history of concomitant hypothyroidism at a young age. Primary adrenal insufficiency is characterized by the destruction of the entire adrenal cortex, thereby resulting in deficiencies in cortisol, the mineralocorticoid aldosterone, and adrenal sex hormones. The resulting clinical manifestations reflect mineralocorticoid deficiency (hypovolemia, salt wasting, hyponatremia, hyperkalemia), glucocorticoid deficiency (fatigue, weight loss, nausea), and adrenal androgen deficiency (loss of pubic and axillary hair). Characteristic laboratory examination results include very low cortisol and aldosterone and very high ACTH and plasma renin activity to reflect physiologic compensation. Patients may also display significant hyperpigmentation. Administration of cosyntropin results in minimal or no cortisol increase, given the destruction of the adrenal cortex. These patients warrant immediate treatment with glucocorticoids, saline expansion, and ultimately mineralocorticoids, to prevent hemodynamic collapse and life-threatening electrolyte abnormalities.

Secondary adrenal insufficiency refers to a disruption at the level of pituitary production of ACTH. In the absence of ACTH, patients manifest glucocorticoid insufficiency; however, mineralocorticoid production (and therefore maintenance of sodium/volume homeostasis and potassium balance) remains intact. When ACTH deficiency is prolonged, the adrenal glands will gradually atrophy and display a diminished response to exogenous ACTH stimulation.

Bornstein SR, Allolio B, Arlt W, et al. Diagnosis and treatment of primary adrenal insufficiency: an Endocrine Society clinical practice guideline. *J Clin Endocrinol Metab.* 2016;101(2):364–389.

18. ANSWER: B. Estradiol 10-μg vaginal pill

Learning objective: Choose appropriate treatment for genitourinary menopausal symptoms.

This patient has genitourinary menopausal symptoms. These are best managed with local therapies. A lubricant with intercourse may be sufficient if the patient has symptoms only with intercourse, but because this patient has symptoms on a daily basis, a local low-dose estradiol formulation will be most effective. Systemic estrogen or gabapentin would be helpful to control the vasomotor symptoms of menopause, but her symptoms are quite mild and probably do not warrant systemic treatment, especially because her risk of breast cancer is elevated due to her prior breast disease and her family history.

Stuenkel CA, Davis SR, Gompel A, et al. Treatment of symptoms of the menopause: an Endocrine Society clinical practice guideline. *J Clin Endocrinol Metab.* 2015;100(11):3975–4011.

19. ANSWER: B. Dexamethasone suppression test

Learning objective: Outline the hormonal evaluation of an incidentally discovered adrenal mass.

The incidental detection of adrenal masses is increasing as the frequency of abdominal imaging expands. Once an adrenal mass is discovered, it is important to assess the mass for malignant potential and hormone functionality because either of these features can result in adverse health sequelae. The vast majority of incidental adrenal masses are *benign* adenomas that are characterized by a lipid-rich density (<10 Hounsfield units on CT scan), such as in the case of this patient; repeat imaging with MRI does not add to the findings described on the basis of the CT scan. Despite the presence of reassuring radiographic features, a benign adenoma may still be functional; excess cortisol, aldosterone, sex hormones, or catecholamines can all result in long-term health complications.

Even when overt features of hypercortisolism (Cushing syndrome) or catecholamine excess (pheochromocytoma) are absent, the prevalence of subclinical cortisol or catecholamine excess is sufficiently high that it is recommended that all patients with a newly discovered adrenal mass be assessed for these hormone excess states. The most efficient and specific testing involves performing a 1-mg dexamethasone suppression test (to assess for cortisol excess) and plasma metanephrines (for catecholamine excess). Serum catecholamines are not reliable indicators, given their variance in the blood; therefore, measurement of intermediates of catecholamine metabolism (metanephrines) is preferred. When high blood pressure, hypokalemia, or hirsutism is present, a serum aldosterone and plasma renin activity, or adrenal androgen profile, should also be assessed.

Young WF Jr. The incidentally discovered adrenal mass. *N Engl J Med.* 2007;356(6):601–610.

20. ANSWER: E. Test for the presence of antiglutamic acid decarboxylase (GAD) antibodies.

Learning objective: Recognize features that should raise the suspicion for type 1 diabetes in adults and choose the correct test to make this diagnosis.

An underlying secondary etiology of diabetes should always be considered in patients with newly diagnosed diabetes, especially if there are features that would be atypical for type 2 diabetes, such as acromegalic or cushingoid findings on exam, rapid failure of oral antidiabetic agents, lean body habitus with no other findings of insulin resistance such as acanthosis nigricans or skin tags, and no other metabolic abnormalities (hypertension, dyslipidemia). The patient described has no physical exam features to suggest Cushing syndrome or acromegaly; thus, a 24-hour urinary free cortisol or IGF-1 level is not needed. The patient does not have symptoms to suggest a pancreatic tumor or chronic pancreatitis as a cause of his hyperglycemia; therefore, a pancreatic MRI is not indicated. Maturity-onset diabetes of youth (MODY) is a monogenic form of diabetes with an autosomal dominant pattern of inheritance. Patients with MODY are usually diagnosed in adolescence and have a strong family history of diabetes, which this patient does not have.

In addition, in the absence of significant weight gain, glycemic control in patients with MODY is unlikely to deteriorate. Testing for MODY is therefore not needed. That leaves the most likely diagnosis of type 1 diabetes. This form of diabetes accounts for 5%–10% of diabetes cases and is a gradually progressive disease that may be diagnosed on the basis of routine screening while patients have only mild hyperglycemia. Type 1 diabetes is usually diagnosed from early childhood to early adulthood, but it may occur at any age. It should therefore be considered even in adult patients, especially those who are lean, who do not have the common metabolic abnormalities usually observed in type 2 diabetes (such as hypertension and dyslipidemia), and who lack a family history of diabetes. In this patient, the rapid failure of oral medications to control blood glucose should increase the suspicion for type 1 diabetes. Autoantibodies such as anti-GAD antibodies, islet cell autoantibodies, and insulin autoantibodies may be used to differentiate type 1 from type 2 diabetes.

Laugesen E, Østergaard JA, Leslie RD; Danish Diabetes Academy Workshop, Workshop Speakeers. Latent autoimmune diabetes of the adult: current knowledge and uncertainty. *Diabet Med.* 2015;32(7):843–852.

21. ANSWER: B. Initiate rosuvastatin 20 mg daily.

Learning objective: Assess and intervene on cardiovascular risk factors in patients with type 2 diabetes.

This patient has diabetes and one risk factor for atherosclerotic cardiovascular disease (ASCVD), namely an LDL level >100 mg/dL. The ADA recommends high-intensity statin treatment, such as rosuvastatin 20 mg, for such individuals. The American Heart Association (AHA) also recommends statin therapy but suggests moderate-intensity statin therapy in patients with diabetes aged 40–75 years with an LDL level of 70–189 mg/dL. A high-intensity statin can be considered if the 10-year risk of ASCVD (as estimated using the AHA ASCVD risk calculator) is above 7.5% or if LDL cholesterol level exceeds 190 mg/dL.

Aspirin for primary prevention is recommended in patients whose 10-year-risk of cardiovascular disease (as estimated using the ASCVD risk calculator) exceeds 10% and can be considered on the basis of individual patient factors for patients whose risk is 5%–10%. In those at lower risk, the risks exceed the benefits. In a woman with diabetes, treatment with aspirin is generally not indicated unless she is over 60 years of age and has at least one other major cardiovascular risk factor (family history of premature atherosclerotic cardiovascular disease, hypertension, smoking, dyslipidemia, or albuminuria). In this patient, the ASCVD 10-year risk is 4.9%; aspirin is therefore not indicated. Even if her risk were >5%, her prior history of gastritis (albeit appropriately treated) should be taken into account before initiating aspirin therapy.

Pharmacologic therapy for hypertension (such as chlorthalidone) is not indicated unless the blood pressure exceeds 140/90 mm Hg. Additional interventions such as insulin to decrease glucose levels that are already very well controlled have not been shown to have a significant effect on cardiovascular outcomes. Routine screening for cardiovascular disease in asymptomatic individuals with, for example, a coronary artery calcium score is not recommended.

American Diabetes Association. Standards of medical care in diabetes—2016 abridged for primary care providers. *Clin Diabetes.* 2017;35(1):5–26.

22. ANSWER: B. Obtain a thyroid scan.

Learning objective: Incorporate radionuclide imaging in the workup of thyrotoxicosis.

When a patient presenting with a thyroid nodule who is not taking levothyroxine is noted to have a suppressed TSH level, a thyroid scan should be checked to determine if the nodule itself is an autonomously functioning toxic adenoma. If there is radioiodine uptake in the nodule on the thyroid scan, it is most likely benign and does not need to be biopsied. If there is no uptake into the nodule, fine-needle aspiration biopsy of the nodule should be performed to guide further management. Treatment of a toxic adenoma or Graves disease with methimazole or radioactive iodine may be indicated, but it should be considered only after it has been determined whether a biopsy is necessary. Referral for thyroid surgery would be indicated only if a biopsy of a cold nodule revealed suspicious or malignant cytopathology or if there were contraindications to treatment of a toxic adenoma with radioactive iodine or methimazole.

Bahn RS, Burch HB, Cooper DS, et al. Hyperthyroidism and other causes of thyrotoxicosis: management guidelines of the American Thyroid Association and American Association of Clinical Endocrinologists. *Endocr Pract.* 2011;17(3):456–520.

23. ANSWER: E. Late-night salivary cortisol

Learning objective: Understand the tests available for diagnosing cortisol excess.

This patient should be screened for Cushing syndrome/hypercortisolism because of a number of concerning clinical signs, including rapid weight gain and new diagnoses of diabetes mellitus, hypertension, and osteoporosis, as well as notable physical examination findings (round face, hirsutism, supraclavicular fat accumulation, pigmented striae, and bruising). After ruling out exogenous glucocorticoid exposure, there are three acceptable first-line screening tests for endogenous hypercortisolism: late-night salivary cortisol, 1-mg overnight dexamethasone suppression test, and 24-hour urine free cortisol with creatinine. The late-night salivary cortisol test takes advantage of the fact that cortisol is secreted in a diurnal rhythm such that nadir levels are usually observed late in the evening in a person without hypercortisolism. Patients with hypercortisolism lose the diurnal variation and show high cortisol levels when they should be at the nadir. The 1-mg overnight dexamethasone suppression test takes advantage of the fact that individuals with normal hypothalamic-pituitary-adrenal (HPA) axis physiology will suppress cortisol secretion when given the synthetic steroid dexamethasone. Individuals with a normal HPA axis and thus normal inhibitory feedback mechanisms should suppress their cortisol level to <1.8 μg/dL at 8:00 a.m. the day following ingestion of 1-mg dexamethasone at 11:00 p.m. the day before. Although cortisol levels vary from minute to minute, patients with Cushing syndrome show generally elevated levels over a 24-hour period. Therefore, patients with Cushing syndrome will have high 24-hour urine free cortisol levels that reflect their overall high continuous cortisol secretion over a 24-hour period. Urinary creatinine should always be checked at the same time as the 24-hour urinary free cortisol to ensure adequacy of the urine collection. These three tests confirm only hypercortisolism/Cushing syndrome and do not indicate the cause of the cortisol hypersecretion. Additional testing with an ACTH level is required to differentiate between ACTH-dependent (most commonly pituitary Cushing disease or ectopic source) and ACTH-independent (likely adrenal source of cortisol overproduction) Cushing syndrome.

An 8:00 a.m. ACTH or cortisol level is not appropriate for screening, because cortisol levels are dynamic over time and influenced by a number of factors, such as acute pain and stress. The 8-mg dexamethasone suppression test (as opposed to the 1-mg dexamethasone suppression test) is used to help distinguish a pituitary source of excess ACTH from an ectopic source; it is not an appropriate initial screening test. A cosyntropin stimulation test is used to diagnose adrenal insufficiency rather than cortisol excess.

Nieman LK, Biller BMK, Findling JW, et al. The diagnosis of Cushing's syndrome: an Endocrine Society clinical practice guideline. *J Clin Endocrinol Metab.* 2008;93(5):1526–1540.

24. ANSWER: B. Medical therapy with a somatostatin analogue

Learning objective: Describe the medical management options for acromegaly.

Multiple treatment modalities exist for recurrent acromegaly. In a case such as this one, medical therapy would be the initial treatment recommendation, particularly because significant residual/recurrent pituitary tumor is not visualized by MRI. There are a number of medical treatment options, but somatostatin analogues are typically the initial treatment of choice in this setting. GH-secreting pituitary tumor cells express somatostatin receptors, and treatment with somatostatin analogues acting via these receptors inhibits somatotrope cellular proliferation and GH secretion, leading to a reduction in IGF-1 levels. Biochemical remission, defined as normalization of IGF-1 and GH levels, is associated with improvement or resolution of acromegaly symptoms. Long-acting somatostatin analogues, such as lanreotide and octreotide LAR, are typically considered the initial medical option in uncontrolled acromegaly. The dopamine agonist cabergoline can be used, especially if there are also elevations in prolactin levels, but it is less efficacious than somatostatin analogues. The GH antagonist pegvisomant is also an option for this patient. This drug tends to be a second-line therapy due to the need for frequent subcutaneous injections and its lack of inhibition of tumor growth. Observation would not generally be advised, because the patient is symptomatic, and biochemical remission is associated with improved clinical outcomes and reduced mortality. Repeat surgery would not be optimal in this case, because a clear surgical target was not identified. Finally, radiation is generally reserved for patients with very aggressive tumors or those for whom medical therapy fails.

Katznelson L, Laws ER Jr, Melmed S, et al. Acromegaly: an Endocrine Society clinical practice guideline. *J Clin Endocrinol Metab.* 2014;99(11):3933–3951.

25. ANSWER: C. Refer the patient to a thyroid surgeon.

Learning objective: Recommend appropriate management of a goiter causing tracheal compression.

A multinodular goiter that has extended substernally to the point of causing tracheal compression should be resected by an experienced thyroid surgeon, regardless of its functional status. The presence of audible stridor and evidence of tracheal narrowing on radiographic images obviates the need for pulmonary function testing with flow–volume loops. Treatment with methimazole might help control hyperthyroidism caused by autonomously functioning thyroid nodules, but it would not help shrink the dominant nodule to any extent. Treatment with ^{131}I might help shrink the dominant nodule over time, but it might cause radiation-induced thyroiditis with expansion of affected tissue that could severely compromise respiratory function. Treatment with levothyroxine to try to suppress further enlargement of thyroid tissue may be marginally effective at best in euthyroid patients, and it would be completely ineffective in a patient presenting with hyperthyroidism.

Newman E, Shaha AR. Substernal goiter. *J Surg Oncol.* 1995;60(3):207–212.

26. ANSWER: E. Start therapy with telmisartan.

Learning objective: Initiate therapy for diabetic nephropathy in a patient with allergy to ACE inhibitors.

This patient has established diabetic nephropathy, as evidenced by an elevated urine albumin-to-creatinine ratio. The benefit of inhibitors of angiotensin, either in the form of angiotensin-converting enzyme (ACE) inhibitors or angiotensin receptor blockers (ARBs) such as telmisartan, has been well established and proven to delay the progression to end-stage renal disease, even in patients with normal blood pressure. The patient's cough when treated with an ACE inhibitor is not a contraindication to ARB therapy. Additional blood pressure control with labetalol is not indicated, because his blood pressure is already at goal. Niacin could raise the HDL but has not been proven to have benefit in preventing complications of diabetes and has side effects that limit its use. The patient only had background retinopathy on the last eye exam; intravitreal bevacizumab is used off-label in the treatment of proliferative diabetic retinopathy. Although the patient should have intensification of his antidiabetic therapy, metformin should be continued unless a contraindication develops.

American Diabetes Association. Standards of medical care in diabetes—2016 abridged for primary care providers. *Clin Diabetes.* 2016;34(1):3–21.

27. ANSWER: A. 1,25-dihydroxy-vitamin D

Learning objective: Describe the mechanism of hypercalcemia in granulomatous diseases.

This patient has sarcoidosis, a granulomatous disorder in which activated macrophages can express the enzyme that converts vitamin D to its active form, calcitriol (1,25-dihydroxyvitamin D). This leads to both hypercalcemia and hypercalciuria. The other choices are all reasonable to check in cases of non–PTH-mediated hypercalcemia but would not explain the underlying pathophysiology of hypercalcemia associated with granulomatous disease. Treatment of the hypercalcemia in sarcoidosis would start with hydration and glucocorticoids.

Carroll MF, Schade DS. A practical approach to hypercalcemia. *Am Fam Physician.* 2003;67(9):1959–1966.

28. ANSWER: C. Karyotyping

Learning objective: Recognize the clinical phenotype of Klinefelter syndrome and obtain appropriate diagnostic evaluation.

This patient has clinical symptoms and signs of male hypogonadism. His biochemical tests reveal primary gonadal failure as the cause of the hypogonadism. Klinefelter syndrome is relatively common among young males with primary hypogonadism. Karyotyping will identify the chromosomal abnormality (XXY). Echocardiogram and renal ultrasound will not uncover the etiology of primary hypogonadism; these may be indicated in a phenotypic woman with Turner syndrome. Pituitary MRI is helpful in patients with hypogonadotropic hypogonadism, but in this case, the FSH and LH would be low (or inappropriately normal). Hemochromatosis, which would be expected if there were signs of iron excess on laboratory evaluation, typically causes hypogonadotropic hypogonadism, not primary gonadal failure.

Dwyer AA, Phan-Hug F, Hauschild M, et al. Transition in endocrinology: hypogonadism in adolescence. *Eur J Endocrinol.* 2015;173(1):R15–R24.

29. ANSWER: A. Hematocrit

Learning objective: Create an appropriate monitoring plan for a patient receiving hormone replacement therapy with testosterone.

According to the Endocrine Society clinical guideline on male hypogonadism, serum total testosterone and hematocrit should be monitored 3–6 months after initiating testosterone treatment. Testosterone levels are measured to allow titration of the testosterone dose to achieve a serum testosterone level in the mid-normal range. The hematocrit is measured to monitor for erythrocytosis, a known side effect of testosterone therapy. If hematocrit is >54%, testosterone therapy is stopped until the hematocrit decreases to a safe level. Measurement of PSA levels is not indicated in men younger than 40 years of age. In men 40 years of age or older, check PSA level before initiating treatment and at 3–6 months. There is no recommendation to order liver function tests or measure prolactin levels.

Bhasin S, Cunningham GR, Hayes FJ, et al. Testosterone therapy in men with androgen deficiency syndromes: an Endocrine Society clinical practice guideline. *J Clin Endocrinol Metab.* 2010;95(6):2536–2559.

30. ANSWER: D. Treatment with levothyroxine

Learning objective: Identify hypothyroidism as a cause of menstrual and laboratory abnormalities.

This woman presents for her annual examination with fatigue, constipation, weight gain, and oligomenorrhea. Although it may be possible that the symptoms are a result of work-related stress and perimenopause, one should keep in mind that hypothyroidism may also present in a similar manner. Her elevated TSH is diagnostic of hypothyroidism. Given that her oligomenorrhea, hyponatremia, hyperprolactinemia, and hyperlipidemia are most likely manifestations of her hypothyroidism, it would be best to treat her hypothyroidism first with levothyroxine before considering treatment for these other clinical abnormalities.

Garber JR, Cobin RH, Gharib H, et al. Clinical practice guidelines for hypothyroidism in adults: cosponsored by the American Association of Clinical Endocrinologists and the American Thyroid Association. *Endocr Pract.* 2012;18(6):988–1028.

31. ANSWER: C. Initiate linagliptin 5 mg daily.

Learning objective: Incorporate patient preference in the choice of antidiabetic agent after failure of metformin monotherapy.

There are various antidiabetic medications available, and the American Diabetes Association, as well as other professional associations, promotes the individualization of the treatment approach, taking into account patient preferences, cost, and potential side effects of each class of medications. In the absence of contraindications, metformin is the preferred initial agent. There is a long-standing evidence base for both the efficacy and safety of metformin; it is not associated with weight gain or hypoglycemia; and it may reduce the risk of cardiovascular events and cancers. When avoiding weight gain is important to the patient, initiation of insulin therapy, sulfonylureas (such as glipizide), meglitinides (such as repaglinide), and thiazolidinediones (such as pioglitazone) should be avoided because these are all associated with weight gain. Linagliptin, an inhibitor of dipeptidyl peptidase-4 (DPP-4), is weight neutral; that is, it is not associated with weight loss or weight gain and is therefore the best option listed. Other options that could promote weight loss include glucagon-like peptide-1 (GLP-1) agonists, sodium/glucose cotransporter 2 (SGLT-2) inhibitors, or pramlintide.

Inzucchi SE, Bergenstal RM, Buse JB, et al. Management of hyperglycemia in type 2 diabetes, 2015: a patient-centered approach: update to a position statement of the American Diabetes Association and the European Association for the Study of Diabetes. *Diabetes Care.* 2015;38(1):140–149.

32. ANSWER: D. Fibroblast growth factor 23 (FGF23)

Learning objective: Recognize the role of FGF23 in phosphate homeostasis.

This patient has severe hypophosphatemia causing osteomalacia. In the absence of a history of poor oral intake, diarrhea, or antacid use, this is most likely resulting from urinary losses, which can be confirmed by a high (or inappropriately normal) urinary phosphate. Vitamin D deficiency and primary hyperparathyroidism are the most common causes of a mild hypophosphatemia, but this patient's vitamin D was normal, as was his calcium. Fanconi syndrome (type 2, or proximal, renal tubular acidosis) is another cause of hypophosphatemia, especially in patients with a paraproteinemic disorder or taking culprit medications, but it is associated with metabolic acidosis and hypokalemia, which were not described here. Hence, this patient is most likely to have tumor-induced osteomalacia, which is caused by FGF23 secretion from a mesenchymal tumor. FGF23 causes phosphate loss in the urine with an elevated urine phosphate. 1,25-dihydroxyvitamin D level is generally low or low-normal in this disorder because the renal tubular defect causing the phosphaturia also impairs synthesis of 1,25-dihydroxyvitamin D. Calcitonin and urinary calcium are not high.

Hamnvik OP, Becker CB, Levy BD, Loscalzo J. Wasting away. *N Engl J Med.* 2014;370(10):959–966.

33. ANSWER: C. Hypothalamic amenorrhea

Learning objective: Identify excessive exercise as a cause of amenorrhea.

This woman is experiencing secondary amenorrhea, defined as an absence of menses for more than three cycles or 6 months in women who had previously been menstruating. The most likely etiology in this case is hypothalamic amenorrhea. This description fits the classic description of the "female athlete triad," which consists of an eating disorder, amenorrhea, and osteoporosis. Although the exact pathophysiology of this disorder is unknown, it is believed that amenorrhea occurs because of a mismatch between nutritional intake and energy expenditure.

Gordon CM, Ackerman KE, Berga SL, et al. Functional hypothalamic amenorrhea: an Endocrine Society Clinical Practice Guideline. *J Clin Endocrinol Metab.* 2017;102(5):1413–1439.

34. ANSWER: D. This cortisol value cannot be adequately interpreted.

Learning objective: Understand the effect of exogenous glucocorticoids on hypothalamic-pituitary-adrenal axis function.

Metastatic solid tumors have been known to metastasize to the hypothalamus or pituitary and result in secondary adrenal insufficiency. Solid tumors can also metastasize to bilateral adrenal glands, although this scenario does not necessarily result in primary adrenal insufficiency. Symptoms of orthostatic hypotension are not pathognomonic for adrenal insufficiency, but this entity should certainly be considered. In the setting of dexamethasone use, cortisol values are reliable only for detecting inappropriately high cortisol states (Cushing syndrome), not when investigating inappropriately low cortisol states (adrenal insufficiency). Dexamethasone is a synthetic glucocorticoid that is not detected by the conventional assay for cortisol; however, like all glucocorticoids, it inhibits the production of ACTH and therefore suppresses endogenous cortisol production. Therefore, a low cortisol level in this patient most likely reflects the expected action of dexamethasone. Whether he may also have concomitant brain metastases that have resulted in secondary adrenal insufficiency by compromising the pituitary apparatus, or concomitant adrenal metastases that have resulted in primary adrenal insufficiency, cannot be ascertained by this single testing performed in the setting of dexamethasone intake.

Bornstein SR, Allolio B, Arlt W, et al. Diagnosis and treatment of primary adrenal insufficiency: an Endocrine Society clinical practice guideline. *J Clin Endocrinol Metab.* 2016;101(2):364–389.

35. ANSWER: E. Wait 6 weeks and recheck a full profile of thyroid hormone levels.

Learning objective: Describe changes in thyroid function with acute nonthyroidal illness.

The shifts in profiles of thyroid hormone levels seen in this patient are characteristic of physiologic changes that may occur during acute illness and subsequent recovery in patients with normal endogenous thyroid function. Initial suppression of TSH, T4, and T3 levels during progression of a nonthyroidal illness may be misinterpreted as evidence of underlying central hypothyroidism caused by hypothalamic or pituitary dysfunction. Subsequent transient elevation of the TSH level during recovery may be misinterpreted as evidence of underlying primary hypothyroidism. In such cases, it is usually prudent to wait until the patient has made a full recovery before attempting to determine whether any thyroid dysfunction is present. A thyroid uptake and scan would not provide any useful information in this setting. Starting treatment with any form of thyroid hormone at this stage would be premature, and doing so would make it difficult to interpret subsequent profiles of thyroid hormone levels. A pituitary MRI scan would be informative only if serial measurement of thyroid hormone levels showed persistent low TSH levels and low free T4 levels consistent with possible central hypothyroidism.

DeGroot LJ. The non-thyroidal illness syndrome [updated 2015 Feb 1]. In: De Groot LJ, Chrousos G, Dungan K, et al., eds, Endotext [Internet]. South Dartmouth, MA: MDText.com, Inc.; 2000. https://www.ncbi.nlm.nih.gov/books/NBK285570/

36. ANSWER: C. Increase levothyroxine dose.

Learning objective: Titrate levothyroxine dose in patients with secondary hypothyroidism based on levels of free T4 and clinical findings.

This patient has central hypothyroidism due to his pituitary macroadenoma. Clinically, he has some symptoms suggestive of inadequately treated hypothyroidism, including fatigue, weight gain, and dry skin. He does not have symptoms or physical examination findings suggestive of hyperthyroidism. His laboratory tests are classic for central hypothyroidism—a low free T4 in combination with either an inappropriately low or normal TSH. This case illustrates how TSH alone cannot be used reliably to assess thyroid hormone replacement in patients with central hypothyroidism and/or hypothalamic/pituitary dysfunction. Clinical findings and peripheral thyroid hormone levels must be used to guide levothyroxine replacement therapy. Therefore, in this case, despite the low TSH, the levothyroxine dose should be increased with the goal of normalizing the free T4.

Garber JR, Cobin RH, Gharib H, et al. Clinical practice guidelines for hypothyroidism in adults: cosponsored by the American Association of Clinical Endocrinologists and the American Thyroid Association. *Endocr Pract.* 2012;18(6):988–1028.

37. ANSWER: D. No further adjustment of her regimen.

Learning objective: Individualize glycemic targets in a patient at high risk of complications from hypoglycemia

The 2012 position statement of the American Diabetes Association (ADA) and the European Association for the Study of Diabetes (EASD) suggests that an HbA_{1c} goal as high as 7.5%–8.0% or even slightly higher is appropriate for patients with a history of severe hypoglycemia; limited life expectancy; advanced complications; extensive comorbid conditions; and those in whom the target is difficult to attain despite intensive self-management education, repeated counseling, and effective doses of multiple glucose-lowering agents, including insulin. The patient described in the question has a long duration of disease with a history of myocardial infarction and appears to have hypoglycemia unawareness. Intensifying therapy in this patient with a sulfonylurea, prandial insulin, or increased basal insulin is likely to be associated with greater risks than benefits. Therefore, maintaining an HbA_{1c} between 7.0% and 7.5% without hypoglycemia is appropriate. A continuous glucose monitor is unlikely to provide any further information.

Inzucchi SE, Bergenstal RM, Buse JB, et al. Management of hyperglycemia in type 2 diabetes, 2015: a patient-centered approach: update to a position statement of the American Diabetes Association and the European Association for the Study of Diabetes. *Diabetes Care.* 2015;38(1):140–149.

38. ANSWER: A. Dietary/lifestyle interventions

Learning objective: Recommend appropriate management of prediabetes.

Prediabetes is a condition in which normal glucose homeostasis is compromised. It is characterized by impaired fasting glucose (fasting plasma glucose of 100–125 mg/dL) and/or impaired glucose tolerance (IGT) (plasma glucose of 140–199 mg/dL 2 hours after a 75-g glucose load), and/or HbA_{1c} levels of 5.7%–6.4%. Prediabetes confers a three- to sevenfold increase in the risk of developing overt type 2 diabetes compared with individuals with normal glucose values. Evidence from numerous studies also suggests that the chronic complications of type 2 diabetes start to develop during the prediabetic state. Therefore, to minimize the burden of complications associated with hyperglycemia, early intervention, before overt diabetes develops, is prudent. However, there are currently no approved pharmacotherapies for prediabetes. Evidence derived from prevention studies supports the hypothesis that early intervention with lifestyle modification or pharmacotherapy may slow the progression to diabetes by delaying the underlying pathophysiology of the disease. In the Diabetes Prevention Program (DPP), in which 3234 individuals with impaired fasting glucose or IGT were enrolled, intensive lifestyle modification, aiming to achieve at least a 7% weight loss and 150 minutes of physical activity per week, reduced the incidence of type 2 diabetes by 58% compared with placebo after 2.8 years of follow-up. Patients randomized to treatment with metformin in the DPP had a 31% reduction in the incidence of type 2 diabetes after 2.8 years of follow-up. There is also evidence derived from randomized clinical trials suggesting potential benefit of other oral hypoglycemic agents, namely acarbose and thiazolidinediones, in preventing the progression from prediabetes to overt diabetes, but these agents are either less effective or have safety and tolerability issues. The most recent position statement issued by the ADA regarding standards of medical care in diabetes, as well as a consensus statement by the American College of Endocrinology (ACE) and the American Association of Clinical Endocrinologists (AACE), recommends lifestyle intervention as the preferred treatment option for prediabetes because it has been shown to be safe and highly effective. Starting metformin therapy, although likely to be effective, is not yet indicated, because current guidelines and available evidence would prioritize initiation/intensification of lifestyle interventions. In this patient, interventions would be directed toward dietary modifications, increased exercise, and weight loss efforts. There is no evidence that insulin or DPP-4 inhibitors have benefit in prediabetes.

Knowler WC, Barrett-Connor E, Fowler SE, et al. Reduction in the incidence of type 2 diabetes with lifestyle intervention or metformin. *N Engl J Med.* 2002;346(6):393–403.

39. ANSWER: E. Starting a gluten-free diet

Learning objective: Recognize calcium malabsorption as a secondary cause of hyperparathyroidism and osteoporosis.

It is important to recognize secondary hyperparathyroidism due to malabsorption and to note that in some disorders, such as celiac disease, calcium malabsorption can occur even in the presence of reasonably normal vitamin D levels. The clues to the diagnosis of celiac disease are the irritable bowel syndrome, weight loss, very low urinary calcium excretion, and a rash that is consistent with dermatitis herpetiformis on physical examination. Increasing calcium and vitamin D will not necessarily correct the secondary hyperparathyroidism, and oral alendronate is unlikely to be absorbed. Parathyroidectomy is clearly inappropriate for secondary hyperparathyroidism because the elevated parathyroid hormone is an appropriate response to calcium malabsorption. A gluten-free diet, after confirming the diagnosis of celiac disease, will improve calcium and nutrient absorption and is the first step in improving this patient's skeletal health.

Cosman F, de Beur SJ, LeBoff MS, et al. Clinician's guide to prevention and treatment of osteoporosis. *Osteoporos Int.* 2014;25(10):2359–2381.

40. ANSWER: A. *CFTR* gene

Learning objective: Distinguish genetic causes of infertility.

About 1%–2% of infertile men have azoospermia due to congenital absence of the vas deferens, and most of these patients have mutations in the *CFTR* gene. Mutations in this gene also causes cystic fibrosis, but men with mutations leading to absent vas deferens do not need to manifest the full clinical picture of cystic fibrosis (such as pulmonary and pancreatic dysfunction). Mutations in the *KISS1, KAL1, FGFR1,* and *TAC3* genes would cause hypogonadotropic hypogonadism with low LH, FSH, and testosterone.

Chillon M, Casals T, Mercier B, et al. Mutations in the cystic fibrosis gene in patients with congenital absence of the vas deferens. *N Engl J Med.* 1995;332(22):1475–1480.

41. ANSWER: A. 24-hour urine free cortisol

Learning objective: Recognize the clinical features of Cushing syndrome and select an appropriate diagnostic test.

Given this patient's presentation, the most likely etiology for her amenorrhea is cortisol excess, possibly resulting from Cushing disease. Therefore, a 24-hour urine free cortisol would be a good screening test to evaluate for cortisol excess. She has a classic presentation for cortisol excess, including progressive weight gain, fatigue, weakness, abdominal striae, and secondary amenorrhea. Cushing disease (pituitary ACTH-dependent Cushing syndrome) is more common in women and typically presents between 25 and 45 years of age. An LH-to-FSH ratio could be helpful in the diagnosis of PCOS, but given her clinical presentation, cortisol excess is more likely. Hyperprolactinemia and hypothyroidism may cause secondary amenorrhea but are less likely, given her clinical presentation.

Nieman LK, Biller BM, Findling JW, et al. The diagnosis of Cushing's syndrome: an Endocrine Society clinical practice guideline. *J Clin Endocrinol Metab.* 2008;93(5):1526–1540.

42. ANSWER: E. Venlafaxine use

Learning objective: Recognize factors that affect measurements of plasma metanephrines.

The assessment of plasma metanephrines should take into account medications that can raise their levels. By the time a catecholamine-producing tumor, such as a pheochromocytoma or paraganglioma, is capable of causing systemic adrenergic symptoms, plasma metanephrine levels are typically greater than fourfold higher than the upper limit of normal. It is not uncommon to see mild elevations in plasma normetanephrines that may represent high sympathetic nervous system tone or medication-induced effects. Medications that inhibit the reuptake of catecholamines in a synapse can increase circulating plasma normetanephrines. These medications include serotonin-norepinephrine reuptake inhibitors (such as venlafaxine), selective serotonin reuptake inhibitors, and tricyclic antidepressants. The discontinuation of venlafaxine is likely to result in normalization of this patient's values.

Neary NM, King KS, Pacak K. Drugs and pheochromocytoma—don't be fooled by every elevated metanephrine. *N Engl J Med.* 2011;364(23):2268–2270.

43. ANSWER: E. Switch to regular insulin, U-500.

Learning objective: Adjust antidiabetic management in patients with severe insulin resistance.

Severe insulin resistance (defined as the need for ≥200 U of insulin per day to achieve glycemic control) is commonly seen with obesity and can complicate diabetes management. The management of patients with diabetes who have severe insulin resistance is difficult and at times frustrating, and it requires a multifaceted approach.

For obese patients, weight loss is the best treatment option, but weight loss can be a challenging task for patients to achieve and maintain. Medications that decrease insulin needs, such as metformin, thiazolidinediones (TZDs), and GLP agonists, might help, but many patients still need high doses of insulin. In addition, treatment with TZDs is generally associated with weight gain, particularly when combined with insulin. Bariatric surgery is highly effective for obese patients with severe insulin resistance.

Delivering an appropriate insulin volume to these patients can be difficult and inconvenient. Most insulin pens can deliver a maximal dose of 60–80 U per injection, whereas patients using a syringe and vial can take up to 100 U per injection. If doses exceed this amount, the patient needs to take several consecutive injections. Furthermore, absorption of insulin from large-volume injections may be less efficient. This has led to the development of concentrated insulins with 200–500 (U-200–U-500) U/mL. This allows for delivery of higher doses of insulin per injection. Improved control may occur because of better compliance with dosing (fewer total daily injections) or better insulin action and absorption. U-500 kinetics are similar to premixed or NPH insulin.

A DPP-4 inhibitor or bromocriptine will not be sufficiently potent to control this patient's hyperglycemia. Increasing the dose of insulin or switching to NPH insulin is not likely to be as effective as switching to regular insulin, U-500.

Lane WS, Cochran EK, Jackson JA, et al. High-dose insulin therapy: is it time for u-500 insulin? *Endocr Pract.* 2009;15(1):71–79.

44. ANSWER: D. Refer for zoledronic acid infusion 5 mg intravenously.

Learning objective: Describe the appropriate treatment for Paget disease based on symptoms and anatomic location of lesions.

This patient has Paget disease, a bone condition of unknown etiology characterized by disordered bone resorption with a secondary increase in osteoblast activity, leading to disorganized bone architecture. Paget disease can be asymptomatic and diagnosed during workup of an incidentally noted increased alkaline phosphatase level. In these asymptomatic cases, if a bone scan does not show lesions in the skull or near joints, treatment may be deferred, and the patient can be monitored for the development of signs and symptoms of progressive disease. However, in this symptomatic patient with lesions close to the hip joint, treatment should be initiated. First-line treatment is a bisphosphonate, but usually at higher doses than for osteoporosis. Oral options are alendronate at a dose of 40 mg by mouth once daily or risedronate 30 mg by mouth once daily. Intravenous options include pamidronate (different dosing regimens; a commonly used regimen is 60 mg every 3 months) or zoledronic acid 5 mg (redosed when there is sign of recurrence after 1–2 years). Calcitonin is no longer recommended as first-line therapy for Paget disease.

Ralston SH. Paget's disease of bone. *N Engl J Med.* 2013; 368(7):644–650.

45. ANSWER: B. Complete blood count

Learning objective: Describe the routine laboratory evaluation for secondary causes of osteoporosis in a patient with newly diagnosed low bone mass.

All patients with osteoporosis should be evaluated for secondary causes of osteoporosis. A medical history and a physical exam should be focused on identifying risk factors and underlying causes of bone loss. In addition, all patients should have a laboratory evaluation for secondary causes. Although the extent of laboratory testing is unclear, the National Osteoporosis Foundation recommends in all patients consideration of sending for a complete blood count; routine chemistry levels, including calcium, phosphorus, magnesium, and renal/liver function tests; a thyroid-stimulating hormone level; a 25-hydroxyvitamin D level; bone turnover markers; and a 24-hour urinary calcium. Men should also have a testosterone level measured. In selected patients, evaluation for primary hyperparathyroidism, multiple myeloma, celiac disease, Cushing syndrome, and systemic mastocytosis may be indicated. In this patient, there are no unusual findings on the physical exam to suggest any of these disorders, and therefore laboratory evaluation beyond the routine tests is not indicated.

Cosman F, de Beur SJ, LeBoff MS, et al. Clinician's guide to prevention and treatment of osteoporosis. *Osteoporos Int.* 2014;25(10):2359–2381.

46. ANSWER: C. Adrenal myelolipoma

Learning objective: Distinguish causes of adrenal masses on the basis of imaging characteristics.

The radiographic phenotype of an adrenal mass can provide valuable clues in distinguishing benign from malignant adrenal processes. Benign adrenal masses are typically lipid-rich and therefore have a low density as measured on noncontrast CT scan by x-ray attenuation (Hounsfield units [HU]). Adipose tissue tends to have a density of approximately −20 to −150 HU. A density of <10 HU (lipid-rich entity) on noncontrast CT scan almost always represents a benign adrenal adenoma, except when the density is very low (less than −40 HU), in which case it almost always represents a myelolipoma. Myelolipomas are benign, lipid-rich growths that are not hormonally active.

Some benign adrenal adenomas may have a lower lipid content and therefore may have a more dense phenotype (>10 HU). Higher-density adrenal masses increase the concern for pheochromocytomas, carcinomas, and other malignant entities.

Young WF Jr. The incidentally discovered adrenal mass. *N Engl J Med.* 2007;356(6):601–610.

47. ANSWER: D. Start levothyroxine at a dose of 25 µg daily.

Learning objective: Safely initiate thyroid hormone replacement therapy in a patient with coronary artery disease.

This patient has primary hypothyroidism based on the elevated TSH and low free T4 and total T4. The treatment is levothyroxine. In view of his coronary artery disease, levothyroxine should be started at a low dose (12.5–25 µg daily) to avoid triggering further ischemia as the metabolic rate starts to increase.

His full replacement dose of 125 µg orally corresponds to an intravenous dose of 60–80 µg. However, starting this dose could exacerbate cardiac ischemia. Similarly, liothyronine (synthetic T3) can rapidly increase metabolic rate and thus worsen cardiac ischemia. Checking antithyroid peroxidase and antithyroglobulin antibodies would not provide any additional information. In the absence of any known history of thyroid surgery or external radiation treatment to the head and neck, it can be presumed that his severe hypothyroidism is due to autoimmune thyroiditis. If the patient had needed an emergent cardiac intervention, it could be performed without waiting for thyroid hormone replacement therapy. However, because this patient does not need the procedure acutely, it would be safer to initiate treatment before revascularization because severe hypothyroidism can increase the risk of complications related to general anesthesia and the use of sedatives.

Garber JR, Cobin RH, Gharib H, et al. Clinical practice guidelines for hypothyroidism in adults: Cosponsored by the American Association of Clinical Endocrinologists and the American Thyroid Association. *Endocr Pract.* 2012;18(6):988–1028.

48. ANSWER: E. Urine pregnancy test

Learning objective: Consider physiologic causes of hyperprolactinemia.

Hyperprolactinemia is a relatively common cause of amenorrhea and is certainly part of the differential diagnosis when a woman presents with missed menstrual cycles. It is important to replicate the laboratory abnormality because performance of the breast examination immediately prior to blood sampling can cause a transient elevation in prolactin. Pregnancy must be excluded as a cause of hyperprolactinemia in all women of childbearing potential because prolactin levels rise as a normal physiologic response during pregnancy. Another physiologic cause is primary hyperparathyroidism because the elevated thyrotropin-releasing hormone (TRH) level seen in this condition stimulates both TSH and prolactin release. Medication-induced hyperprolactinemia is another cause to consider. A pituitary MRI to assess for the presence of a pituitary adenoma is indicated only after other causes of hyperprolactinemia have been excluded. If a mass is seen that impinges on the optic apparatus, visual fields should be formally assessed. Although dopamine is a regulator of prolactin release, serum levels are not helpful, because they do not reflect levels in the hypothalamo-hypophyseal portal system. A pelvic ultrasound does not have a role in the workup of hyperprolactinemia.

Melmed S, Casanueva FF, Hoffman AR, et al. Diagnosis and treatment of hyperprolactinemia: an Endocrine Society clinical practice guideline. *J Clin Endocrinol Metab.* 2011;96(2):273–288.

49. ANSWER: B. Increase the dose of levothyroxine to nine pills per week once she is pregnant.

Learning objective: Advise appropriate dose adjustment of thyroid hormone replacement in a woman pursuing pregnancy.

Levothyroxine requirements increase in pregnancy due to the increased levels of thyroid-binding proteins under the influence of estrogen. A similar effect is seen when initiating the combined oral contraceptive pill. In pregnancy, a dose increase of 30% is usually required even early in pregnancy. Therefore, women with hypothyroidism who are of childbearing age should be advised to increase the dose of levothyroxine from seven pills per week to nine pills per week (so take two pills on 2 days of the week) as soon as they are pregnant. There is no need to increase the dose before the patient is pregnant or to measure monthly TSH values while she is attempting pregnancy, because her last TSH was normal. Women attempting pregnancy should not take agents that contain T3, because T3 does not cross the placenta, and therefore the fetus may be relatively hypothyroid. Fetal thyroid ultrasound is recommended in certain cases if the mother has had Graves disease.

Alexander EK, Pearce EN, Brent GA, et al. 2017 Guidelines of the American Thyroid Association for the Diagnosis and Management of Thyroid Disease During Pregnancy and the Postpartum. *Thyroid.* 2017;27(3):315–389.

50. ANSWER: A. Medical therapy with a dopamine agonist

Learning objective: Choose appropriate therapies for a prolactin-secreting pituitary adenoma.

Medical therapy with a dopamine agonist is considered the first-line initial therapy for symptomatic prolactinomas. Dopamine agonists have both antiproliferative and antisecretory effects on prolactin-producing pituitary cells and typically result in both decreased prolactin secretion and tumor shrinkage. Cabergoline is preferred over bromocriptine for most patients due to its increased efficacy and tolerability. Somatostatin analogues are used in the treatment of acromegaly. Transsphenoidal surgery is reserved for patients who do not tolerate or are not responsive to the dopamine agonists. Radiation would be considered only in very rare cases of advanced or progressive prolactinomas for which medical or surgical interventions have failed. Observation alone would not be the preferred approach in a patient with a macroadenoma (size >10 mm), because control of tumor growth would be desired.

Melmed S, Casanueva FF, Hoffman AR, et al. Diagnosis and treatment of hyperprolactinemia: an Endocrine Society clinical practice guideline. *J Clin Endocrinol Metab.* 2011;96(2):273–288.

Acknowledgment

The author and editors gratefully acknowledge the contributions of the previous authors, Carolyn Becker, Amir Tirosh, Le Min, Klara Rosenquist, Anand Vaidya, Whitney W. Woodmansee, Bindu Chamarthi, and Matthew Kim.

6 Nephrology and Hypertension

MEGAN PROCHASKA AND ERNEST I. MANDEL

1. A 55-year-old man with a history of stage 3 chronic kidney disease secondary to hypertensive nephropathy presents with ongoing hypertension and mild bilateral lower extremity swelling. His blood pressure was previously controlled with hydrochlorothiazide. Laboratory results reveal an estimated glomerular filtration rate (GFR) of 30 mL/min/1.73 m2. Complete blood count, transaminases, albumin, and coagulation studies are all normal. Urinalysis is normal. A recent echocardiogram was normal.

   What is the next step in managing the patient's hypertension?

   A. Start amlodipine.
   B. Start lisinopril.
   C. Change hydrochlorothiazide to chlorthalidone.
   D. Change hydrochlorothiazide to furosemide.
   E. Low-salt diet

2. A 30-year-old man presents to the emergency department with a 3-week history of headaches and blurry vision and is found to have a blood pressure of 270/140 mm Hg. Physical examination is notable for retinal hemorrhages. The complete blood count reveals a white blood cell count of 5500/mm^3, hemoglobin of 8 g/dL, and platelets of 50,000/µL. Serum creatinine is 19 mg/dL. Coagulation studies are normal. Fibrinogen is elevated. Lactate dehydrogenase (LDH) is elevated, reticulocyte index is calculated to be elevated, and haptoglobin is low. A review of the peripheral smear reveals schistocytes. The urine sediment is remarkable for several red blood cell casts. Electrocardiography reveals the presence of left ventricular hypertrophy.

   What is the diagnosis?

   A. Atypical hemolytic uremic syndrome
   B. Glomerulonephritis
   C. Hypertensive emergency
   D. Thrombotic thrombocytopenic purpura
   E. Disseminated intravascular coagulation

3. A 42-year-old man with a history of HIV on antiretroviral therapy (ART) and with hypertension presents with a 1-week history of polyuria and progressive muscle weakness. Medications include lamivudine, tenofovir disoproxil, efavirenz, lisinopril, and amlodipine. His laboratory values are notable for sodium 135 mEq/L, potassium 2.5 mEq/L, chloride 110 mEq/L, bicarbonate 19 mEq/L, blood urea nitrogen 24 mg/dL, creatinine 1.0 mg/dL, glucose 95 mg/dL, and phosphorus 1.5 mg/dL. Urinalysis reveals pH 6.0, 2+ glucose, and 2+ protein.

   Which of the following is the likely cause of his clinical presentation?

   A. Lamivudine
   B. Tenofovir disoproxil
   C. Efavirenz
   D. Lisinopril
   E. Amlodipine

4. A 65-year-old woman with a history of stage 4 chronic kidney disease, hypertension, stroke, and recently diagnosed lung cancer presents to the clinic for evaluation of asymptomatic anemia. Hemoglobin is 9 g/dL. Iron stores are normal. Vitamin B_{12} and folate levels are found to be normal.

   What is the next step?

   A. Start an erythropoietin-stimulating agent.
   B. Transfuse packed red blood cells.
   C. Transfuse packed red blood cells and start an erythropoietin-stimulating agent.
   D. Start oral iron therapy.
   E. Counsel the patient on vascular access for dialysis.

5. A 72-year-old woman with three-vessel coronary artery disease returns from the operating room after undergoing coronary artery bypass grafting with the intraoperative use of cardiopulmonary bypass, with postoperative laboratory tests revealing acute kidney injury and hyperkalemia with a potassium of 6.5 mEq/L. EKG shows peaked T waves and widened QRS complexes. Calcium, insulin, and dextrose are administered.

   What is the next best management step for definitive treatment of hyperkalemia?

   A. Furosemide
   B. Sodium polystyrene sulfonate
   C. Sodium polystyrene sulfonate with sorbitol
   D. Sodium bicarbonate
   E. Hemodialysis

6. A 47-year-old African American man with recently diagnosed HIV infection in the setting of esophageal candidiasis is referred for evaluation of bilateral lower extremity edema associated with a serum creatinine of 2 mg/dL and 3+ albumin by urine dipstick. A 24-hour urine collection reveals 6 g of proteinuria. Testing for hepatitis B and C is negative. After confirming the suspected diagnosis by kidney biopsy, which of the following treatment options should be pursued in addition to an angiotensin-converting enzyme (ACE) inhibitor?
   A. Steroids alone
   B. ART alone
   C. ART + steroids
   D. Steroids + mycophenolate mofetil
   E. Plasmapheresis

7. A 71-year-old man with chronic kidney disease presents for a routine visit. He is currently asymptomatic. On physical examination, his jugular vein is not distended and he has no peripheral edema. Laboratory data are remarkable for serum sodium of 130 mEq/L, potassium 4 mEq/L, chloride 104 mEq/L, bicarbonate 24 mEq/L, blood urea nitrogen 28 mg/dL, creatinine 3 mg/dL, and glucose 90 mg/dL. An osmolality gap is present. Urine dipstick analysis is negative for protein. Of the following, which is the most likely explanation of the patient's hyponatremia?
   A. Hypovolemia
   B. Low solute intake
   C. Multiple myeloma
   D. Syndrome of inappropriate antidiuretic hormone (SIADH)
   E. Hypothyroidism

8. A 26-year-old woman is referred to the emergency department for evaluation of acute kidney injury. Physical examination is remarkable for a blood pressure of 130/80 mm Hg, diffuse skin thickening, and sclerodactyly. Laboratory tests reveal an acute rise in creatinine from 1 mg/dL to 4.5 mg/dL. White blood cell count is 4500/μL, hemoglobin is 7 g/dL, and platelets are 110,000/μL. LDH is elevated and haptoglobin is low. Schistocytes are present on peripheral smear.
   What is the next best step?
   A. Renal biopsy
   B. Plasmapheresis
   C. Captopril
   D. Intravenous immunoglobulin therapy (IVIG)
   E. Methylprednisolone

9. A 41-year-old man presents with resistant hypertension and hypokalemia. Physical examination is remarkable for a blood pressure of 180/110 mm Hg despite three antihypertensive agents at maximal doses. There is no peripheral edema on examination. Secondary hypertension workup reveals an aldosterone-to-plasma renin activity ratio of 35, with a serum aldosterone level of 30 ng/dL. After confirmatory testing is performed to demonstrate inappropriately high aldosterone secretion, CT imaging of the abdomen and pelvis with contrast is performed and reveals no evidence of adrenal pathology.
   What is the next step?
   A. Adrenal vein sampling
   B. MRI with gadolinium contrast
   C. Addition of spironolactone
   D. Renal artery stenting
   E. Renal sympathetic denervation

10. A 48-year-old woman with rheumatoid arthritis and Crohn disease presents to the clinic with bloody diarrhea and abdominal pain, suspected to be related to Crohn flare. She is initiated on steroids in the clinic and sent to the emergency department. Laboratory tests reveal sodium 135 mEq/L, potassium 3.0 mEq/L, chloride 110 mEq/L, bicarbonate 16 mEq/L, blood urea nitrogen 20 mg/dL, and creatinine 1.2 mg/ dL. Urinalysis is within normal limits. Urine pH is 6.5. The urine anion gap is positive.
   What is the likely cause of the patient's hypokalemia?
   A. Loss of potassium and bicarbonate in stool
   B. Hypokalemia resulting from corticosteroid administration
   C. Distal (type 1) renal tubular acidosis (RTA)
   D. Proximal (type 2) RTA
   E. Type 4 RTA

11. A 29-year-old woman with lupus presents with a new onset of 3+ proteinuria on urine dipstick. A spot urine protein-to-creatinine ratio is 5. Serum creatinine is stable at 0.9 mg/dL. The patient has low C3 and C4, elevated dsDNA titers, and evidence of red blood cell casts on urine microscopy. Renal biopsy is performed, and histopathology demonstrates focal lupus nephritis (WHO class III).
   What is the next step?
   A. No therapy, continue close monitoring.
   B. ACE inhibitor and prednisone
   C. ACE inhibitor and rituximab
   D. ACE inhibitor, prednisone, and mycophenolate mofetil
   E. ACE inhibitor, prednisone, and cyclophosphamide

12. An 88-year-old man with a history of uncontrolled hypertension and stroke was recently seen in the clinic and started on amlodipine 5 mg daily and benazepril 20 mg daily. He now presents to the clinic with blood pressure of 140/70 mm Hg.

What is the next step in management?

A. Add chlorthalidone 12.5 mg daily.
B. Increase benazepril to 40 mg daily.
C. Increase amlodipine to 10 mg once daily.
D. Counsel on low-salt diet.
E. Perform a workup for secondary causes of hypertension.

13. A 52-year-old woman presents to the emergency room after a motor vehicle accident in which she sustained a crush injury and is found to have acute kidney injury 3 days after admission to the hospital. Laboratory data reveal sodium 137 mEq/L, potassium 4.3 mEq/L, chloride 105 mEq/L, bicarbonate 25 mEq/L, creatinine 3 mg/dL, calcium 6.5 mg/dL, and phosphorus 6 mg/dL. Creatine kinase is found to be 10,000 U/L.

What is the most appropriate treatment?

A. Isotonic bicarbonate
B. Isotonic saline
C. Furosemide
D. Hemodialysis
E. Mannitol

14. An 18-year-old man presents with acute kidney injury 3 days after an upper respiratory tract infection, with rise in creatinine from 0.9 to 1.6 mg/dL. The patient's urinalysis reveals 2+ blood and 2+ protein. C3 and C4 are normal. Serologic workup is negative for antineutrophil cytoplasmic antibody (ANCA) and antibodies against glomerular basement membrane (anti-GBM). Serum protein electrophoresis (SPEP) and urine protein electrophoresis (UPEP) are within normal limits.

What is the likely diagnosis?

A. IgA nephropathy
B. Postinfectious glomerulonephritis
C. Thin basement membrane disease
D. Alport syndrome
E. Granulomatous polyangiitis

15. A 71-year-old man with a history of chronic obstructive pulmonary disease (COPD), smoking, and chronic hyponatremia attributed to SIADH presents to the emergency department with altered mental status, tongue biting, and urinary incontinence. Serum sodium is found to be 105 mEq/L, down from 125 mEq/L, which was noted on laboratory testing approximately 2 weeks prior to presentation. Therapy is initiated with hypertonic saline, and a repeat serum sodium in 10 hours is found to be 120 mEq/L. His mental status has now improved back to baseline.

What is the next step in therapy?

A. Continue hypertonic saline.
B. Stop hypertonic saline and start D5W and DDAVP.
C. Stop hypertonic saline and monitor closely.
D. Switch fluids to isotonic saline.
E. Switch fluids to half-normal saline.

16. A 44-year-old woman with a history of asthma and gastroesophageal reflux disease (GERD) and chronic cough presents with a fever, rash, and a newly noted eosinophilia, associated with acute kidney injury. Urinalysis is remarkable for cellular casts. She has been on inhaled steroids for treatment of her asthma and was recently initiated on treatment for GERD in the setting of a persistent cough. The patient monitors her peak flows, and these have been normal. She otherwise has no symptoms.

What is the likely cause of the patient's acute kidney injury?

A. Acute tubular necrosis
B. Acute interstitial nephritis
C. Acute glomerulonephritis
D. Henoch-Schönlein purpura
E. Drug reaction with eosinophilic and systemic symptoms (DRESS) syndrome

17. A 70-year-old man with a history of congestive heart failure, coronary artery disease, hypertension, and total body volume overload presents with recurrent admissions for pulmonary edema. His outpatient blood pressures are well controlled on a combination of furosemide, carvedilol, amlodipine, and lisinopril. He is compliant with his medications. Secondary workup of the patient's hypertension reveals unilateral atherosclerotic renal artery stenosis.

What is the next step?

A. Percutaneous renal artery angioplasty with stent placement
B. Renal artery surgical revascularization
C. Adding a thiazide diuretic
D. Increasing the dose of furosemide
E. Referring for heart transplant

18. A 55-year-old woman with a history of long-standing diabetes with macroalbuminuria and hypertension presents to the clinic with ongoing hypertension. She takes lisinopril 40 mg daily for management of hypertension, but her blood pressure remains at 150/85 mm Hg. She reports compliance with a low-salt diet. Urine microalbumin-to-creatinine ratio reveals ongoing macroalbuminuria.

What is the next best agent to add?

A. Add valsartan.
B. Add chlorthalidone.
C. Add metoprolol.
D. Add aliskiren.
E. Add benazepril.

19. A 32-year-old man returns from travel to India with symptoms of productive cough, night sweats, chill, and unintentional weight loss. He does not initially seek medical care and develops worsening malaise, nausea, and lightheadedness. When he presents to the emergency department, his blood pressure

is 84/45 mm Hg. Laboratory data are remarkable for sodium 122 mEq/L and potassium 6.1 mEq/L. Serum creatinine is 1.1 mg/dL.

What is the next step in management?

A. Fluid restriction
B. Hypertonic saline
C. Isotonic saline alone
D. Isotonic saline with hydrocortisone
E. Tolvaptan

20. A 30-year-old woman presents to the clinic for evaluation of an enlarging jaw mass. Laboratory results reveal potassium 5.5 mEq/L, calcium 6.5 mg/dL, phosphorus 11 mg/ dL, and creatinine 1.4 mg/dL. Uric acid is 15 mg/dL.

In addition to intravenous fluids, what is the next step in the appropriate management of this condition?

A. Rasburicase
B. Allopurinol
C. Febuxostat
D. Sodium polystyrene sulfonate
E. Hemodialysis

21. A 62-year-old man with a history of type 2 diabetes mellitus, coronary artery disease, peripheral artery disease, and hypertension presents to the clinic for routine follow-up. He is currently on three antihypertensive agents. His blood pressure is 130/70 mm Hg. Serum creatinine is 0.7 mg/dL. There is no evidence of microalbuminuria. Serum aldosterone and plasma renin activity are mildly elevated. A renal duplex study reveals bilateral renal artery stenosis.

What is the next step in managing this patient?

A. Percutaneous renal artery angioplasty with stent placement
B. Renal artery surgical revascularization
C. Adding an additional antihypertensive
D. Stopping an antihypertensive to permissively raise the systolic blood pressure closer to 140 mm Hg
E. Do nothing

22. A 56-year-old man presents for evaluation of anxiety, depression, and peripheral neuropathy. He has been employed as a painter for most of his adult life. Laboratory testing reveals an estimated GFR of 25 mL/min/1.73 m^2, nongap metabolic acidosis associated with a positive urine anion gap, and microcytic anemia. A serum lead level was found to be elevated.

What would a renal biopsy be expected to demonstrate in this patient?

A. Acute interstitial nephritis
B. Acute tubular necrosis
C. Glomerulonephritis
D. Glomerular hypertrophy
E. Chronic interstitial nephritis

23. A 60-year-old patient with autosomal dominant polycystic kidney disease underwent a living unrelated kidney transplant 10 years ago. He had been on stable doses of tacrolimus, mycophenolate mofetil, and prednisone, but he accidentally took double the dose of tacrolimus over the past 2 weeks.

Which of these findings is associated with calcineurin inhibitor toxicity?

A. Hypokalemia
B. Acute interstitial nephritis
C. Hypomagnesemia
D. Hypercalcemia
E. Rhabdomyolysis

24. A 38-year-old woman presents with newly diagnosed Hodgkin lymphoma associated with bilateral lower extremity edema. Laboratory workup reveals 10 g of proteinuria on a 24-hour urine collection.

Which of the following pathologic entities most likely explains the presence of proteinuria in this patient?

A. Membranous nephropathy
B. Minimal change disease
C. Focal segmental glomerulosclerosis
D. IgA nephropathy
E. Amyloidosis

25. A 49-year-old man with untreated hepatitis C viral infection develops persistent proteinuria.

Which of the following is a renal manifestation associated with hepatitis C viral infection?

A. Acute interstitial nephritis
B. Focal segmental glomerulosclerosis
C. Polyarteritis nodosa
D. Nephrogenic diabetes insipidus
E. Fanconi syndrome

26. A 43-year-old man presents with bilateral lower extremity edema associated with 3 g/d of proteinuria with preserved renal function. He undergoes renal biopsy, which demonstrates membranous nephropathy. Infectious workup for hepatitis B and C virus and syphilis is negative. Complements are normal. Lupus serologies are unremarkable. Age-appropriate cancer screening is unremarkable. In addition to an ACE inhibitor, what therapy should be offered?

A. Nothing
B. Steroids
C. Steroid
D. Steroids and cyclophosphamide
E. Rituximab

27. A 92-year-old woman presents to the emergency department with symptoms of right-sided weakness and slurred speech that were noted upon awakening from sleep. MRI confirms an acute ischemic stroke. Her initial blood pressure on presentation was 240/120 mm Hg, but it has since come down to 200/100 mm Hg. She continues to have slurred speech and right-sided weakness but appears to be alert and following commands.

Which of the following is the most appropriate blood pressure goal in this setting?

A. Less than 220/120 mm Hg
B. Less than 180/105 mm Hg
C. Less than 150/90 mm Hg
D. Less than 140/90 mm Hg
E. Less than 120/80 mm Hg

28. A 77-year-old man with hypertension, restrictive cardiomyopathy, recently diagnosed diabetes, and peripheral neuropathy develops 10 g/d of proteinuria as measured by a 24-hour urine collection. The onset of peripheral neuropathy preceded the diagnosis of diabetes. Physical examination is remarkable for periorbital purpura and lateral scalloping of the tongue.

What is the likely explanation for the patient's nephrotic range proteinuria?

A. AA amyloid
B. AL amyloidosis
C. Focal segmental glomerulosclerosis (FSGS)
D. Diabetic nephropathy
E. Hypertensive nephropathy

29. An 18-year-old man presents with hemolytic anemia, thrombocytopenia, and acute kidney injury, in the absence of a diarrheal prodrome. C3 is low, and C4 is normal. CH50 is <10%, and AH50 is <10%. ADAMTS13 activity is somewhat low at 40%.

How should this condition be treated?

A. Plasmapheresis
B. IVIG
C. Steroids
D. Rituximab
E. Eculizumab

30. A 36-year-old woman with a history of lupus nephritis presents with a rising creatinine level and worsening proteinuria. She recently completed a course of treatment with steroids and mycophenolate mofetil for International Society of Nephrology/Renal Pathology Society (ISN/RPS) class IV and class V lupus nephritis. A repeat biopsy is performed and reveals class VI nephropathy.

What is the most appropriate treatment?

A. Rituximab
B. Steroids and mycophenolate mofetil
C. Steroids and cyclophosphamide
D. Steroids and tacrolimus
E. Discuss dialysis and transplant

31. A 62-year-old woman presents with a rise in creatinine from 1 to 6 mg/L in the span of 1 week, associated with a new onset of hemoptysis. Serologic workup reveals positive c-ANCA and anti-PR3 antibody.

What is the appropriate treatment?

A. Steroids
B. Steroids and cyclophosphamide
C. Plasmapheresis, steroids, and cyclophosphamide
D. Rituximab
E. Dialysis

32. A 65-year-old man with a family history of autosomal dominant polycystic kidney disease is diagnosed with polycystic kidney disease on the basis of CT imaging.

Which of the following treatments could be expected to reduce the annual increase in kidney size?

A. Vasopressin receptor antagonism
B. Antihypertensive therapy
C. Statin therapy
D. Low-protein diet
E. Steroid therapy

33. A 54-year-old woman with a history of stage 4 chronic kidney disease secondary to uncontrolled diabetes mellitus presents with the following laboratory values: calcium 7.1 mg/dL, phosphorus 6.3 mg/dL, PTH 1000 pg/mL, and normal 25-hydroxy-vitamin D level. In addition to starting a phosphorus binder, what is the next step in management?

A. Start 25-hydroxyvitamin D supplementation.
B. Start 1,25-hydroxyvitamin D supplementation.
C. Start cinacalcet, a calcimimetic.
D. Start calcium supplementation.
E. Refer for parathyroidectomy.

34. A 25-year-old man presents to clinic for follow-up after a recent attack of gout. His serum uric acid is 6.7 mg/dL, and his creatinine is 1.4 mg/dL. His brother also has gout and was diagnosed with end-stage kidney disease at the age of 41; his mother died at age 59 after 10 years on dialysis.

What is the most likely diagnosis?

A. Uromodulin kidney disease
B. Lead nephropathy
C. Acute uric acid nephropathy
D. Chronic urate nephropathy
E. Diabetic nephropathy

35. A 42-year-old man with a diagnosis of hypertension, coronary artery disease, congestive heart failure, and obstructive sleep apnea presents for evaluation of ongoing hypertension. The patient is already on three antihypertensives. A secondary workup for causes of hypertension is performed. Endocrine workup is negative. Serum aldosterone and plasma renin activity are within normal limits. A renal ultrasound duplex study reveals no evidence of renal artery stenosis.

What is the best next step in management?

A. Add a fourth antihypertensive medication.
B. Recommend continuous positive airway pressure (CPAP) at night.
C. Refer for renal sympathetic denervation.
D. Counsel on DASH diet.
E. Counsel on low-salt diet.

36. A 68-year-old man with a history of coronary artery disease with multiple prior myocardial infarctions, peripheral artery disease, and diabetes mellitus presents with ongoing hypertension despite the use of benazepril.

Which of the following agents should be added next for the management of this patient's hypertension?
A. Hydrochlorothiazide
B. Amlodipine
C. Furosemide
D. Amiloride
E. Minoxidil

37. A 58-year-old woman with no known medical history is sent to the emergency department for evaluation of hypertension with a blood pressure of 210/110 mm Hg. The patient currently has no complaints. Laboratory test results are unremarkable, with the exception of urinalysis that reveals trace protein. Electrocardiogram reveals left ventricular hypertrophy.

What is the next step in management?
A. Oral chlorthalidone and lisinopril and follow-up as an outpatient
B. Intravenous labetalol
C. Intravenous nitroprusside
D. Intravenous nitroglycerin
E. Intravenous hydralazine and transition to oral hydralazine

38. A 64-year-old woman with a long-standing history of bipolar disorder managed on lithium for 20 years is referred to the nephrology department for evaluation of chronic kidney disease (CKD) and concern for lithium nephrotoxicity. In addition to diabetes insipidus, renal tubular acidosis (RTA), and chronic interstitial nephritis, which of the following is a manifestation of lithium nephrotoxicity?
A. Hypercalciuria
B. Hypoparathyroidism
C. Hyperphosphatemia
D. Hypocalcemia
E. Nephrotic syndrome

39. A 42-year-old man with a history of alcohol abuse presents to the emergency department with a seizure in the setting of alcohol withdrawal. He is initiated on a lorazepam intravenous drip and transferred to the intensive care unit. Weaning the drip results in recurrent seizures, so lorazepam is restarted. Serum chemistries reveal sodium 138 mEq/L, potassium 3.6 mEq/L, chloride 98 mEq/L, bicarbonate 22 mEq/L, blood urea nitrogen 13 mg/dL, creatinine 0.9 g/dL, and glucose 90 mg/dL. Ethanol level is undetectable. Measured serum osmolality is 298 mOsm/kg. Serum ketones are negative. Serum lactic acid is within normal limits. Urinalysis is within normal limits.

What is the likely cause of the patient's anion gap acidosis?
A. Lorazepam
B. Rhabdomyolysis related to seizure
C. Alcoholic ketoacidosis
D. Uremia
E. D-Lactic acidosis

40. A 35-year-old woman presents with a new onset of hypertension, and a secondary workup of hypertension is performed. Renal ultrasound with duplex is notable for an increased peak velocity and tortuosity in the middle and distal renal arteries in the left kidney.

Which of the following statements is true about this condition?
A. The condition is more common in men.
B. Extracranial cerebrovascular involvement is common.
C. MR angiogram is the preferred diagnostic study.
D. Surgical management is the preferred treatment for the renal lesions.
E. Atherosclerosis is the primary cause of the disease.

41. A 55-year-old man with a history of cirrhosis resulting from fatty liver disease presents with a gastrointestinal bleed, followed by the development of oliguric acute kidney injury with no proteinuria and a normal urine sediment. Urine sodium is less than 10 mEq/L. Volume repletion with blood products and crystalloid solution results in no improvement in the patient's renal function.

Which of the following is true about the likely clinical diagnosis?
A. Octreotide and midodrine can be used for definitive management of this condition.
B. Liver transplant is contraindicated.
C. Hemodialysis, if indicated, is typically well tolerated.
D. Renal biopsy would be expected to reveal a normal kidney
E. If evaluating the patient for a liver transplant, a kidney transplant would also be indicated.

42. A 28-year-old man presents with arm and leg cramps and polyuria and is found to have a blood pressure of approximately 90/50 mm Hg associated with a serum potassium level of 3.1 mEq/L and a magnesium level of 0.9 mEq/L. Urinary calcium is low, and urinary chloride is elevated.

What is the likely diagnosis?

A. Surreptitious vomiting
B. Bartter syndrome
C. Gitelman syndrome
D. Primary hyperaldosteronism
E. Cushing syndrome

43. An 18-year-old man with a history of deafness and hematuria presents with a progressively rising creatinine level. His sister, mother, and father are all healthy, though he does recall a maternal grandfather who died as a result of complications of kidney disease.

What is the likely diagnosis?
A. Thin basement membrane disease
B. Alport syndrome
C. Fabry disease
D. Amyloidosis
E. Tubulointerstitial nephritis with uveitis

44. A 47-year-old woman with a history of Roux-en-Y gastric bypass surgery 6 years ago presents with acute onset of right-flank pain and gross hematuria. Abdominal imaging with a CT scan demonstrates a kidney stone.

Which of the following is the most likely type of kidney stone?
A. Calcium phosphate
B. Calcium oxalate
C. Uric acid
D. Cystine
E. Struvite

45. A 19-year-old man with a history of stroke in the absence of hypertension, left ventricular hypertrophy, and angiokeratomas (vascular cutaneous lesions) presents for evaluation of chronic kidney disease. Renal imaging demonstrates multiple renal sinus cysts.

What is the likely diagnosis?
A. Thin basement membrane disease
B. Alport syndrome
C. Fabry disease
D. Amyloidosis
E. Tubulointerstitial nephritis with uveitis

46. A 39-year-old man with newly diagnosed Hodgkin lymphoma develops dyspnea and is noted to have Kussmaul respirations. Serum chemistries and blood gas reveal anion gap acidosis. Blood, urine, and sputum cultures are sent, and he is started on empiric broad-spectrum antimicrobial therapies. Despite negative culture data and several days of antibiotics, the anion gap acidosis is persistent.

How would you classify this patient's anion gap acidosis?
A. Type A lactic acidosis
B. Type B lactic acidosis
C. D-Lactic acidosis
D. Ketoacidosis
E. Ethylene glycol acidosis

47. A 53-year-old woman with a history of alcohol abuse presents to the emergency department in an inebriated state after drinking antifreeze solution. Laboratory test results are remarkable for a negative ethanol level, sodium 137 mEq/L, bicarbonate 8 mEq/L, chloride 101 mEq/L, glucose 110 mg/dL, BUN 18 mg/dL, and serum osmolality 312 mOsm/kg. Urinalysis reveals calcium oxalate crystals.

What is the next step in management?
A. Start isotonic saline.
B. Perform gastric lavage.
C. Administer furosemide.
D. Administer activated charcoal.
E. Administer fomepizole and prepare for dialysis.

48. A 56-year-old woman with type 2 diabetes and hypertension currently on losartan and amlodipine presents for follow-up. Blood pressure is 130/80 mm Hg, and physical exam is otherwise notable for clear lungs and trace lower extremity edema. Laboratory test results are notable for creatinine 2.4 mg/dL, potassium 5.2 mEq/L, and bicarbonate 20 mmol/L. Urine studies are notable for pH 5.5 and microalbumin-to-creatinine ratio of 64 mg/g.

What is the most appropriate next step in management?
A. Add spironolactone 12.5 mg daily.
B. Discontinue losartan and replace with chlorthalidone 12.5 mg daily.
C. Start oral sodium bicarbonate therapy.
D. Start oral potassium citrate therapy.
E. Start fludrocortisone 0.1 mg daily.

49. A 65-year-old man with a history of diabetes mellitus, hypertension, and gout presents with new-onset abdominal pain. He takes metformin, lisinopril, and allopurinol. His electrolytes are within the reference range. His uric acid is 5.7 mg/dL, and his creatinine is 1.2 mg/dL. He has a noncontrast CT scan that shows a 9-mm kidney stone on the right and multiple smaller kidney stones on the left. He passes one of the stones, and the stone analysis reveals 100% uric acid.

Which of the following is the target urinary pH for treatment of uric acid kidney stones?
A. pH 5.0–5.5
B. None; pH is not a factor in the management of uric acid kidney stones.
C. pH greater than 7.5
D. pH 6.5–7.0
E. pH less than 5.0

50. An 84-year-old woman presents for follow-up of CKD. Since her last visit 6 months ago, she has become increasingly dependent after experiencing an influenza-like illness, now with a 10-lb weight loss and poor nutrition. Three months ago, she moved into a nursing home. Past medical history includes

CKD stage 3 with baseline creatinine 1.3 mg/dL presumed to be secondary to long-standing hypertension as well as past NSAID use for osteoarthritis. Current medications include amlodipine 10 mg daily, metoprolol 50 mg daily, furosemide 40 mg daily, lisinopril 10 mg daily, and acetaminophen 975 mg three times daily. Blood pressure is 142/74 mm Hg, and physical exam reveals a thin woman with clear lungs and no lower extremity edema. Laboratory testing reveals Cr 1.4 mg/dL, sodium 134 mEq/L, chloride 99 mg/dL, bicarbonate 17 mmol/L, and albumin 2.9 mg/dL. Lactate and ketones are normal.

Which of the following is the most appropriate next step in management of the patient's acidosis?

A. Start oral bicarbonate therapy.
B. Discontinue acetaminophen.
C. Start parenteral nutrition.
D. Discontinue lisinopril.
E. Start midodrine to optimize perfusion.

Chapter 6 Answers

1. **ANSWER: D. Change hydrochlorothiazide to furosemide.**

Amlodipine is incorrect because it may worsen the patient's lower extremity edema. Though angiotensin-converting enzyme (ACE) inhibitors such as lisinopril are recommended in patients with proteinuric chronic kidney disease, they do not provide a preferential benefit in treating patients with nonproteinuric chronic kidney disease. Though chlorthalidone has been purported to be more effective than hydrochlorothiazide on the basis of meta-analyses (due to a longer duration of action), thiazide diuretics are less effective than loop diuretics in chronic kidney disease. For this reason, the correct answer is to switch the thiazide to a loop diuretic (furosemide) to treat the patient's apparent volume expansion. A low-salt diet should always be recommended because a high-salt diet can lead to diuretic resistance, but in this patient it is not likely the reason for the patient's diuretic resistance.

2. **ANSWER: C. Hypertensive emergency**

The presence of markers of hemolysis (anemia, elevated LDH, low haptoglobin, and elevated reticulocyte index), combined with the presence of schistocytes in the peripheral smear, raises concern for microangiopathic hemolytic anemia. Although these findings, in combination with thrombocytopenia, raise concern for hemolytic uremic syndrome and thrombotic thrombocytopenic purpura, the renal disease seen is usually much milder, and hypertension of this severity is not typical. On the other hand, hypertensive emergency can cause thrombotic microangiopathy and is the likely explanation for this patient's clinical presentation. The presence of left ventricular hypertrophy on an electrocardiogram (EKG) suggests that the hypertension has been long-standing. Atypical hemolytic uremic syndrome describes a variant of hemolytic uremic syndrome (HUS) that occurs in the absence of diarrhea and can be explained by other infections or complement dysregulation. Though red blood cell casts are seen in glomerulonephritis, they can also be seen in thrombotic microangiopathies. Disseminated intravenous coagulopathy (DIC) is less likely in the setting of normal coagulation studies and an elevated fibrinogen level.

3. **ANSWER: B. Tenofovir disoproxil**

This patient's clinical presentation is consistent with Fanconi syndrome resulting from tenofovir disoproxil therapy. Fanconi syndrome is a disorder of the proximal tubule characterized by low serum bicarbonate resulting from reduced proximal bicarbonate reabsorption, low serum phosphate resulting from phosphaturia, glucosuria with normal serum glucose, and proteinuria. Fanconi syndrome can be inherited or acquired. Tenofovir in general is associated with acquired Fanconi syndrome, which is significant because an estimated 84% of U.S. residents on therapy for HIV infection take a formulation of tenofovir, and this drug is also used to treat chronic hepatitis B infection. Since 2015 there have been two different formulations of tenofovir available as part of antiretroviral regimens for HIV infection: tenofovir disoproxil (which was approved by the FDA in 2001) and tenofovir alafenamide (which was approved by the FDA in 2015). Both are prodrugs of the same active antiviral medication, but tenofovir alafenamide achieves high intracellular concentrations of the active drug, thereby allowing for lower doses of the prodrug and diminished renal toxicity. As the use of tenofovir alafenamide rises, the occurrence of Fanconi syndrome associated with tenofovir would be expected to decline.

Sax PE, Wohl D, Yin MT, et al. Tenofovir alafenamide versus tenofovir disoproxil fumarate, coformulated with elvitegravir, cobicistat, and emtricitabine, for initial treatment of HIV-1 infection: two randomised, double-blind, phase 3, non-inferiority trials. *Lancet.* 2015;385(9987):2606–2615.

Walensky RP, Horn TH, Paltiel AD. The Epi-TAF for tenofovir disoproxil fumarate? *Clin Infect Dis.* 2016;62(7):915–918.

4. **ANSWER: E. Counsel the patient on vascular access for dialysis.**

On the basis of the 2012 Kidney Disease Improving Global Outcomes (KDIGO) guidelines, there should be careful consideration of whether erythropoietin-stimulating agent (ESA) therapy should be started for hemoglobin values >10 g/dL. The risks and benefits should be weighed. Risks of ESAs include hypertension, thrombosis, stroke, and the observation of increased mortality in patients with malignancy. In patients with hemoglobin values <10 g/dL, ESA therapy needs to be individualized. The absence of anemic symptoms and the presence of lung cancer would both argue against the use of ESA therapy. Though packed red blood cell transfusion would be safe to administer from the standpoint of malignancy, there is no clear indication for transfusion in the absence of symptoms. Iron therapy is not warranted in the setting of normal iron stores. All patients with stage 4 CKD should be counseled on vascular (and peritoneal) access for dialysis, so this is the correct answer.

Kidney Disease: Improving Global Outcomes (KDIGO) Chronic Kidney Disease Work Group. KDIGO 2012 Clinical Practice Guideline for the Evaluation and Management of Chronic Kidney Disease. *Kidney Int* (Suppl). 2013;3:1–150.

5. **ANSWER: E. Hemodialysis**

In this patient with hyperkalemia with peaked T waves and widened QRS complexes, temporizing measures and definitive management of hyperkalemia are strongly indicated. Sodium polystyrene sulfonate with or without sorbitol carries a risk of intestinal necrosis, which is greatest in the postoperative setting and thus should be avoided in this patient. Sodium bicarbonate may aid in shifting potassium intracellularly, but it does not remove potassium from the body. Although a loop diuretic could be considered with less severe hyperkalemia, the evidence of cardiotoxicity on an EKG warrants hemodialysis for correction of hyperkalemia. Indeed, furosemide takes several hours to be effective and will not resolve this patient's EKG changes acutely.

Kovesdy CP. Management of hyperkalemia: an update for the internist. *Am J Med.* 2015;128(12):1281–1287.

6. **ANSWER: B. ART alone**

HIV-associated nephropathy (HIVAN) is seen most commonly in African Americans, especially in the setting of advanced HIV with a low CD4 count associated with acute kidney injury and nephrotic-range proteinuria. Renal biopsy is required to confirm the diagnosis because nearly 40% of individuals with suspected HIVAN will have an alternate diagnosis by biopsy. Antiretroviral therapy (ART) is the mainstay of treatment. Steroids are not typically indicated, but they may be considered if renal function worsens despite the initiation of ART along with renin-angiotensin system (RAS) inhibition. Steroid-sparing agents are not indicated. Steroids plus mycophenolate mofetil are also not indicated. Plasmapheresis plays no role in the management of HIVAN. Though HIV can be associated with a thrombotic microangiopathy, the suspected diagnosis in this patient is HIVAN. Furthermore, plasmapheresis should not be combined with an ACE inhibitor, because the combination can result in a syndrome of abdominal pain, flushing, and hypotension.

7. **ANSWER: C. Multiple myeloma**

The first step in analyzing a patient with hyponatremia is to differentiate pseudohyponatremia from true hyponatremia by evaluating the serum osmolality. Though this patient's calculated serum osmolality ([2 × Na] + [BUN/2.8] + [glucose/18]) is on the lower end of normal at 275 mOsm/kg, the presence of an osmolality gap suggests that the measured osmolality is actually normal to elevated, raising concern for pseudohyponatremia. Combined with a low anion gap, which can be seen with hypercalcemia or a positively charged immunoglobulin, these findings are strongly suggestive of a diagnosis of multiple myeloma. Urine protein by dipstick is specific for albumin and would not be expected to reveal the presence of a paraprotein. All other answer choices reflect causes of true hyponatremia.

8. **ANSWER: C. Captopril**

Scleroderma renal crisis (SRC) develops in 10%–20% of patients with diffuse systemic sclerosis. Clinically, it resembles thrombotic thrombocytopenic purpura–hemolytic-uremic syndrome (TTP-HUS) and can present with hemolytic anemia, mild thrombocytopenia, and thrombotic microangiopathy on renal biopsy, but the physical examination features of scleroderma help distinguish this entity from TTP-HUS. Renal biopsy is not helpful, because it will not distinguish SRC from TTP-HUS. The use of high-dose steroids is a risk factor for the development of SRC. The mainstay of therapy is ACE inhibition (captopril), even in advanced renal failure requiring dialysis, because there is a much greater chance of renal recovery with discontinuation of dialysis and improved mortality observed in patients treated with ACE inhibitors.

Denton CP, Lapadula G, Mouthon L, Müller-Ladner U. Renal complications and scleroderma renal crisis. *Rheumatology (Oxford).* 2009;48(Suppl 3):iii32–iii35.

9. **ANSWER: A. Adrenal vein sampling**

In this patient with an elevated aldosterone to plasma renin activity (PRA) ratio (>30) and elevated serum aldosterone (>20 ng/dL) with positive confirmatory testing, the diagnosis is primary hyperaldosteronism. In cases of hyperaldosteronism with normal adrenal imaging, the possibilities include a nonvisualized adrenal mass and bilateral adrenal hyperplasia. The only way to distinguish between these in the face of normal CT imaging is to pursue adrenal vein sampling. CT imaging has superior spatial resolution compared with MRI in the visualization of adrenal glands, so an MRI study would not be helpful. Spironolactone would be appropriate only if bilateral adrenal hyperplasia were confirmed by adrenal vein sampling. The other answers are not treatments for primary hyperaldosteronism.

10. ANSWER: C. Distal (type 1) renal tubular acidosis (RTA)

A positive urine anion gap (urine $Na^+ + K^+ - Cl$) suggests that impaired renal excretion of ammonium (which is an unmeasured cation in the urine) is the cause of the patient's metabolic acidosis, as opposed to loss of bicarbonate in the stool, which would result in a negative urine anion gap. The presence of a low serum bicarbonate with a normal anion gap favors a diagnosis of RTA as opposed to a steroid-induced hypokalemia, which would be expected to be associated with a metabolic alkalosis from mineralocorticoid receptor binding by the corticosteroid. Type 4 RTA is associated with hyperkalemia. Absence of glycosuria on urinalysis argues against Fanconi syndrome, which often accompanies a proximal RTA from injury to the proximal tubule. Distal RTA (seen with urine pH >5.5 and hypokalemia) related to rheumatoid arthritis is the likely explanation of the hypokalemia.

11. ANSWER: D. ACE inhibitor, prednisone, mycophenolate mofetil

Renal biopsy is required in most patients with known lupus and evidence of renal involvement because the severity on clinical presentation may be discordant with the true degree of renal involvement by biopsy, and because the histologic subtype along with indices of activity and chronicity help guide the treatment. Once the pathological classification is determined, therapy may be initiated. ACE inhibitor is an important adjunctive therapy for patients with proteinuria. The Joint European League Against Rheumatism and European Renal Association-European Dialysis and Transplant Association (EULAR/ERA-EDTA) guideline recommends immunosuppression for patients with class III lupus nephritis. Prednisone along with mycophenolate mofetil is the recommended initial treatment. Prednisone and cyclophosphamide is an appropriate treatment option but poses a greater risk of infertility in this patient. Glucocorticoid monotherapy is not recommended. On the basis of the LUNAR trial, there is insufficient evidence to support the use of rituximab as an initial immunosuppressive therapy for class III lupus nephritis.

Bertsias GK, Tektonidou M, Amoura Z, et al. Joint European League Against Rheumatism and European Renal Association-European Dialysis and Transplant Association (EULAR/ERA-EDTA) recommendations for the management of adult and paediatric lupus nephritis. *Ann Rheum Dis.* 2012;71(11):1771–1782.

Rovin BH, Furie R, Latinis K, et al. Efficacy and safety of rituximab in patients with active proliferative lupus nephritis: the Lupus Nephritis Assessment with Rituximab study. *Arthritis Rheum.* 2012;64(4):1215–1226.

12. ANSWER: D. Counsel on low-salt diet.

In the very elderly (patients older than 80 years of age), the benefits of controlling blood pressure aggressively are not known. The SPRINT trial demonstrated a decreased risk of the composite cardiovascular outcome when targeting systolic blood pressures less than 120 mm Hg compared with less than 140 mm Hg. However, SPRINT excluded individuals with prior stroke, so it cannot be directly applied in this case. On the basis of the HYVET trial, it is known that treating systolic blood pressure to less than 150 mm Hg decreases the risk of fatal stroke, heart failure, and all-cause mortality. The ACCOMPLISH trial demonstrated that nonobese individuals at higher risk for cardiovascular events may particularly benefit from the combination of a dihydropyridine calcium channel blocker and ACE inhibitor therapy. Because this patient's systolic blood pressure is already under 150 mm Hg, medications should not be intensified, and a secondary workup should not be performed. It is always reasonable to counsel hypertensive patients on a low-salt diet.

Jamerson K, Weber MA, Bakris GL, et al. Benazepril plus amlodipine or hydrochlorothiazide for hypertension in high-risk patients. *N Engl J Med.* 2008;359(23):2417–2428.

SPRINT Research Group. A randomized trial of intensive versus standard blood-pressure control. *N Engl J Med.* 2015;373(22):2103–2116.

13. ANSWER: B. Isotonic saline

Isotonic saline is the mainstay of therapy for management of rhabdomyolysis. Isotonic bicarbonate should not be used in the setting of hypocalcemia, because the use of bicarbonate can reduce the ionized fraction of calcium as a result of increased albumin binding of calcium, leading to symptomatic hypocalcemia. Loop diuretics such as furosemide can be used if there is volume overload, but they can also worsen hypocalcemia and should not be used as first-line therapy. The role of mannitol in the management of rhabdomyolysis remains uncertain.

14. ANSWER: A. IgA nephropathy

IgA nephropathy can present as a rapidly progressing glomerulonephritis (biopsy with crescentic IgA nephropathy), as a latent finding of hematuria and proteinuria, or in the setting of an upper respiratory tract infection ("synpharyngitic hematuria"), as is the case in this patient. IgA nephropathy typically occurs 1–3 days after an upper respiratory tract infection, as opposed to postinfectious glomerulonephritis (GN), which occurs 7–21 days after an infection. The presence of normal complements also helps distinguish IgA nephropathy from postinfectious GN. Thin basement membrane disease can be associated with some hematuria but does not fit the clinical picture. Alport syndrome can be associated with proteinuria, hearing loss, and progression to end-stage renal disease, but it does not fit the clinical picture. Granulomatous polyangiitis (formerly known as *Wegener granulomatosis*) is unlikely with a negative ANCA.

15. ANSWER: B. Stop hypertonic saline and start D5W and DDAVP.

Rapid overcorrection of chronic hyponatremia (rise in Na^+ >10 mEq/24 h) can result in osmotic demyelination syndrome. The symptoms of osmotic demyelination typically do not occur for 2–6 days after the sodium has been overcorrected. Animal models show a decreased incidence of osmotic demyelination when sodium that has been overcorrected is relowered. Human studies show that relowering is safe. The best answer in this patient would be to stop the hypertonic saline and to relower the sodium using D5W and DDAVP.

Sterns RH. Disorders of plasma sodium—causes, consequences, and correction. *N Engl J Med* 2015;372(1):55–65.

16. ANSWER: B. Acute interstitial nephritis

Though the triad of fever, eosinophilia, and rash is seen in only a small percentage of patients with allergic interstitial nephritis (AIN), any combination of these signs should raise suspicion for it. Allergic interstitial nephritis (causing acute interstitial nephritis) is the likely diagnosis in this patient, and a proton pump inhibitor for treatment of the patient's GERD is the likely culprit. Cellular casts raise concern for glomerulonephritis, but the type of cells was not specified in the question stem. White blood cell casts can be seen in AIN, whereas typically red blood cell casts are seen in glomerulonephritis. DRESS can result from a drug hypersensitivity as well, but the absence of other systemic symptoms makes this diagnosis unlikely.

Geevasinga N, Coleman PL, Webster AC, Roger SD. Proton pump inhibitors and acute interstitial nephritis. *Clin Gastroenterol Hepatol.* 2006;4(5):597–604.

17. ANSWER: A. Percutaneous renal artery angioplasty with stent placement

Though the largest trial comparing renal artery stenting with medical management (ASTRAL trial) found that stenting conferred little benefit and much risk in the management of renal artery stenosis, the enrollment criteria for the study excluded all patients whose physicians felt they would "definitely" benefit from stenting. Though stenting should not generally be performed in asymptomatic patients, refractory heart failure or recurrent flash pulmonary edema is an ACC/AHA class I indication for renal artery revascularization. The safest way to achieve this is via percutaneous angioplasty and stent placement, with surgical revascularization reserved for patients with complex anatomy. The other options are not appropriate at this time.

ASTRAL Investigators. Revascularization versus medical therapy for renal-artery stenosis. *N Engl J Med.* 2009;361(20):1953–1962.

18. ANSWER: B. Add chlorthalidone.

In patients with diabetes, compelling medications for hypertensive management include thiazides, beta-blockers angiotensin-converting-enzyme inhibitors (ACEIs), angiotensin receptor blockers (ARBs), and calcium channel blockers. Though the COOPERATE trial suggested a benefit of dual RAS blockade with ACEIs and ARBs (such as valsartan), it was later found that the authors had engaged in serious scientific misconduct, resulting in retraction of the paper from *The Lancet.* The ONTARGET trial demonstrated no benefit to combination therapy with an ACEI and an ARB. Diabetic proteinuria tends to improve with lowering of blood pressure, and the addition of chlorthalidone would be a reasonable choice for a second antihypertensive. Metoprolol is unlikely to lower the patient's blood pressure as much as a diuretic.

Mann JF, Schmieder RE, McQueen M, et al. Renal outcomes with telmisartan, ramipril, or both, in people at high vascular risk (the ONTARGET study): a multicentre, randomised, double-blind, controlled trial. *Lancet.* 2008;372(9638):547–553.

19. ANSWER: D. Isotonic saline with hydrocortisone

The patient's symptomatology is highly concerning for tuberculosis, and the acute development of hypotension, hyponatremia, and hypokalemia are all concerning for adrenal crisis likely resulting from tuberculous infiltration of the adrenal glands. Though the patient will ultimately benefit from multidrug therapy for tuberculosis, the acute management should be focused on volume resuscitation and steroid administration for management of acute adrenal crisis. Fluid restriction is inappropriate in a patient who appears hypovolemic. Hypertonic saline should be reserved for patients with symptomatic hyponatremia and sodium values less than 120 mEq/L. Tolvaptan is contraindicated in hypovolemic patients because it induces a free water diuresis that may worsen hypovolemia.

20. ANSWER: A. Rasburicase

This patient has spontaneous tumor lysis syndrome secondary to Burkitt lymphoma. Intravenous fluids are important in preventing this condition when administered with chemotherapy, but rasburicase is the safest and fastest way to break down uric acid (to the water-soluble compound allantoin) to enhance its clearance. Allopurinol and febuxostat would not be helpful in the acute setting. The hyperkalemia is being driven by breakdown of tumor cells and is not likely to respond significantly to sodium polystyrene sulfonate. Indications for hemodialysis in tumor lysis syndrome include severe oliguria, persistent hyperkalemia, and hyperphosphatemia-induced symptomatic hypocalcemia, none of which are present at this time.

Alakel N, Middeke JM, Schetelig J, et al. Prevention and treatment of tumor lysis syndrome, and the efficacy and role of rasburicase. *Onco Targets Ther.* 2017;10:597–605.

Criscuolo M, Fianchi L, Dragonetti G, et al. Tumor lysis syndrome: reviewof pathogenesis, risk factors and management of a medical emergency. *Expert Rev Hematol.* 2016;9(2): 197–208.

21. ANSWER: E. Do nothing.

In the absence of renovascular disease (given normal creatinine) and refractory hypertension, there is no acute indication to pursue renal artery revascularization. There are considerable risks with both percutaneous angioplasty and surgical revascularization, so these procedures should be reserved for patients with compelling indications. A blood pressure of 130/70 mm Hg in a patient with diabetes is appropriate and requires no adjustment of antihypertensives.

22. ANSWER: E. Chronic interstitial nephritis

Lead nephropathy can present acutely with Fanconi syndrome resulting from injury to the proximal tubules with intranuclear inclusion bodies made up of lead–protein complexes. Chronic injury is characterized by the finding of chronic interstitial nephritis. Glomerulosclerosis may also be seen on biopsy.

23. ANSWER: C. Hypomagnesemia

Acute kidney injury, thrombotic microangioathy, hyperkalemia, hypomagnesemia, and hyperlipidemia are all associated with the use of calcineurin inhibitors such as tacrolimus. Hypercalcemia, hypokalemia, acute interstitial nephritis, and rhabdomyolysis are not typically associated with tacrolimus toxicity.

24. ANSWER: B. Minimal change disease

The most common cause of nephrotic syndrome in patients with Hodgkin lymphoma is minimal change disease, though focal segmental glomerulosclerosis has also been described. The other conditions listed do not share an association with Hodgkin disease. Approximately 0.4% of patients with Hodgkin lymphoma develop minimal change disease, and the degree of proteinuria typically parallels the course of the malignancy.

Peces R, Sánchez L, Gorostidi M, et al. Minimal change nephrotic syndrome associated with Hodgkin's lymphoma. *Nephrol Dial Transplant.* 1991;6(3):155–158.

25. ANSWER: C. Polyarteritis nodosa

Hepatitis C–associated renal diseases include mixed cryoglobulinemia, membranoproliferative glomerulonephritis (MPGN), membranous nephropathy, and polyarteritis nodosa (PAN). Membranous nephropathy, MPGN, and PAN can also be observed in hepatitis B.

26. ANSWER: A. Nothing

Phospholipase A2 receptor (PLA2R) has been identified as a key pathogenic antigen in idiopathic membranous nephropathy, which appears to be the diagnosis in this patient without a clear secondary cause. Treatment of idiopathic membranous nephropathy is stratified by the clinical severity. Patients with normal renal function and proteinuria <4 g/d (such as in the patient in this case) can be safely observed without immunosuppression because they often undergo spontaneous partial or complete remission. Glucocorticoids in combination with either cyclophosphamide or a calcineurin inhibitor may be effective in treating patients at moderate and higher risk for progression of renal disease. Rituximab may be used in refractory cases.

Beck Jr LH, Bonegio RG, Lambeau G, et al. M-type phospholipase A2 receptor as target antigen in idiopathic membranous nephropathy. *N Engl J Med.* 2009;361(1):11–21.

27. ANSWER: A. Less than 220/120 mm Hg

In a patient experiencing an acute ischemic stroke, the blood pressure goal is determined by candidacy for thrombolytic therapy. Because the patient's stroke symptoms occurred while she was asleep, the timing of symptom onset cannot be determined. Thus systemic thrombolytic therapy cannot be safely offered. In a patient who is not a candidate for thrombolytic therapy (such as the patient in this case), most consensus guidelines suggest lowering the blood pressure only if it is above 220/120 mm Hg. This strategy is described as permissive hypertension. In candidates for thrombolytic therapy, blood pressure must be maintained at <180/105 mm Hg to minimize the risk of hemorrhagic conversion. After the acute stroke episode has resolved, a systolic blood pressure goal of 150 mm Hg may be appropriate in this very elderly patient (>80 years of age) as per the HYVET trial.

Beckett NS, Peters R, Fletcher AE, et al. Treatment of hypertension in patients 80 years of age or older. *N Engl J Med.* 2008;358(18):1887–1898.

28. ANSWER: B. AL amyloidosis

Amyloidosis typically presents with a combination of symptoms, signs, and laboratory abnormalities, including nephrotic syndrome, restrictive cardiomyopathy, peripheral neuropathy, hepatomegaly, macroglossia, purpura, and abnormal bleeding. The presence of lateral scalloping of the tongue as seen in this patient can be a result of the lateral edges of the tongue being flattened by the teeth in the setting of macroglossia. AA amyloid tends to occur secondarily to chronic inflammation, which does not appear to be present in this patient. AL amyloidosis refers to a monoclonal gammopathy complicated by the formation of fibrils made up of light chain fragments. The presence of purpura, especially in the periorbital area, is characteristic of AL amyloidosis. Diabetes mellitus can cause both a peripheral neuropathy and nephrotic-range proteinuria but usually needs to be present for several years prior to onset of these complications. Hypertensive nephropathy is not associated with nephrotic-range proteinuria. FSGS can be associated with nephrotic syndrome but cannot explain the patient's associated symptoms.

Wechalekar AD, Gillmore JD, Hawkins PN. Systemic amyloidosis. *Lancet.* 2016;387(10038):2641–2654.

29. ANSWER: E. Eculizumab

The patient's diagnosis is hemolytic uremic syndrome (HUS) without diarrhea, also known as *atypical HUS.* Atypical HUS is characterized by a low C3 level. When it is caused by factor H or I deficiency, it is associated with low CH50 and AH50. ADAMTS13 activity may be low but is typically greater than 10%, which helps distinguish this condition from thrombotic thrombocytopenic purpura. Blocking the terminal complement cascade is the most effective therapy for this condition, which can be achieved with eculizumab.

Legendre CM, Licht C, Muus P, et al. Terminal complement inhibitor eculizumab in atypical hemolytic-uremic syndrome. *N Engl J Med.* 2013;368(23):2169–2181.

30. ANSWER: E. Discuss dialysis and transplant.

ISN/RPS class VI lupus nephritis denotes a biopsy with global sclerosis noted on more than 90% of the glomeruli. In this setting, the kidney is "burned out," and immunosuppressive therapy is not warranted. The appropriate course of action in this setting would be to discuss dialysis and transplant, which are likely in the patient's near future, even if no acute indications for dialysis exist at this time.

Bertsias GK, Tektonidou M, Amoura Z, et al. Joint European League Against Rheumatism and European Renal Association-European Dialysis and Transplant Association (EULAR/ERA-EDTA) recommendations for the management of adult and paediatric lupus nephritis. *Ann Rheum Dis.* 2012;71(11):1771–1782.

31. ANSWER: C. Plasmapheresis, steroids, and cyclophosphamide

Based on the results of the MEPEX trial, in patients with ANCA-associated vasculitis and a creatinine level greater than 5.8 mg/dL, an approach of plasma exchange, prednisolone, and cyclophosphamide was superior to an approach of a methylprednisolone pulse followed by prednisolone and cyclophosphamide with regard to mortality and renal function. All of the patients in the MEPEX trial were switched to azathioprine for maintenance therapy after 3 months. Dialysis may ultimately be needed, but based on the information provided in the question, it is not emergently indicated.

Jayne DR, Gaskin G, Rasmussen N, et al. Randomized trial of plasma exchange or high-dosage methylprednisolone as adjunctive therapy for severe renal vasculitis. *J Am Soc Nephrol.* 2007;18(7):2180–2188.

32. ANSWER: A. Vasopressin receptor antagonism

Chronic kidney disease (CKD) is a risk factor for cardiovascular disease, so control of hypertension and lipids is certainly important. However, the only therapy listed above that has been shown (in the TEMPO trial) to reduce the annual increase in total kidney volume and slow the decline in kidney function is tolvaptan, a vasopressin receptor antagonist. A low-protein diet can slow the progression of CKD. Steroid therapy has no role in the treatment of polycystic kidney disease.

Torres VE, Chapman AB, Devuyst O, et al. Tolvaptan in patients with autosomal dominant polycystic kidney disease. *N Engl J Med.* 2012;367(25):2407–2418.

33. ANSWER: B. Start 1,25-hydroxyvitamin D supplementation

This patient has secondary hyperparathyroidism associated with chronic kidney disease, in which the elevation in PTH results from chronically high phosphorus and low calcium concentrations. The goal of reducing PTH is to prevent high-turnover renal bone disease. Overreduction of PTH may result in a low-turnover bone disease, so PTH is not typically lowered all the way down to normal. The first line of therapy in lowering PTH is to control high phosphorus via institution of a low-phosphorus diet and a phosphorus-binding agent. The next line of therapy is to correct for deficiencies in 25-hydroxyvitamin D levels. The next line of therapy would be to use 1,25-hydroxyvitamin D to suppress PTH. Cinacalcet is reserved for refractory cases, often as a bridge to parathyroidectomy.

Cunningham J, Locatelli F, Rodriguez M. Secondary hyperparathyroidism: pathogenesis, disease progression, and therapeutic options. *Clin J Am Soc Nephrol.* 2011;6(4):913–921.

34. ANSWER: A. Uromodulin kidney disease

Uromodulin kidney disease (UKD), sometimes referred to as *familial juvenile hyperuricemic nephropathy* (FJHN), is the most common subtype of a broader category of autosomal dominant tubulointerstitial kidney diseases (ADTKD). UKD is characterized by mutations in the *UMOD* gene encoding uromodulin (also known as *Tamm-Horsfall protein*). Clinical manifestations include gout, hyperuricemia, and progressive renal disease. The early onset of renal disease distinguishes UKD from gout and other uric acid renal diseases. Acute uric acid nephropathy is typically associated with overproduction and underexcretion of uric acid from rapid cell lysis as occurs in the treatment of certain myeloproliferative disorders, leukemias, and lymphomas. Lead nephropathy can occur in association with gout, though it usually includes some history of workplace, water supply, or moonshine exposure. Chronic urate nephropathy is associated with impaired renal function, but the early onset of renal disease and family history make UKD more likely.

Eckardt KU, Alper SL, Antignac C, et al. Autosomal dominant tubulointerstitial kidney disease: diagnosis, classification, and management—a KDIGO consensus report. *Kidney Int.* 2015;88(4):676–683.

35. ANSWER: B. Recommend continuous positive airway pressure (CPAP) at night

Obstructive sleep apnea (OSA) is a known secondary cause of hypertension. The severity of sleep apnea correlates with the severity of hypertension, and approximately three-fourths of patients referred with resistant hypertension who were referred for sleep studies were found to have OSA. Treating the OSA with CPAP may result in a modest improvement in blood pressure. A DASH diet and a low-salt diet may also be helpful, but the OSA needs to be addressed first.

36. ANSWER: B. Amlodipine

Based on the results of the ACCOMPLISH trial published in the *New England Journal of Medicine* in 2008, the combination of benazepril and amlodipine was superior to the combination of benazepril and hydrochlorothiazide in reducing cardiovascular events in patients with hypertension with a high risk for such events. The other agents would not be first- or second-line therapies for hypertension. Furosemide can be used as a diuretic in the presence of chronic kidney disease when thiazide diuretics lose their potency, which is not the case in this patient.

Jamerson K, Weber MA, Bakris GL, et al. Benazepril plus amlodipine or hydrochlorothiazide for hypertension in high-risk patients. *N Engl J Med.* 2008;359(23):2417–2428.

37. ANSWER: A. Oral chlorthalidone and lisinopril and follow-up as an outpatient

Hypertensive urgency is defined by severe hypertension in the relative absence of symptoms, which is the diagnosis in this patient. As opposed to hypertensive emergency, the management of hypertensive urgency involves the use of oral hypertensives to achieve a reduction of blood pressure to goal over hours to days. Given the severe elevation of blood pressure, a two-drug regimen should be started, and a thiazide-type diuretic combined with an ACE inhibitor would be a reasonable regimen. Hydralazine is not a first-line antihypertensive, and intravenous hydralazine is not indicated.

Kessler CS, Joudeh Y. Evaluation and treatment of severe asymptomatic hypertension. *Am Fam Physician.* 2010;81(4):470–476.

Stafford EE, Will KK, Brooks-Gumb AN. Management of hypertensive urgency and emergency. *Clin Rev.* 2012;22(10):20.

38. ANSWER: E. Nephrotic syndrome

Nephrogenic diabetes insipidus (and central diabetes insipidus), chronic interstitial nephritis, and distal RTA can occur in patients with lithium nephrotoxicity. Nephrotic syndrome (related to minimal change disease and focal segmental glomerulosclerosis) has also been described in patients with lithium nephrotoxicity. Hyperparathyroidism with resultant hypercalcemia has been described in patients taking lithium therapy. Other associated findings in this setting include normal serum phosphorus level and hypermagnesemia.

39. ANSWER: A. Lorazepam

The salient features in this patient's clinical presentation include an anion gap acidosis and an osmolality gap (measured osmolality 298 mOsm/kg vs. calculated osmolality 285 mOsm/kg). This suggests an unmeasured osmole. This occurs most commonly with ethylene glycol and methanol poisoning. Propylene glycol toxicity can also present this way, with most reported cases occurring due to administration of medications that contain a propylene glycol solvent, including lorazepam and phenobarbital. The other answer choices would not cause an osmolality gap. Though acute alcohol poisoning can result in an osmolality gap, the negative ethanol level suggests that the ethanol is not directly responsible for the osmolality gap.

Tsao YT, Tsai WC, Yang SP. A life-threatening double gap metabolic acidosis. *Am J Emerg Med.* 2008;26(3):385.e5–6.

40. ANSWER: B. Extracranial cerebrovascular involvement is common.

In patients with established renal fibromuscular dysplasia (FMD), as many as 65% of patients can be found to have carotid and vertebral artery involvement. FMD is more common in women. Though CT angiogram has excellent diagnostic utility, MR angiography is poorly sensitive for the diagnosis of FMD due to poor spatial resolution. In patients with newly diagnosed hypertension as a result of FMD, percutaneous transluminal angioplasty is the preferred approach if opting for definitive therapy. Unlikely atherosclerotic renal artery stenosis, the pathology of the lesion most commonly found in FMD is medial fibroplasia.

41. ANSWER: D. Renal biopsy would be expected to reveal a normal kidney.

Hepatorenal syndrome (HRS) is a feared complication of end-stage liver disease that carries a great degree of morbidity and mortality. Hepatorenal syndrome is a disorder marked by splanchnic vasodilation and renal artery vasoconstriction, with a decrease in renal perfusion causing reductions in glomerular filtration rate and sodium excretion. It can be precipitated by infections or bleeding. The renal parenchyma would be expected to be preserved early in the diagnosis. If a liver transplant were being considered, a kidney transplant would not be indicated early in the process, because there should be no irreversible injury present. Octreotide and midodrine are temporizing measures at best because liver transplant is the only cure for type 1 HRS unless there is spontaneous improvement in the underlying liver function. Hemodialysis may be difficult to perform in patients with HRS because they are frequently hypotensive at baseline. Continuous venovenous hemofiltration may be needed as a bridge to liver transplant if renal replacement therapy is required.

Ginès P, Schrier RW. Renal failure in cirrhosis [Published erratum appears in *N Engl J Med.* 2011 Jan 27;364(4):389]. *N Engl J Med* 2009;361:1279–1290.

42. ANSWER: C. Gitelman syndrome

Gitelman syndrome is the most likely diagnosis in this patient. Although both Gitelman and Bartter syndromes are associated with hypotension and hypokalemia, the presence of low urine calcium favors a diagnosis of Gitelman syndrome. If one can remember that Gitelman syndrome resembles the administration of thiazide diuretics (whereas Bartter syndrome resembles loop diuretics), it is easy to remember that Gitelman syndrome is associated with a low urine calcium because it is precisely this property of thiazide diuretics that makes them useful for the treatment of calcium oxalate stone disease by minimizing calcium excretion in the urine. Surreptitious vomiting would be expected to result in a low urinary chloride resulting from volume depletion. Both primary hyperaldosteronism and Cushing syndrome are associated with hypokalemia, and these patients are typically hypertensive. In the case of Cushing syndrome, physical examination findings may also be readily apparent.

43. ANSWER: B. Alport syndrome

Alport syndrome is an inherited form of glomerular dysfunction associated with sensorineural hearing loss that is most frequently X-linked in transmission. The syndrome affects males out of proportion to females. Symptoms may begin with episodes of gross hematuria but ultimately progress to proteinuria, hypertension, chronic kidney disease, and end-stage renal disease. The other diagnoses would not account for the patient's hearing loss.

Kruegel J, Rubel D, Gross O. Alport syndrome—insights from basic and clinical research. *Nat Rev Nephrol.* 2013;9(3):170–178.

44. ANSWER: B. Calcium oxalate

Calcium oxalate is the most common stone type for all patients who form kidney stones. Patients with a history of gastric bypass surgery are at increased risk of calcium oxalate stones, primarily due to increased risk of hyperoxaluria. Bariatric surgery can lead to malabsorption of free fatty acids. Fatty acids in the intestinal lumen bind to free calcium, resulting in an increase in free oxalate, which is absorbed and subsequently excreted in the urine. In addition, patients with malabsorption may have lower urine volume due to fluid losses resulting from diarrhea and low urinary citrate due to chronic metabolic acidosis resulting from diarrhea. Both low urine volume and low urinary citrate are risk factors for kidney stone formation. Low urine citrate is a risk factor for calcium oxalate stones because citrate is an inhibitor of calcium oxalate formation.

Gonzalez, RD, Canales BK. Kidney stone risk following modern bariatric surgery. *Curr Urol Rep.* 2014;15(5):401.

45. ANSWER: C. Fabry disease

Fabry disease is an X-linked lysosomal storage disorder that may be associated with renal dysfunction in half of patients by the age of 35 years. Fabry disease should be suspected in young adult patients with the following findings: chronic kidney disease of unclear etiology, multiple renal sinus and parapelvic cysts, decreased perspiration, cutaneous vascular lesions, left ventricular hypertrophy of unclear etiology, and stroke of unclear etiology.

Zarate YA, Hopkin RJ. Fabry's disease. *Lancet.* 2008; 372(9647):1427–1435.

46. ANSWER: B. Type B lactic acidosis

Type A lactic acidosis is the type most commonly seen and occurs as a result of cell breakdown resulting from tissue hypoperfusion, as is present in septic shock. This patient has no clinical signs of septic shock, which is documented on the basis of negative culture data and lack of response to broad-spectrum antibiotics. Type B lactic acid can be seen with medications (e.g., metformin and certain HIV medications), malignancy, and alcoholism. D-Lactic acidosis may be seen in patients with short gut syndrome as a result of bacterial metabolism in the gut. This patient most likely has type B lactic acidosis related to Hodgkin lymphoma, which may respond to chemotherapy.

47. ANSWER: E. Administer fomepizole and prepare for dialysis

This patient is likely experiencing ethylene glycol intoxication, which causes a large anion gap and osmolality gap. Calcium oxalate crystaluria can be found in ethylene glycol toxicity because oxalate is a metabolite of ethylene glycol. Treatment of ethylene glycol toxicity includes stabilization of the airway and circulatory systems. Inhibition of alcohol dehydrogenase with fomepizole (or ethanol if fomepizole is not available) will block ethylene glycol from being metabolized to toxic metabolites. Dialysis will remove ethylene glycol and toxic metabolites and is fundamental to management of severe intoxication. Sodium bicarbonate can be used to correct severe acidemia, which will also reduce the diffusion of toxic metabolites across cell membranes and into end-organ tissues. There is a limited role for gastric lavage or activated charcoal because ethylene glycol is absorbed quickly.

48. ANSWER: C. Start oral sodium bicarbonate therapy

This patient has hyporeninemic hypoaldosteronism, which is a common renal manifestation of diabetes mellitus. It manifests as mild hyperkalemia that leads to decreased ammonia production, resulting in decreased urinary acid excretion and metabolic acidosis; this is also known as type IV RTA. Management of type IV RTA can include both hyperkalemia and acidosis management. Hyperkalemia can be managed by diuretic therapy, especially when the patient has volume overload, or by fludrocortisone when volume overload is not present and blood pressure is not elevated. In this patient with relatively mild hyperkalemia and otherwise controlled blood pressure with signs of mild volume overload, one could consider a diuretic, though not in place of an angiotensin receptor blocker, which is indicated for diabetic nephropathy. With underlying hypertension and mild volume overload, fludrocortisone would not be indicated. Oral bicarbonate therapy could be considered to increase buffering capacity and prevent bone demineralization. Additionally, there is some evidence that treating metabolic acidosis in CKD may prevent progression; in that case, the goal bicarbonate would be >22 mmol/L. Likewise, spironolactone could enhance the hypoaldosterone state and exacerbate hyperkalemia. Although potassium citrate would provide base supplementation, it would not be appropriate to administer potassium salts to this patient. An alternative option not offered could also be dietary potassium restriction.

49. ANSWER: D. pH 6.5–7.0

Although most kidney stones are calcium oxalate stones, uric acid stones still account for 5%–10%. Clinical risk factors for uric acid stones include gout, chronic diarrhea, diabetes, and metabolic syndrome. The most important biochemical risk factor for uric acid stones is low urinary pH. In addition to increased fluid intake, management of uric acid stones should be focused on urine alkalinization. The target urinary pH for management is 6.5–7.0. At a urine pH of 6.75, greater than 90% of the urinary uric acid will be present as the soluble urate salt. For this reason, uric acid stones can be dissolved by increasing urinary volume and using therapies (such as potassium citrate) to increase urine pH to 6.5–7.0. A urine pH less than 5.5 would increase the risk of uric acid stones. A urine pH greater than 7.5 will add little additional risk reduction for uric acid stones but may increase the risk of calcium phosphate stones (which form in alkaline urine). Urine pH is not a factor for calcium oxalate stones, but it is an important factor for uric acid stones.

Coe FL, Evan A, Worcester E. Kidney stone disease. *J Clin Invest.* 2005;115(10):2598–2608.

50. ANSWER: B. Discontinue acetaminophen

This elderly patient likely has 5-oxoprolinemia (also known as *pyroglutamate*), which is a metabolite of acetaminophen that can accumulate and cause an anion gap metabolic acidosis. Risk factors include malnutrition and CKD, both of which this patient has. Owing to concerns regarding NSAID and opiate use in the elderly, acetaminophen use has become more common, with standing regimens introduced especially in nursing home patients in an effort to manage pain proactively. Discontinuing acetaminophen, assuming such a decision would be acceptable to the patient from a pain management perspective, is the correct choice in this case to resolve the acidosis, with some experts recommending *N*-acetylcysteine despite a lack of evidence of efficacy. Eliminating the cause of the acidosis is preferable to starting alkali therapy. Because the patient's lactate is normal and blood pressure is stable, midodrine is not indicated. Although her albumin is low, parenteral nutrition would not be first-line therapy for malnutrition. Lisinopril is not relevant to the patient's acidosis.

Fenves AZ, Kirkpatrick HM 3rd, Patel VV, et al. Increased anion gap metabolic acidosis as a result of 5-oxoproline (pyroglutamic acid): a role for acetaminophen. *Clin J Am Soc Nephrol.* 2006;1(3):441–447.

Acknowledgment

The authors and editors gratefully acknowledge the contributions of the previous authors, Karandeep Singh and Ajay K. Singh.

7

Gastroenterology

MUTHOKA L. MUTINGA, MOLLY PERENCEVICH, AND ROBERT BURAKOFF

1. A 54-year-old man with a long history of gastroesophageal reflux disease but no other medical conditions undergoes an esophagogastroduodenoscopy (EGD), which reveals a 6-cm-long segment of salmon-colored mucosa extending proximally from the gastroesophageal junction. Biopsies demonstrate the presence of Barrett esophagus (intestinal metaplasia of the esophagus), but no dysplasia is noted. Surveillance biopsies obtained 1 year later reveal no dysplasia.

What is the current recommended surveillance guideline for this patient?

A. Biopsy of the Barrett segment every 3 months
B. Biopsy of the Barrett segment every 6–12 months
C. Biopsy of the Barrett segment every 3–5 years
D. Biopsy of the Barrett segment every 10 years
E. No further biopsies are necessary.

2. A 24-year-old woman with a long history of nonbloody diarrhea and bloating, but with no systemic symptoms such as weight loss, is seen in your office for further management. Her quality of life has been adversely affected by these symptoms. Prior evaluation including stool and laboratory tests, imaging, and colonoscopic biopsies as well as inspection of the terminal ileum have been unrevealing.

Which of the following treatment options is most likely to result in significant improvement of symptoms?

A. Hyoscyamine
B. Prednisone
C. Rifaximin
D. Mesalamine
E. Psyllium

3. A 67-year-old man with a history of congestive heart failure and peripheral vascular disease presents with 48 hours of left lower quadrant pain, diarrhea with intermittent bleeding, and low-grade fever. Stool cultures are negative for infection, and ischemic colitis is considered as a possible cause of his symptoms.

Which one of the following is true of this disorder?

A. Digoxin may predispose patients to bowel ischemia.
B. Urgent angiography is useful for identifying a culprit blood vessel.
C. This disorder has the highest mortality rate of the ischemic gut disorders.
D. The diagnosis can be definitively made on the basis of CT imaging.
E. Serum lactate levels are markedly elevated in this disorder.

4. A 46-year-old man with a long history of intravenous drug abuse is noted to have persistent elevation of liver transaminases despite a long period of sobriety from alcohol and illicit drug use. An extensive workup for causes of liver blood test abnormalities, including a hepatitis C antibody test, is negative. However, in light of his risk factors, you obtain a hepatitis C viral load, which confirms that he does actually have hepatitis C infection.

Which of the following conditions could result in a false-negative hepatitis C virus (HCV) antibody test result?

A. Autoimmune hepatitis
B. Lupus
C. HIV infection
D. Rheumatoid arthritis

5. A 57-year-old man with cirrhosis due to alcoholism, who is currently undergoing biweekly therapeutic paracentesis to manage refractory ascites, is seen in follow-up. He is compliant with a low-sodium diet and diuretic therapy. Recently, ultrasound imaging revealed patent hepatic and portal veins, and there is no evidence of hepatocellular carcinoma. Ascites fluid analysis is not suggestive of spontaneous bacterial peritonitis.

Which of the following statements is true regarding nonselective beta-blocker therapy in patients with cirrhosis?

A. It is indicated for management of acute variceal bleeding.
B. It does not alter the risk of developing spontaneous bacterial peritonitis.
C. It increases mortality in patients with decompensated cirrhosis.
D. It is indicated to prevent variceal formation in patients with early cirrhosis.

6. A 52-year-old woman presents for evaluation of symptoms of dry eyes and mouth. She is not taking any medications that could cause these symptoms and is otherwise asymptomatic. A thorough history and physical examination are unrevealing. Results of laboratory tests for primary Sjögren syndrome are negative.

   Which of the following gastrointestinal disorders is often associated with secondary Sjögren syndrome?
   A. Gastroesophageal reflux disease
   B. Small intestinal bacterial overgrowth
   C. Gallstone pancreatitis
   D. Primary biliary cirrhosis
   E. Ulcerative colitis

7. A 34-year-old with intermittent postprandial bloating and pain undergoes abdominal ultrasound imaging to evaluate for gallstones. No gallstones are found, and the gallbladder appears normal. However, she is noted to have a 2.5-cm solid lesion in the right lobe of the liver. She has no history of malignancy and no risk factors for chronic hepatitis B. She has been on oral contraceptives for 10 years.

   Which of the following liver lesions is most strongly associated with long-term use of oral contraceptives?
   A. Cavernous hemangioma
   B. Focal nodular hyperplasia
   C. Gastrointestinal stromal tumor
   D. Hepatic adenoma
   E. Nodular regenerative hyperplasia

8. A 62-year-old farmer presents for a second opinion after unrevealing extensive workup of migrating joint pain for the past 2 years and chronic diarrhea, postprandial abdominal cramping, and weight loss for the past 6 months. Your suspicion for Whipple disease is high.

   Which of the following statements regarding this disease is true?
   A. Chronic diarrhea is common, but extraintestinal symptoms are rare.
   B. Prolonged antibiotic treatment is required to eradicate the causative organism.
   C. The causative organism, *Tropheryma whipplei,* is easily cultured.
   D. The disease is more common in women than in men.
   E. Colonoscopy with biopsy is the diagnostic test of choice.

9. A 39-year-old man with long-standing gastroesophageal reflux disease on long-term proton pump inhibitor (PPI) therapy undergoes an upper endoscopy for evaluation of recent exacerbation of symptoms. No Barrett esophagus, hiatal hernia, or reflux esophagitis is noted. However, many small to medium-sized gastric polyps are found and removed. The pathology report confirms that they are all fundic gland polyps.

   Which of the following statements regarding gastric polyps is true?
   A. Fundic gland polyps and adenomas are the most common epithelial gastric polyps.
   B. Hyperplastic gastric polyps have no malignant potential.
   C. Fundic gland polyps in familial adenomatous polyposis syndrome (FAP) have no malignant potential.
   D. PPI-associated fundic gland polyps are not associated with an increased risk of cancer.

10. A 22-year-old man returned early from a volunteer trip to Mexico 3 weeks ago, where he and his two friends developed watery diarrhea and a fever. Although the diarrhea and fever resolved, the man subsequently developed painful swelling of his left knee. Testing for gonorrhea is negative. Reactive arthritis associated with the recent enteric infection is suspected.

    Which of the following is true about this condition?
    A. Intestinal infection with ameba has been associated with this syndrome.
    B. There is a higher prevalence of HLA-DQ2 antigen.
    C. It is more common in women than in men.
    D. It may be associated with a triad of arthritis, conjunctivitis, and esophagitis.
    E. Synovial fluid shows an elevated leukocyte count.

11. A 57-year-old man is referred to your clinic for evaluation of symptoms of dysphagia. He was asymptomatic until 6 months ago, when he began developing proximal upper and lower extremity muscle weakness, double vision, and drooping of his eyelids, more noticeable at the end of the day than at other times. He was recently admitted to the hospital when he developed a cough and fever and was found to have a right middle lobe pneumonia thought to be likely due to aspiration. He endorses a sensation of difficulty chewing and swallowing. He denies a sensation of food getting stuck after he swallows.

    What is his likely diagnosis?
    A. Goiter
    B. Early hypopharyngeal cancer
    C. Anxiety disorder
    D. Myasthenia gravis
    E. Gastroesophageal reflux disease

12. A 33-year-old woman is seen in your office for evaluation of fatigue, malaise, and mild right upper quadrant discomfort, ongoing for the past 1 month. Her medical history is notable for hypothyroidism, and her only medication is levothyroxine. Her examination result is notable only for mildly tender hepatomegaly. On further questioning, she reports no

risk factors for viral hepatitis. She does not consume alcohol or illicit drugs, nor does she take herbs or supplements. Her mother has lupus, and a maternal aunt has rheumatoid arthritis. Laboratory test results are notable for ALT 480 U/L, AST 211 U/L, total bilirubin 0.4 mg/dL, alkaline phosphatase 89 U/L, total protein 9.1 g/dL, albumin 4.1 g/dL, and TSH 2.1 μIU/mL. Her antismooth muscle antibody titer is 1:320.

Which of the following statements about her likely diagnosis is true?

A. This condition most often occurs in men.
B. The treatment of choice is prednisone with or without azathioprine.
C. The presence of other autoantibodies is uncommon.
D. There is a very low risk of developing cirrhosis.
E. It does not recur after liver transplant.

13. A 41-year-old man with ulcerative colitis, well controlled for several years with mesalamine, presents with a 1-week history of up to 15 foul-smelling, watery stools per day. Laboratory workup reveals mild leukocytosis with mild elevation in the baseline serum creatinine level. He tests positive for *Clostridium difficile* and is started on oral vancomycin, which results in quick improvement in symptoms.

Which of the following statements regarding *C. difficile* infection is true?

A. Stool testing for cure should be performed after completion of treatment.
B. There is a hypervirulent strain associated with lower clinical cure rates and increased recurrence rates.
C. Testing of all patients with inflammatory bowel disease (IBD) who are hospitalized with a disease flare is not recommended.
D. Repeat testing after a negative test should be performed.
E. Hand hygiene with an alcohol-based hand sanitizer soap is more effective than soap-and-water sanitizers.

14. A 79-year-old man presents with a 9-month history of difficulty swallowing with a sensation of a lump in his throat. His son, who accompanied him for the office appointment, also notes that he frequently experiences regurgitation and coughing while eating and that he has noticed over the same period that his father has had a foul breath odor.

Based on your clinical suspicion, what is the best test to diagnose a Zenker diverticulum?

A. Esophagogastroduodenoscopy (EGD)
B. Barium esophagram
C. CT scan
D. Esophageal motility study
E. Laryngoscopy

15. A 22-year-old Caucasian man with end-stage cystic fibrosis is being evaluated for a lung transplant. He was diagnosed with cystic fibrosis after presenting with meconium ileus as a newborn. Since then, he has experienced a variety of gastrointestinal complications of cystic fibrosis.

Which of the following are the most common gastrointestinal complications of cystic fibrosis (CF)?

A. Small intestinal bacterial overgrowth and dysphagia
B. Gastroesophageal reflux disease and constipation
C. Gastroesophageal reflux disease and diarrhea
D. Pancreatic insufficiency and gallstones
E. Gallstones and dysphagia

16. A 28-year-old man with eczema undergoes an urgent upper endoscopy in the emergency room to dislodge an esophageal food impaction. Examination of his esophagus after removal of the food bolus reveals multiple thin rings and linear furrows along most of the esophagus. No hiatal hernia, visible esophageal inflammation, mass, or luminal narrowing is seen. Biopsies from the middle and distal esophagus are obtained.

Further questioning reveals a several years' history of intermittent dysphagia for solids with several prior episodes of food impaction that resolved without need for medical attention. The patient has not experienced weight loss or frequent heartburn. His hematocrit is normal.

What is his likely diagnosis?

A. Esophageal lichen planus
B. Schatzki ring
C. Eosinophilic esophagitis
D. Peptic stricture
E. Plummer-Vinson syndrome

17. A 64-year-old obese woman with a history of chronic *Salmonella typhi* is noted to have a 3-cm gallstone. Her daughter did some research about her mother's condition and was quite alarmed about what she discovered. She decided to accompany her mother to her next appointment and asked a number of questions. One of these was related to concern about the increased risk for what type of cancer?

A. Hepatocellular cancer
B. Sarcoma
C. Breast cancer
D. Gallbladder cancer
E. Colorectal cancer

18. A 31-year-old man with AIDS and a CD4 count of 35 undergoes an esophagogastroduodenoscopy (EGD) for evaluation of odynophagia that failed to respond to empiric therapy for candidal esophagitis. Several small, shallow ulcers are noted in the middle and distal esophagus, and biopsies are obtained for further evaluation.

Which of the following is the most likely diagnosis?
A. Pill-induced esophageal ulcer
B. Idiopathic esophageal ulcer
C. Herpes simplex virus (HSV)–associated ulcer
D. Cytomegalovirus (CMV)-associated ulcer
E. Mycobacterium avium complex (MAC)–associated ulcer

19. A 52-year-old woman with a 30-year history of pancolitis due to ulcerative colitis is seen for routine follow-up in the office. Her ulcerative colitis has been under good control for most of the duration of the disease.

Which of the following statements regarding screening for colonic dysplasia in patients with inflammatory bowel disease is true?
A. Screening colonoscopy examinations for patients who have ulcerative proctitis should begin after 10–12 years of disease.
B. Patients with isolated Crohn ileitis have an increased risk of developing colorectal cancer.
C. Patients with left-sided ulcerative colitis are not at an increased risk of developing colorectal cancer compared with the general population.
D. Patients who are noted to have high-grade dysplasia, confirmed by a second pathologist, should undergo more intensive surveillance colonoscopies every 6 months.
E. Patients with inflammatory bowel disease and primary sclerosing cholangitis (PSC) should undergo surveillance colonoscopy every 1–2 years following the diagnosis of PSC.

20. A 72-year-old man with a history of coronary artery disease and arthritis presents to the emergency department with melena. His wife reports that he takes both aspirin and ibuprofen. She also noticed that he seemed confused today. A physical examination reveals that his heart rate is 98 beats per minute and his blood pressure is 85/43 mm Hg. His laboratory findings are notable for a hematocrit of 26% (baseline, 42%), normal INR, and normal platelet count, as well as a normal albumin level and other components of the comprehensive metabolic panel, except for an elevated blood urea nitrogen (BUN) level. His calculated AIMS65 score is 3.

Which of the following is a criterion used to calculate the AIMS65 score?
A. Presence of melena
B. Age >45 years
C. Systolic blood pressure <120 mm Hg
D. INR >2.0
E. Albumin <4.0

21. A 23-year-old woman with anorexia nervosa is seen in your office for evaluation of a rash. Her examination is notable for a symmetric erythematous, pruritic, blistering rash on exposed skin resembling a sunburn, even though it is late winter. She reports intermittent diarrhea, and her parents have noted that she appears disoriented at times. She denies use of laxatives, illicit drugs, or over-the-counter medications. Her food intake has been very poor over the past few months.

What vitamin deficiency is she likely to have?
A. Vitamin C deficiency
B. Niacin deficiency
C. Thiamine deficiency
D. Vitamin A deficiency
E. Vitamin K deficiency

22. A 77-year-old man with a remote history of a transient ischemic attack and atrial fibrillation, currently maintained on warfarin, presents with brisk, painless hematochezia began 4 hours earlier. He does not take aspirin or nonsteroidal antiinflammatory drugs (NSAIDs) and has no history of gastrointestinal bleeding. He last had a colonoscopy at age 70 but does not recall the findings, and the procedure report is not accessible. He has no history of prior operations, including vascular surgery. On presentation he was normotensive, but he became lightheaded and orthostatic with mild tachycardia when standing up. His hematocrit is 34% (baseline hematocrit was 42% 3 months ago), INR is 1.4, platelet count is 256,000/μL, BUN is 28 mg/dL, and creatinine is 0.8 mg/dL. After fluid resuscitation with 1 L of normal saline, he is no longer tachycardic or orthostatic, but he continues to pass blood from the rectum.

Which of the following statements regarding his management is correct?
A. An unprepped colonoscopy should be performed next.
B. Fresh frozen plasma should be administered while awaiting the next intervention.
C. Angiography to localize and treat the source of bleeding should be performed next.
D. An upper esophagogastroduodenoscopy should be performed next.

23. A 53-year-old man who underwent a Roux-en-Y gastric bypass surgery 1 year ago is seen for evaluation of fatigue. He has not experienced melena, hematochezia, or any gastrointestinal symptoms, and he does not take aspirin or NSAIDs. He takes a proton pump inhibitor once per day and an iron supplement, but he has not been taking a multivitamin that had been prescribed following the surgery. Mild muscle weakness is noted on examination of his upper and lower extremities. Laboratory tests are notable for microcytic anemia and mild neutropenia. A colonoscopy performed 1 year ago was normal.

What is the likely cause of his anemia?
A. Folate deficiency
B. Iron deficiency
C. Copper deficiency
D. Vitamin B_{12} deficiency
E. Calcium deficiency

24. A 19-year-old college student presents with a 6-month history of abdominal bloating, diarrhea, and unexplained weight loss. She recently also noticed a rash on her elbows. Her medical history is notable for type 1 diabetes mellitus. In addition, she was recently diagnosed with vitamin D deficiency despite frequent sun exposure. Considering her likely diagnosis, which of the following may also be noted?
   A. Pericarditis
   B. Paget disease of the bone
   C. Hypersplenism
   D. Idiopathic pulmonary hypertension
   E. Abnormal liver function test results

25. A 62-year-old man with chronic hepatitis C–associated cirrhosis presents to the emergency room with confusion and abdominal pain. He is noted to have ascites, peripheral and scrotal edema, and asterixis.
   Which statement is true regarding care of patients with cirrhosis and potential complications?
   A. Bare stents are preferred for transjugular intrahepatic portosystemic shunts (TIPS).
   B. Patients with ascites fluid total protein <1.1 g/dL and serum bilirubin >2.5 mg/dL should receive prophylactic antibiotics.
   C. Endoscopic variceal sclerotherapy is the preferred option for secondary prophylaxis of variceal hemorrhage.
   D. Ambulatory patients who have an ascites fluid polymorphonuclear count >150 cells/mm^3 should receive empiric antibiotics within 24 hours of their test result.
   E. The Model for End-Stage Liver Disease (MELD) score is based on albumin, INR, and total bilirubin.

26. A 29-year-old woman with a history of several episodes of severe acute abdominal pain lasting several days is seen in your office for further evaluation. Review of laboratory test results during episodes of pain is notable for elevated lipase (greater than three times the upper limit of normal), but her liver biochemical test results and triglyceride level are normal. Results of toxic screens, including tests for alcohol, are negative. Ultrasound imaging during at least one episode of pain reveals a normal gallbladder without stones or sludge, as well as a normal bile duct size. She does not smoke or drink alcohol, and she has no family history of pancreatitis. She is referred for consideration of Oddi sphincter manometry.
   Which of the following medications may reduce the risk of postendoscopic retrograde cholangiopancreatography (post-ERCP) pancreatitis?
   A. *N*-acetylcysteine
   B. Octreotide
   C. Rectal indomethacin
   D. Allopurinol
   E. Pentoxifylline

27. A 23-year-old medical student with frequent heartburn since starting medical school 2 years ago is seen in your office for further management. His symptoms are mostly nocturnal, and he reports frequently eating fast food at night shortly before going to bed.
   Which statement regarding gastroesophageal reflux disease (GERD) is true?
   A. Surgical therapy should be considered in patients who do not respond to proton pump inhibitor (PPI) therapy.
   B. Routine biopsies from the distal esophagus are recommended to diagnose GERD.
   C. The treatment of choice for symptomatic relief and healing of erosive esophagitis is an 8-week course of a proton pump inhibitor.
   D. Barium radiographs are useful for the diagnosis of GERD.
   E. Obesity is not associated with increased risk for development of GERD.

28. A 65-year-old woman is noted to have a 1.2-cm solitary cyst with a central scar in the head of the pancreas on an abdominal CT scan obtained to evaluate acute left lower quadrant pain. In addition to being prescribed antibiotics for confirmed acute uncomplicated sigmoid diverticulitis, she is advised to follow up with a gastroenterologist regarding the newly diagnosed pancreatic cyst. She has had no prior abdominal imaging for comparison.
   Which of the following cystic pancreatic lesions has the lowest malignant potential?
   A. Mucinous cystic neoplasm
   B. Main-branch intraductal papillary mucinous neoplasm
   C. Solid pseudopapillary neoplasm
   D. Serous cystadenoma
   E. Side-branch intraductal papillary mucinous neoplasm

29. A 36-year-old man is referred for colonoscopy to evaluate occasional rectal bleeding and mild iron deficiency. A colonoscopy examination reveals 15 small to medium-sized polyps, which are all removed. The pathology report indicates that all the polyps are tubular adenomas. The patient has no family history of colon cancer or other malignancies.
   Which of the following intestinal polyposis syndromes is characterized by multiple adenomatous polyps?
   A. Peutz-Jeghers syndrome
   B. MUTYH-associated polyposis
   C. Juvenile polyposis syndrome
   D. Cowden syndrome
   E. Cronkhite-Canada syndrome

30. A 35-year-old man with idiopathic cardiomyopathy is noted to have mild hypoalbuminemia, mild liver biochemical test abnormalities, and a small amount of ascites on ultrasound imaging of the abdomen. He has no history of alcoholism, and test results for chronic liver disease are negative.

Which of the following clinical or laboratory findings is typical of congestive heart failure (CHF)–associated liver disease?

A. Presence of portosystemic shunts such as esophageal varices
B. Normal total protein (>2.5 g/dL) in ascites
C. Presence of clinically overt jaundice
D. Serum-to-ascites albumin gradient (SAAG) <1.1 g/dL
E. Absence of hepatojugular reflux

31. A 26-year-old woman with prior history of IV drug abuse resulting in HIV and hepatitis C coinfection is seen in a prenatal clinic for routine care. She is in the third trimester of pregnancy with her first child.

Which of the following statements regarding vertical transmission of hepatitis C virus (HCV) is true?

A. Cesarean section reduces the risk of transmission to a greater degree than vaginal delivery.
B. HIV coinfection does not alter the risk of transmission.
C. Breastfeeding is not associated with increased risk of transmission.
D. Patients with HCV genotype 1 have a greater risk of transmission than other genotypes.

32. A 46-year-old man is referred for upper endoscopy for evaluation of a 1-month history of nausea, epigastric pain, diarrhea, and weight loss. He is noted to have bilateral lower extremity edema. Marked diffuse thickening of gastric folds is noted on upper endoscopic evaluation. Histologic examination of biopsies of the gastric folds reveals extreme foveolar hypertrophy and glandular atrophy suggestive of Ménétrier disease.

Which of the following is true regarding Ménétrier disease in adults?

A. The disease is generally self-limited.
B. Hypoalbuminemia results primarily from diminished protein absorption.
C. It occurs more frequently in women than in men.
D. Treatment with an H_2 receptor blocker may provide symptomatic relief.
E. Superficial biopsies of the stomach are generally sufficient to establish the diagnosis.

33. A previously healthy 33-year-old man with no known underlying medical conditions presents with malaise and jaundice ongoing for the past week or more. Laboratory test results are notable for marked elevation of bilirubin and transaminases as well as mild coagulopathy. Neurologic examination reveals that he has grade I encephalopathy. The results of evaluation for infectious, toxic, autoimmune, and vascular causes of acute liver failure are negative.

Which of the following metabolic liver diseases may result in acute liver failure?

A. Nonalcoholic steatohepatitis
B. Hemochromatosis
C. Alpha-1 antitrypsin deficiency
D. Wilson disease
E. Glycogenic hepatopathy

34. A 27-year-old man with ulcerative colitis was recently diagnosed with primary sclerosing cholangitis (PSC) after undergoing evaluation of isolated elevation of alkaline phosphatase. His transamines, albumin, and bilirubin levels, as well as his prothrombin time, are all normal. He has done some research regarding PSC and learned that cholestatic liver diseases such as primary biliary cirrhosis (PBC) and PSC may result in fat-soluble vitamin deficiencies, especially in the setting of more advanced liver disease. Symptoms of which fat-soluble vitamin may result in loss of proprioception?

A. Vitamin A
B. Vitamin D
C. Vitamin E
D. Vitamin K
E. Vitamin B_{12}

35. You are asked for advice regarding consideration of transjugular intrahepatic portosystemic shunt (TIPS) placement in a 54-year-old man with cirrhosis complicated by refractory hepatic hydrothorax. He has no history of hepatic encephalopathy and is compliant with diuretics and a low-sodium diet. Your colleague wants to learn more about situations in which a TIPS procedure may be useful and when it is contraindicated.

In which of the following conditions should a TIPS procedure be avoided?

A. Refractory ascites in a patient with right heart failure
B. Acute refractory variceal bleeding not controlled with pharmacologic and endoscopic therapy
C. Hemorrhage from inaccessible gastric or intestinal varices
D. Bleeding from portal hypertensive gastropathy
E. Refractory hepatic hydrothorax

36. A 52-year-old man with a history of heartburn and cardiomyopathy presents with difficulty swallowing solids and liquids for the past 7 months. An upper endoscopy shows reflux esophagitis but no strictures or masses. Esophageal manometry shows low-amplitude contractions in the distal esophagus and incompetence of the lower esophageal sphincter. The skin of his hands has become thicker, which he thinks is from spending more time at work. He is originally from Brazil but has been living in the United States for the last 20 years and works as a mechanic.

Which test result is most likely to be found in this patient?

A. Barium esophagram with distal "bird's beak" narrowing
B. Positive *Trypanosoma cruzi* antibody
C. Positive anti–Scl-70 antibody
D. Adenocarcinoma on biopsies of the stomach
E. Lung mass on chest CT scan

37. A 45-year-old woman presents with postprandial epigastric pain for the past 8 months. She does not have dysphagia, anemia, nausea, or weight loss. A *Helicobacter pylori* stool antigen test result is negative. An empiric trial of a proton pump inhibitor for 8 weeks does not improve her symptoms. The result of esophagogastroduodenoscopy (EGD) is unremarkable, including gastric biopsies. Laboratory and imaging findings are not suggestive of biliary or pancreatic disease.

Which of the following is the most appropriate next step in management?

A. A low-fat diet
B. Ranitidine
C. Metoclopramide
D. Amitriptyline
E. Probiotics

38. A 69-year-old man with coronary artery disease status after myocardial infarction and percutaneous coronary intervention 2 years ago presents with melena and anemia. Esophagogastroduodenoscopy (EGD) identifies an 8-mm clean-based ulcer in the duodenal bulb. In addition to his usual aspirin, he recently started taking ibuprofen daily for back pain. In addition to stopping the ibuprofen and prescribing omeprazole to facilitate ulcer healing, what do you recommend at this time?

A. Start sucralfate
B. Lifelong use of omeprazole to prevent ulcer recurrence
C. Repeat EGD in 8 weeks
D. Stopping his aspirin
E. Testing for *H. pylori* infection

39. A 24-year-old woman from Algeria is pregnant with her first child. Routine screening identifies her as having a positive HBsAg. Additional testing shows negative HBsAb, negative HBeAg, and positive HBeAb. Her hepatitis B viral load is 1186 IU/mL at the end of the second trimester. Liver enzymes, INR, and abdominal ultrasound findings are normal. In addition to following her liver enzymes and providing the infant with hepatitis B immune globulin (HBIG) and hepatitis B vaccination, which of the following would you recommend with regard to her hepatitis B infection?

A. No treatment at this time
B. Tenofovir
C. Pegylated interferon
D. Cesarean delivery at term
E. Lamivudine

40. A 32-year-old woman with ulcerative colitis comes to your office for evaluation of symptoms. She was diagnosed with mild to moderate pancolitis last year. She initially responded well to induction and maintenance therapy with mesalamine. However, 2 months ago, she developed bloody diarrhea occurring six times per day, as well as lower abdominal cramping. Treatment with prednisone 40 mg daily resulted in improved symptoms, but symptoms recurred when the prednisone dose was tapered to 10 mg daily. A physical examination reveals her vital signs are normal, and she has minimal left lower quadrant tenderness. Laboratory studies reveal a white blood cell count of 11,000/μL and hematocrit of 34.5%, and the result of stool testing for *Clostridium difficile* is negative.

Which of the following is the most appropriate next step in treating this patient?

A. Switch to balsalazide.
B. Add budesonide.
C. Increase prednisone to 20 mg daily and continue indefinitely.
D. Increase prednisone to 20 mg/day and add azathioprine.
E. Add ciprofloxacin.

41. A 61-year-old woman presented to the hospital with new-onset abdominal distention and jaundice. She has a long history of drinking two or three glasses of wine per day and has been drinking more than this for the past few months in the context of social stressors. She denies abdominal pain, rectal bleeding, melena, confusion, fever, or chills. A physical examination reveals her vital signs are normal. She is mildly jaundiced and appears to have ascites, but she has no leg edema, spider angiomas, or asterixis. Her laboratory studies show ALT 66 U/L, AST 424 U/L, alkaline phosphatase 285 U/L, total bilirubin 6.3 mg/dL, albumin 3 g/dL, white blood cell count 15,000/μL, hematocrit 35%, platelets 345,000/μL, and INR 1.3. Her test result for viral hepatitis is negative. An abdominal ultrasound reveals moderate ascites and fatty liver with Doppler measurements suggesting portal hypertension, but she has no splenomegaly or evidence of portosystemic shunts. Paracentesis shows ascites fluid albumin of 0.9 g/dL and WBC 195/mm^3.

Which of the following is the most appropriate next step in management?
A. Cefotaxime
B. Supportive care
C. Prednisolone
D. Nadolol
E. Pentoxifylline

42. A 54-year-old man is hospitalized with pancreatitis related to alcohol use. Five days after admission, he continues to have epigastric pain and nausea, and he has not been able to tolerate much oral intake. A physical examination reveals his vital signs are normal, but he has diffuse abdominal pain with palpation. Laboratory studies show a white blood cell count of 14,300/μL, ALT 89 U/L, AST 345 U/L, alkaline phosphatase 176 U/L, and total bilirubin 2.3 mg/dL. Abdominal CT with intravenous contrast shows a diffusely edematous pancreas with multiple small peripancreatic fluid collections, no pancreatic necrosis, and no gallstones or biliary dilation.

Which of the following is the most appropriate next step in management?
A. Parenteral nutrition
B. Enteral nutrition with a nasojejunal tube
C. Imipenem
D. Pancreatic debridement
E. Interventional radiology drainage of fluid collection

43. A 34-year-old woman with autoimmune thyroiditis presents with recurrent episodes of pancreatitis. Abdominal ultrasound shows no evidence of gallstones, and she denies significant alcohol use. Abdominal CT shows a diffusely enlarged pancreas with no focal lesions. A serum IgG4 test result is elevated.

Which of the following therapies is most likely to prevent additional episodes of pancreatitis?
A. Prednisone
B. Alcohol cessation
C. Cholecystectomy
D. Pancreaticoduodenectomy (Whipple procedure)
E. Fibrate

44. A 73-year-old woman presents with persistent diarrhea for the past 6 months. The diarrhea is watery, occurs 8–10 times per day, including at night, and does not improve with fasting. She also reports episodes of flushing as well as fatigue and dyspnea on exertion. Stool study results are negative for infection, and her white blood cell count is normal. An electrocardiogram shows low-voltage QRS, a chest x-ray shows cardiomegaly, and an echocardiogram shows moderate to severe tricuspid regurgitation.

Which of the following tests is most likely to be diagnostic in this patient?
A. Serum vasoactive intestinal peptide
B. Serum calcitonin
C. Serum gastrin
D. Urinary 5-hydroxyindoleacetic acid
E. Fat pad biopsy with Congo red staining

45. A 67-year-old man with cirrhosis due to hepatitis C presents to the emergency department with hematemesis and hematochezia. He is initially hypotensive, but he is stabilized with intravenous fluids and blood transfusions. A physical examination reveals he is jaundiced and moderately encephalopathic, has spider angiomas on his chest, and has moderate ascites. Concurrently with intravenous octreotide infusion and PPI therapy, which of the follow treatments should be initiated at this time?
A. Penicillin
B. Intravenous albumin
C. Ceftriaxone
D. *N*-acetylcysteine
E. Vasopressin

46. A 78-year-old man with hypertension and diabetes presents for evaluation of ongoing anemia for the past 5 months. He denies abdominal pain, acid reflux, nausea, rectal bleeding, or melena. He has felt more tired and short of breath with exertion, but he has not had chest pain, cough, or lightheadedness. His medications are lisinopril, insulin, and aspirin.

A physical examination shows his vital signs are normal. He has no scleral icterus, lymphadenopathy, or cardiac murmurs. His lungs are clear, and his abdomen is soft, nontender, and nondistended with no organomegaly. Laboratory testing shows a hematocrit of 28% (his prior baseline was 40%) with a mean corpuscular volume of 72 fL, as well as normal white blood cell count, normal platelet count, and normal coagulation studies. His ferritin level is 7 μg/L. The result of fecal occult blood testing is positive. A colonoscopy and esophagogastroduodenoscopy (EGD) did not reveal a bleeding source. The result of CT enterography was unremarkable. He received 2 U of blood transfusion for symptomatic anemia.

Which of the following is the next most appropriate step in evaluation?
A. Push enteroscopy
B. CT angiography
C. Wireless capsule endoscopy
D. Double-balloon enteroscopy
E. Tagged red blood cell scan

47. A 53-year-old woman with chronic pancreatitis and diabetes presents for evaluation of loose stool for the past 4 months. She reports four or five bowel movements per day, including occasional nocturnal symptoms. She has bloating and chronic abdominal pain but no rectal bleeding or nausea. Her medical history includes chronic pancreatitis due to prior alcoholism, diabetes mellitus, and seasonal allergies. She takes lisinopril, insulin, aspirin, oxycodone, pancreatic enzyme supplementation, and loratadine. Her sister has celiac disease. She reports no change in diet or increase in fatty food consumption.

A physical examination reveals her vital signs are normal. She has mild epigastric pain with palpation but is otherwise not distended and has no organomegaly. She has no rashes. Laboratory studies reveal normal liver enzymes and lipase, hematocrit 33% with mean corpuscular volume 102 fL, and normal white blood cell count and platelets. Her vitamin B_{12} level is 198 pg/mL; her folate level is 31 ng/mL; and her tissue transglutaminase IgA antibody is normal (with normal total serum IgA level). Test results for stool culture, ova and parasite examinations, and Giardia antigen are negative. The result of a colonoscopy including the terminal ileum is normal, including random biopsies of the colon. The result of an esophagogastroduodenoscopy (EGD) including biopsies of the duodenum is normal. Abdominal imaging shows stable features of chronic pancreatitis but no intestinal inflammation or strictures. An increase in the dose of her pancreatic enzyme supplementation does not improve her symptoms.

Which of the follow is the most likely diagnosis?

A. Steatorrhea due to pancreatic exocrine dysfunction
B. Irritable bowel syndrome
C. Celiac disease
D. Small intestinal bacterial overgrowth
E. Crohn disease

48. A 29-year-old woman with Crohn disease and prior small bowel resections presented with severe left flank pain. Urinalysis reveals 100–200 red blood cells per high-power field and no bacteria. A kidney stone is identified on a CT scan. She reports no recent change in her medications (infliximab, calcium, vitamin D), but she has been eating more spinach salads recently. In addition to increasing her fluid intake, what recommendations would you give this patient to prevent additional stone formation?

A. Low-oxalate diet and stop the calcium supplementation
B. Low-oxalate diet and continue the calcium supplementation
C. High-oxalate diet and stop the calcium supplementation
D. High-oxalate diet and continue the calcium supplementation
E. Potassium citrate

49. A 61-year-old woman with a history of hypertension and low back pain presents to the emergency department with epigastric pain for the past 36 hours. The pain is constant and radiates to her back. She also has nausea, vomiting, and decreased oral intake. Her medications are hydrochlorothiazide and occasional acetaminophen. A physical examination reveals her temperature is 100.3°F, heart rate 95 beats per minute, blood pressure 136/84 mm Hg, respiration rate 14 per minute, and BMI 31 kg/m^2. She has scleral icterus and dry mucous membranes. Her abdomen is tender in the epigastrium and right upper quadrant, but there is no rebound or guarding. She does not have ascites or spider angiomas. Laboratory testing reveals a white blood cell count of 13,600/μL, lipase 3578 U/L, alanine aminotransferase 347 U/L, aspartate aminotransferase 266 U/L, alkaline phosphatase 272 U/L, and total bilirubin 5.2 mg/dL. Abdominal ultrasonography shows cholelithiasis and a dilated common bile duct to 11 mm but no choledocholithiasis. Twelve hours later, her pain remains unchanged, her total bilirubin is 5.8 mg/dL, and her temperature is 101.1°F.

Which of the following is the most appropriate next step in management?

A. Abdominal CT
B. Magnetic resonance cholangiopancreatography
C. Cholecystectomy
D. Ursodiol
E. Endoscopic retrograde cholangiopancreatography

50. A 35-year-old woman is being evaluated for chronic abdominal pain and constipation for the past 3 years. The pain is located in the lower abdomen, occurs approximately once per week, and improves after defecation. She reports having a bowel movement approximately every 3 days, although the frequency varies. The stools are hard, and she often has a sense of incomplete evacuation. She denies nausea, vomiting, rectal bleeding, weight loss, or neurologic symptoms. She has one child. Her mother had colorectal cancer at age 59.

A physical examination reveals her vital signs are normal. Her abdominal examination is unremarkable, and her rectal tone is normal. Laboratory evaluation shows normal renal function, electrolytes, complete blood count, and thyroid-stimulating hormone. The results of a colonoscopy and radiopaque marker study are normal.

What is the most likely diagnosis for this patient?

A. Colonic inertia
B. Dyssynergic defecation
C. Constipation-predominant irritable bowel syndrome
D. Multiple sclerosis
E. Chronic intestinal pseudoobstruction

Chapter 7 Answers

1. **ANSWER: C. Biopsy of the Barrett segment every 3–5 years**

Current Barrett esophagus surveillance guidelines recommend EGD with biopsies every 3–5 years if the initial biopsies followed by surveillance biopsies obtained 1 year later do not reveal dysplasia. Barrett esophagus surveillance every 3 months is recommended for patients with high-grade dysplasia who do not wish to undergo ablative or surgical therapy. A surveillance interval of every 6–12 months is recommended for patients with low-grade dysplasia. No subsequent surveillance and surveillance every 10 years are not acceptable for this patient, who may be at long-term risk of developing adenocarcinoma of the esophagus.

Spechler SJ, Sharma P, Souza RF, et al. American Gastroenterological Association medical position statement on the management of Barrett's esophagus. *Gastroenterology.* 2011;140:1084–1091.

2. **ANSWER: C. Rifaximin**

Irritable bowel syndrome (IBS) is a functional bowel disorder characterized by episodic abdominal discomfort and altered bowel habits. Bloating, nausea, and fatigue may also be present. Visceral hypersensitivity is thought to play a role. Treatment options, including stool bulking agents such as psyllium, dietary modification, and antispasmodic agents such as hyoscyamine, may result in variable improvement of symptoms in some patients. Mesalamine, though effective for treatment of inflammatory bowel disease (IBD), is not useful for management of IBS. A 2-week course of rifaximin, a poorly absorbed, topically acting antibiotic, has been shown to result in significant reduction in irritable bowel syndrome–related symptoms such as bloating, loose stools, and abdominal pain.

Pimentel M, Lembo A, Chey WD, et al. Rifaximin therapy for patients with irritable bowel syndrome without constipation. *N Engl J Med.* 2011;364(1):22–32.

3. **ANSWER: A. Digoxin may predispose patients to bowel ischemia.**

Ischemic colitis is a form of gut ischemia most often affecting the descending and sigmoid colon. It results from low vascular flow to a colonic segment rather than from an embolic process or vascular thrombosis. It is generally associated with low mortality and rarely causes hemodynamically significant bleeding. Digoxin, a splanchnic vasoconstrictor, can predispose to both mesenteric ischemia and ischemic colitis. CT imaging may show colonic thickening, but it cannot distinguish ischemic colitis from other inflammatory or infectious processes. Angiography is of limited value in ischemic colitis and is more useful for evaluation of suspected acute mesenteric ischemia. Elevation of serum lactate is uncommon in patients with ischemic colitis and, if present, suggests the presence of bowel infarction and necrosis.

Flynn AD, Valentine JF. Update in the diagnosis and management of colonic ischemia. *Curr Treat Options Gastroenterol.* 2016;14(1):128–139.

4. **ANSWER: C. HIV infection**

A false-negative HCV antibody test result may occur in patients who have immunocompromised states such as HIV or renal failure or who have malignancies such as lymphoma. Clarification of a suspected false-positive or false-negative HCV antibody test result can be made by performing an HCV RNA (viral load) test. A false-positive HCV antibody test result may occur in patients with a variety of autoimmune disorders, such as autoimmune hepatitis, lupus, and rheumatoid arthritis, possibly related to the hypergammaglobulinemia.

Smith BD, Teshale E, Jewett A, et al. Performance of premarket rapid hepatitis C virus antibody assays in 4 National Human Immunodeficiency Virus Behavioral Surveillance System sites. *Clin Infect Dis.* 2011;53(8):780–786.

5. **ANSWER: C. It increases mortality in patients with decompensated cirrhosis.**

Researchers in recent studies have noted *increased* mortality in patients with decompensated cirrhosis who are treated with nonselective beta blockers. Nonselective beta blockers are indicated for both primary and secondary prophylaxis of variceal bleeding but not in the acute management of variceal bleeding. Use of nonselective beta blockers decreases the risk of spontaneous bacterial peritonitis and bleeding from portal hypertensive gastropathy. Nonselective beta blockers are not indicated for prevention of variceal formation in early cirrhosis.

Ge PS, Runyon BA. The changing role of beta-blocker therapy in patients with cirrhosis. *J Hepatol.* 2014;60(3):643–653.

6. **ANSWER: D. Primary biliary cirrhosis**

Secondary Sjögren syndrome may develop in as many as 40%–65% of patients with primary biliary cirrhosis (PBC). Typical symptoms include dry mouth (xerostomia) and dry eyes (keratoconjunctivitis) and may precede PBC-related symptoms. Gastroesophageal reflux disease, small intestinal bacterial overgrowth, and gallstone pancreatitis are not associated with Sjögren syndrome. Ulcerative colitis is associated with several extraintestinal manifestations, such as uveitis, but secondary Sjögren syndrome is not one of them.

Uddenfeldt P, Danielsson A, Forssell A, et al. Features of Sjögren's syndrome in patients with primary biliary cirrhosis. *J Intern Med.* 1991;230(5):443–448.

7. **ANSWER: D. Hepatic adenoma**

Hepatic adenomas are a common focal hepatic lesion seen predominantly in young women with a history of prolonged oral contraceptive use, and they sometimes undergo malignant transformation. They are typically found incidentally on imaging. Gastrointestinal tumors (GISTs) are generally benign tumors, but they are most often found in the stomach and small intestine, not in the liver. The remaining benign liver lesions mentioned have not been definitively linked to the use of oral contraceptives. Cavernous hemangiomas are the most common benign focal hepatic lesions. Focal nodular hyperplasia (FNH), 90% of which occur in women, are the second most common benign liver tumors. FNH lesions may be responsive to estrogen, but the development of FNH has not been conclusively linked to oral contraceptive use. Nodular regenerative hyperplasia is uncommon and is characterized by development of multiple small regenerative nodules.

Algarni AA, Alshuhri AH, Alonazi MM, et al. Focal liver lesions found incidentally. *World J Hepatol.* 2016;8(9):446–451.

8. **ANSWER: B. Prolonged antibiotic treatment is required to eradicate the causative organism.**

Whipple disease requires prolonged antibiotic therapy, usually for 12 months. Most cases occur in middle-aged men of European ancestry. Extraintestinal symptoms are common and may include rheumatologic, cardiac, and central nervous system involvement, for example. The causative organism, *Tropheryma whipplei,* a gram-positive bacillus related to actinomycetes, is difficult to culture. It is believed to be acquired from soil and animals, making this rare disease more common in farmers. Esophagogastroduodenoscopy (EGD) with small bowel biopsy, not colonoscopy, is the diagnostic test of choice. The diagnosis can usually be made by identification of characteristic PAS staining of macrophages in the lamina propria of the small intestine or with electron microscopy.

Marth T, Moos V, Müller C, et al. *Tropheryma whipplei* infection and Whipple's disease. *Lancet Infect Dis.* 2016;16(3): e13–e22.

9. **ANSWER: D. PPI-associated fundic gland polyps are not associated with an increased risk of cancer.**

Fundic gland polyps may develop in people who are on long-term PPI therapy, and in this setting, they are *not associated* with an increased risk of malignancy. However, in patients with FAP, fundic gland polyps *are associated* with an increased risk of cancer. The most common types of gastric polyps are fundic gland polyps and hyperplastic polyps, representing 70%–90% of gastric polyps. Dysplastic tissue can be found in 5%–19% of hyperplastic polyps. Some guidelines recommend resection of gastric hyperplastic polyps larger than 0.5–1 cm. Adenomatous gastric polyps should be resected due to risk of malignancy, and a surveillance endoscopy should be performed 1 year after resection followed by surveillance every 3–5 years thereafter.

Evans JA, Chandrasekhara V, Chathadi KV, et al. The role of endoscopy in the management of premalignant and malignant conditions of the stomach. *Gastrointest Endosc.* 2015;82(1):1–8.

10. **ANSWER: E. Synovial fluid shows an elevated leukocyte count.**

Postenteric reactive arthritis (formerly known as *Reiter syndrome)* typically develops 2–4 weeks after an acute diarrheal illness. It is an immune-mediated synovitis, so the synovial fluid shows an elevated leukocyte count despite the absence of infection. Gonococcal arthritis is important to exclude in a young person presenting with acute monoarticular arthritis. *Shigella* sp. is the most commonly associated enteric organism associated with this syndrome, although *Salmonella* sp., *Campylobacter jejuni, Yersinia enterocolitica,* and even *Clostridium difficile* have been implicated. Amebic intestinal infections are not associated with reactive arthritis. People who develop this syndrome have a higher prevalence of *HLA-B27* antigen, not HLA-DQ2, which is associated with celiac disease. This syndrome is more common in men and classically is associated with the triad of arthritis, conjunctivitis, and *urethritis,* not esophagitis.

Morris D, Inman RD. Reactive arthritis: developments and challenges in diagnosis and treatment. *Curr Rheumatol Rep.* 2012;14(5):390–394.

11. **ANSWER: D. Myasthenia gravis**

This patient exhibits classic features of myasthenia gravis, including muscle fatigue and ocular-bulbar symptoms. Myasthenia gravis can cause oropharyngeal dysphagia due to muscle weakness, which can be a risk for aspiration. The globus sensation, which refers to a sensation of a lump or foreign body in the throat in the absence of dysphagia and odynophagia, is not a feature of myasthenia gravis. Gastroesophageal reflux, goiter, early hypopharyngeal cancer, and anxiety disorders all can be associated with globus sensation, unlike myasthenia gravis.

Binks S, Vincent A, Palace J. Myasthesia gravis: a clinical-immunological update. *J Neurol.* 2016;263(4):826–834.

12. **ANSWER: B. The treatment of choice is prednisone with or without azathioprine.**

The patient's elevated hepatic enzymes, female sex, elevated globulin levels (total protein, albumin), lack of risk factors for chronic viral hepatitis, personal history of hypothyroidism that could be autoimmune in nature, family history of autoimmune disorders, and high-titer anti–smooth muscle antibody test are strong clues suggesting autoimmune hepatitis. Autoimmune hepatitis usually presents in the fourth decade of life and is more common in women than in men. Several autoantibodies may be present, such as antinuclear antibody (ANA), antisoluble liver antigen (SLA), antiliver kidney microsomal type 1 (anti-LKM-1) antibodies, and antineutrophil cytoplasmic antibodies (ASCA), for example. Treatment consists of a glucocorticoid (such as prednisone) with or without azathioprine. Undiagnosed and untreated autoimmune hepatitis may lead to the development of cirrhosis. Autoimmune hepatitis recurs in 20%–30% of patients after liver transplant despite the immunosuppression regimen.

Liberal R, Vergani D, Mieli-Vergani G. Update on autoimmune hepatitis. *J Clin Transl Hepatol.* 2015;3(1):42–52.

13. **ANSWER: B. There is a hypervirulent strain associated with lower clinical cure rates and increased recurrence rates.**

A hypervirulent strain of *C. difficile* (NAP1/BI/027) that is associated with lower clinical cure rates and increased recurrence rates has been described. The *C. difficile* toxin and PCR assay results may remain positive after resolution of symptoms; hence, testing for cure after symptoms resolution is not advised. There has been a significant increase in the incidence of *C. difficile* infection in patients with IBD. Hence, all patients with IBD who are hospitalized with a disease flare should undergo testing. Repeat *C. difficile* testing after a negative test result is positive <5% of the time, and furthermore, repeat testing increases the likelihood of a false-positive result. Hand hygiene with soap and water is more effective than alcohol-based hand sanitizers for eradicating *C. difficile* spores and is therefore recommended when caring for a patient with *C. difficile* infection.

Ofosu A. *Clostridium difficile* infection: a review of current and emerging therapies. *Ann Gastroenterol.* 2016;29(2):147–154.

14. **ANSWER: B. Barium esophagram**

Zenker diverticulum is an outpouching of the mucosa immediately above the upper esophageal sphincter. The best test to perform to diagnose a Zenker diverticulum is a barium esophagram. EGD may not identify them, and there is a risk of inadvertent perforation of the diverticulum. A CT scan may show a large Zenker diverticulum. Laryngoscopy is not an ideal method for identifying a Zenker diverticulum. An esophageal motility study would not diagnose a Zenker diverticulum, but it may provide information regarding the underlying pathogenesis.

Law R, Katzka DA, Baron TH. Zenker's diverticulum. *Clin Gastroenterol Hepatol.* 2014;12(11):1773–1782.

15. **ANSWER: B. Gastroesophageal reflux disease and constipation**

Cystic fibrosis (CF) is an inherited disease characterized by a mutation in the cystic fibrosis transmembrane conductance regulator (CFTR). CFTR is found in all epithelia of the gastrointestinal tract, including the pancreas and liver. Constipation and obstipation rather than diarrhea are common in patients with CF, and they are related to intestinal dysmotility and decreased water secretion due to the CFTR defect. GERD is reported in 30% of adult patients with CF, and it occurs primarily due to inappropriate lower esophageal sphincter relaxation. Intestinal dysmotility, use of acid-suppressing agents, and chronic antibiotic therapy predispose patients with CF to develop small intestinal bacterial overgrowth (SIBO). Although SIBO occurs in 30%–55% of patients with CF, dysphagia is not a typical symptom of CF. More than 85% of patients with CF have pancreatic insufficiency related to pancreatic ductal obstruction caused by thick pancreatic fluid secretions. Gallstones are not typically associated with CF. Liver disease in patients with CF can include asymptomatic elevation in liver enzyme tests, hepatosplenomegaly, steatosis, and cirrhosis.

Assis DN, Freedman SD. Gastrointestinal disorders in cystic fibrosis. *Clin Chest Med.* 2016;37(1):109–118.

16. **ANSWER: C. Eosinophilic esophagitis**

Eosinophilic esophagitis typically occurs in young men with a history of atopic disorders such as eczema and asthma. Endoscopic findings include multiple thin rings with linear furrows. Eosinophilic esophagitis is a chronic inflammatory, immune-mediated condition in which dense eosinophilic infiltrates are seen on esophageal biopsies (>15/high-power field).

Esophageal lichen planus can cause dysphagia due to stricture formation, but the disease occurs mostly in middle-aged women, and strictures tend to be located in the proximal esophagus. A Schatzki ring is solitary and located in the distal esophagus, often in association with a hiatal hernia. Peptic strictures generally occur in the distal esophagus and cause focal luminal narrowing. In addition, signs of acid-induced injury such as reflux esophagitis and ulceration are commonly seen. Plummer-Vinson syndrome is characterized by proximal esophageal webs causing dysphagia, atrophic glossitis, and iron-deficiency anemia.

Zhang M, Li Y. Eosinophilic gastroenteritis: a state-of-the-art review. *J Gastroenterol Hepatol.* 2017;32(1):64–72.

17. **ANSWER: D. Gallbladder cancer**

Risk factors for gallbladder cancer include obesity, gallstones, "porcelain" gallbladder, and chronic *Salmonella typhi* infection. Gallstones are present in 70%–90% of patients with gallbladder cancer. Large, solitary stones (>2.5 cm) are associated with the greatest risk. A "porcelain" gallbladder is characterized by intramucosal calcification due to chronic inflammation and is associated with a 2%–3% incidence of gallbladder cancer.

Kanthan R, Senger JL, Ahmed S, et al. Gallbladder cancer in the 21st century. *J Oncol.* 2015;2015:967472.

18. ANSWER: C. Herpes simplex virus (HSV)–associated ulcer

Herpes simplex virus is usually associated with multiple small, shallow ulcers rather than a solitary, large ulcer. Certain antiretroviral medications such as didanosine (ddI) and zidovudine (AZT) can cause pill esophagitis. These ulcers *are typically solitary* and are often found in the proximal to middle esophagus. CMV and idiopathic ulcers are the most common causes of esophageal ulceration in patients with AIDS and are usually large, solitary, and well circumscribed. MAC can occasionally cause esophageal ulceration in patients with AIDS.

O'Rourke A. Infective oesophagitis: epidemiology, cause, diagnosis and treatment options. *Curr Opin Otolaryngol Head Neck Surg.* 2015;23(6):459–463.

19. ANSWER: E. Patients with inflammatory bowel disease and primary sclerosing cholangitis (PSC) should undergo surveillance colonoscopy every 1–2 years following the diagnosis of PSC.

Colorectal cancer is one of the most dreaded complications of inflammatory bowel disease (IBD), accounting for 15% of IBD-related deaths. Patients with IBD and PSC have a higher risk of developing colorectal cancer, so it is recommended that they undergo surveillance colonoscopy every 1–2 years from the time of diagnosis of PSC.

Patients with ulcerative proctitis (rectal involvement only) are not considered at increased risk of developing colorectal cancer. Long-standing Crohn colitis is associated with an increased risk of colorectal cancer. However, Crohn disease limited to the ileum is not associated with an increased risk of developing colon cancer. Patients with long-standing ulcerative colitis, including left-sided disease as well as pancolitis, are at increased risk of developing colorectal cancer. Screening for dysplasia and cancer should begin after 8 years of disease in patients who have pancolitis and after 10–12 years for those with left-sided colitis, and who are surgical candidates, per current guidelines. Colectomy is recommended if high-grade dysplasia is detected and confirmed by a second pathologist. Such patients have a 43% risk of synchronous malignancy.

Farraye FA, Odze RD, Eaden J, et al. AGA technical review on the diagnosis and management of colorectal neoplasia in inflammatory bowel disease. *Gastroenterology.* 2010;138(2):746–774.

20. ANSWER: A. Presence of melena

The AIMS65 score is used to predict inpatient mortality in patients with upper gastrointestinal bleeding. The score is easy to calculate and relies on data readily obtainable in the emergency department.

The presence of melena is not a variable used to calculate the score. A score of 1 point is given to each of the following five risk factors: **A**lbumin <3.0 mg/dL, **I**NR >1.5, Altered **m**ental status, **S**ystolic blood pressure <90 mm Hg, and age >**65**. A patient with an upper gastrointestinal bleed who has an AIMS65 score of 3, such as in this case, has an estimated inpatient mortality rate of 9%, compared with a mortality rate of 0.3% for those with a score of 0.

Saltzman JR, Tabak YP, Hyett BH, et al. A simple risk score accurately predicts in-hospital mortality, length of stay, and cost in acute upper GI bleeding. *Gastrointest Endosc.* 2011;74(6):1215–1224.

21. ANSWER: B. Niacin deficiency

This patient has pellagra, a common manifestation of niacin deficiency. It is uncommon in the Western world except as a complication of anorexia nervosa, alcoholism, and some malabsorptive disorders. The classic clinical features are diarrhea, pigmented dermatitis (as described in this patient), and dementia. Vitamin C deficiency, known as *scurvy,* causes perifollicular hemorrhage, gingivitis, anemia, and joint pain. Thiamine deficiency may cause a variety of symptoms, such as polyneuropathy (dry beriberi) and high-output cardiac failure (wet beriberi), as well as ataxia, nystagmus, confabulation, memory loss, and ophthalmoplegia (Wernicke-Korsakoff syndrome). Vitamin A deficiency can cause night blindness, corneal drying, and follicular hyperkeratosis. Vitamin K deficiency causes easy bruising and bleeding.

Barsell A, Norton SA. Pellagra's three Ds: dermatology, death and Dracula. *JAMA Dermatol.* 2015;151(9):951.

22. ANSWER: D. An upper esophagogastroduodenoscopy should be performed next.

An upper gastrointestinal source of bleeding should be considered in patients presenting with brisk hematochezia and hemodynamic instability. The elevated blood urea nitrogen/creatinine ratio also suggests an upper gastrointestinal source of bleeding in this case. For further evaluation, an esophagogastroduodenoscopy (upper endoscopy) should be performed urgently prior to beginning the bowel preparation for a colonoscopy examination because it is important to exclude an upper gastrointestinal source of the significant bleeding, such as a peptic ulcer. An unprepped flexible sigmoidoscopy or colonoscopy has low diagnostic yield and is not recommended for evaluation of lower GI bleeding. Fresh frozen plasma (FFP) would not be indicated in this case, because endoscopic hemostasis can be adequately achieved with an INR <1.5. In patients with an INR of 1.5–2.5, endoscopic hemostasis may be considered before or concomitant with giving reversal agents such as FFP. Reversal agents should be administered prior to endoscopy in patients with an INR >2.5. Angiography and other radiographic interventions should be considered in patients with ongoing bleeding *and a negative upper endoscopy* who also fail to adequately respond to hemodynamic resuscitation. In this setting, angiography may localize the source of bleeding in 25%–70% of examinations.

Strate LL, Gralnek IM. ACG clinical guideline: management of patients with acute lower gastrointestinal bleeding. *Am J Gastroenterol.* 2016;111:459–474.

23. ANSWER: C. Copper deficiency

Bariatric surgery is the most common cause of acquired copper deficiency. Microcytic, hypochromic anemia and neutropenia are typical hematologic manifestations. Muscle weakness, skin depigmentation, abnormally formed hair, hepatosplenomegaly, and even ataxia and neuropathy, mimicking vitamin B_{12} deficiency, have been described.

Folate, iron, and vitamin B_{12} deficiencies can occur in up to 40% of patients who have undergone Roux-en-Y gastric bypass surgery and who do not take multivitamin with mineral supplements. Lack of gastric acid impairs iron and vitamin B_{12} absorption. Bypassing the duodenum and proximal jejunum impairs folate and iron absorption as well. Folate and vitamin B_{12} deficiency cause macrocytic anemia. Although iron deficiency may cause a microcytic anemia, muscle weakness and neutropenia are not typical. Poor calcium absorption can occur after gastric bypass, but it usually causes secondary hyperparathyroidism and metabolic bone disease.

Gletsu-Miller N, Broderius M, Frediani JK, et al. Incidence and prevalence of copper deficiency following Roux-en-Y gastric bypass surgery. *Int J Obes (Lond).* 2012;36:328–335.

24. ANSWER: E. Abnormal liver function test results

This patient has celiac disease, a small intestinal disorder resulting from a gluten allergy. This disease is characterized by the gastrointestinal symptoms described. In addition, some patients may develop a dermatologic manifestation—dermatitis herpetiformis—as described in this case. Celiac disease has been associated with Down syndrome, selective IgA deficiency, type 1 diabetes mellitus, thyroid disease, autoimmune liver disease, and *idiopathic liver enzyme elevations.*

Osteoporosis may develop from calcium and vitamin D malabsorption. Paget disease of the bone has not been directly associated with celiac disease. Some studies suggest that patients with celiac sprue may be at increased risk of ischemic heart disease, but pericarditis has not been reported to be associated with celiac sprue. Hyposplenism, not hypersplenism, has been described in some patients with celiac sprue, though the mechanisms are unknown. Patients with hyposplenism should receive pneumococcal vaccination. The Lane-Hamilton syndrome, characterized by the coexistence of celiac sprue and idiopathic pulmonary hemosiderosis (not idiopathic pulmonary hypertension), has been reported in some patients. Adherence to a gluten-free diet has led to resolution of pulmonary symptoms in a few patients.

Kelly CP, Bai JC, Liu E, et al. Advances in diagnosis and management of celiac disease. *Gastroenterology.* 2015;148(6):1175–1186.

25. ANSWER: B. Patients with ascites fluid total protein <1.1 g/dL and serum bilirubin >2.5 mg/dL should receive prophylactic antibiotics.

Patients with cirrhosis who have low total protein levels in ascites fluid and advanced liver disease are at increased risk of developing spontaneous bacterial peritonitis and should therefore receive prophylactic antibiotics. Covered stents are preferred to bare stents for TIPS procedures, owing to lower risk of shunt occlusion and dysfunction. A *combination* of a nonselective beta blocker plus endoscopic variceal band ligation (not sclerotherapy) is the preferred method for secondary prophylaxis of variceal hemorrhage. The threshold for empiric antibiotic treatment for suspected spontaneous bacterial peritonitis is a polymorphonuclear count >250. The Model for End-Stage Liver Disease (MELD) score is based on creatinine, INR, and total bilirubin (albumin is not included).

Pericleous M, Sarnowski A, Moore A, et al. The clinical management of abdominal ascites, spontaneous bacterial peritonitis and hepatorenal syndrome: a review of current guidelines and recommendations. *Eur J Gastroenterol Hepatol.* 2016;28(3):e10–e18.

26. ANSWER: C. Rectal indomethacin

Meta-analyses of several randomized controlled studies have demonstrated that rectally administered indomethacin significantly reduces the incidence of post-ERCP pancreatitis. In addition, recent data suggest that rectally administered indomethacin alone may be more effective than no prophylaxis and pancreatic duct stent placement in preventing post-ERCP pancreatitis.

N-acetylcysteine has not been shown to be beneficial in preventing post-ERCP pancreatitis. Octreotide may reduce serum amylase elevation, but the results of studies evaluating its effect on the incidence of post-ERCP pancreatitis are mixed. Studies of allopurinol and pentoxifylline have not supported their use for the prevention of post-ERCP pancreatitis.

Thiruvengadam NR, Forde KA, Ma GK, et al. Rectal indomethacin reduces pancreatitis in high- and low-risk patients undergoing endoscopic retrograde cholangiopancreatography. *Gastroenterology.* 2016;151(2):288–297.e4.

27. ANSWER: C. The treatment of choice for symptomatic relief and healing of erosive esophagitis is an 8-week course of a proton pump inhibitor.

PPI therapy is associated with superior healing rates and lower relapse rates compared with H_2 blockers in patients with erosive esophagitis. The greatest response to antireflux surgery is seen primarily in patients with typical symptoms of heartburn and/or regurgitation, who demonstrate good response to PPI therapy, or those who have abnormal ambulatory pH monitoring studies with good symptom correlation. On the basis of current literature, the use of routine biopsies of the esophagus to diagnose GERD cannot be recommended. The overall sensitivity of a barium esophagram to diagnose GERD is low; hence, it is not recommended for diagnosis. Last, obesity is a risk factor for GERD, and indeed modest weight loss is one of the more effective lifestyle modifications that may be beneficial for GERD management.

Anderson WD 3rd, Strayer SM, Mull SR. Common questions about the management of gastroesophageal reflux. *Am Fam Physician.* 2015;91(10):692–697.

28. ANSWER: D. Serous cystadenoma

Serous cystadenomas are more common in women, usually occur in people aged 60 or older, predominate in the pancreatic head, and are almost always benign. They are usually small lesions, calcify more than any other pancreatic neoplasm, and may contain a classic central stellate scar.

Mucinous cystic neoplasms are found almost exclusively in women, tend to occur at a younger age, predominate in the pancreatic tail, are solitary, and have a moderate malignant potential. Intraductal papillary cystic neoplasms (IPMNs) occur with similar frequency in men and women and usually arise in the head of the pancreas. They appear to be more common in cigarette smokers, patients with familial adenomatous polyposis (FAP) and Peutz-Jegher syndromes, and in patients with familial pancreatic carcinoma. Main-branch IPMNs have a higher malignant potential than side-branch IPMNs. Solid pseudopapillary neoplasms predominantly affect women and occur at a young age (median age of 30–38 years). They contain solid and cystic components and may be difficult to differentiate from cystic pancreatic endocrine neoplasms on fine-needle aspiration (FNA) cytologic analysis. Although most solid pseudopapillary neoplasms are benign, some may exhibit vascular and perineural invasion, and these variants are thought to have moderate to high malignant potential.

Stark A, Donahue TR, Reber HA, et al. Pancreatic cyst disease: a review. *JAMA.* 2016;315(17):1882–1893.

29. ANSWER: B. MUTYH-associated polyposis

MUTYH-associated polyposis (MAP) is an autosomal recessive disorder associated with biallelic mutations of the *MUTYH* gene and is characterized by multiple adenomatous polyps. It is currently the only known autosomal recessive hereditary colon cancer syndrome. MAP may be phenotypically indistinguishable from attenuated familial polyposis syndrome (AFAP) and, in a few cases, classic familial adenomatous polyposis syndrome (FAP).

The other syndromes mentioned are characterized by hamartomatous polyps as detailed below.

Peutz-Jeghers syndrome is an autosomal dominant disorder due to a germline mutation of a serine threonine kinase (STK11 or LKB1) characterized by multiple hamartomatous polyps, predominantly in the small intestine. Patients with Peutz-Jeghers syndrome have distinctive mucocutaneous pigmentation (brown macules) not only on the lips and perioral/buccal mucosa but also on the hands and feet in some cases.

Juvenile polyposis syndrome is an autosomal dominant disorder associated with germline mutations of one of three genes (*BMPR1A, SMAD4,* and *ENG).* Patients with juvenile polyposis syndrome have multiple hamartomatous polyps in the colon and have an increased risk of developing colorectal cancer.

Cowden syndrome is an autosomal dominant disorder associated with a germline mutation of the *PTEN* gene. Patients with Cowden syndrome have multiple gastrointestinal hamartomatous polyps as well as some characteristic dermatologic manifestations, including oral fibromas, cutaneous verrucous papules known as *trichilemmomas,* and punctate palmoplantar keratosis.

Cronkhite-Canada syndrome is a rare nonfamilial disorder of unknown etiology with features including hamartomatous gastrointestinal polyposis. Other features of this syndrome include alopecia, onychodystrophy, cutaneous hyperpigmentation, diarrhea, weight loss, and abdominal pain.

Jasperson K, Burt RW. The genetics of colorectal cancer. *Surg Oncol Clin N Am.* 2015;24(4):683–703.

30. ANSWER: B. Normal total protein (>2.5 g/dL) in ascites

Patients with CHF-associated liver disease generally have preserved hepatic synthetic function and thus higher protein levels (usually >2.5 g/dL) than patients with primary liver disease. In addition, patients with CHF-associated liver disease rarely have evidence of portosystemic shunts such as esophageal varices and lack clinically overt jaundice, though up to 70% may have a mild increase in unconjugated bilirubin. Just as in patients with primary liver disease, patients with CHF-associated liver disease who have ascites have a SAAG >1.1 g/dL as a result of portal hypertension. Hepatojugular reflux is generally present and can be useful in distinguishing hepatic congestion from primary intrahepatic liver disease.

Weisberg IS, Jacobson IM. Cardiovascular diseases and the liver. *Clin Liver Dis.* 2011;15(1):1–20.

31. ANSWER: C. Breastfeeding is not associated with increased risk of transmission.

The mode of delivery (vaginal versus cesarean section), breastfeeding, and viral genotype are not associated with increased risk of vertical transmission of hepatitis C virus (HCV). Vertical transmission of HCV is estimated to be 20% in women coinfected with hepatitis C and HIV, compared with a 4%–7% risk in patients with HCV monoinfection. Vertical transmission occurs almost exclusively among women who have detectable HCV viremia.

Checa Cabot CA, Stoszek SK, Quarleri J, et al. Mother-to-child transmission of hepatitis C virus (HCV) among HIV/HCV-coinfected women. *J Pediatric Infect Dis Soc.* 2013;2(2):126–135.

32. ANSWER: D. Treatment with an H_2 receptor blocker may provide symptomatic relief.

In adults, Ménétrier disease is four times more common in men than in women. Symptoms of postprandial epigastric pain and weight loss are common. Patients may develop anemia due to gastrointestinal occult blood loss. The etiology of the disorder is unknown. Patients often experience relief of epigastric pain with the use of H_2 receptor blockers. In adults, Ménétrier disease typically is associated with *chronic symptoms,* whereas in children, it is usually a self-limited disease. Hypoalbuminemia, peripheral edema, and ascites may occur as a result of protein loss from the hypersecretory gastric mucosa. Esophagogastroduodenoscopy (EGD) will show thickened gastric folds. A full-thickness biopsy of the stomach is usually required for diagnosis.

Lambrecht NW. Ménétrier's disease of the stomach: a clinical challenge. *Curr Gastroenterol Rep.* 2011;13(6):513–517.

33. ANSWER: D. Wilson disease

Wilson disease presents on rare occasions with acute liver failure, which is uniformly fatal without liver transplant. Wilson disease is a rare disorder of copper transport with a prevalence of 1 in 30,000 people. It typically presents in the second to fourth decades of life. Early in the disease, hepatic steatosis may be present, and chronic liver disease is common if it goes unrecognized and untreated. Neurologic symptoms such as tremors and choreic movements, as well as psychiatric problems, hemolytic anemia, and other extrahepatic manifestations, may be present. Undiagnosed Wilson disease sometimes presents with acute liver failure, as in this case.

Nonalcoholic steatohepatitis (NASH) is now increasingly recognized as a major cause of cryptogenic cirrhosis. Associated medical conditions include hypertension, dyslipidemia, obesity, insulin resistance, or frank diabetes. It is not associated with acute liver failure.

Hemochromatosis is the most common inherited disorder among Caucasians of Northern European descent, with a prevalence of 1 in 200 people. Untreated patients may develop cirrhosis, cardiac dysfunction, or diabetes, but acute liver failure has not been reported. Early detection and treatment with phlebotomy may result in a normal lifespan for affected patients.

Alpha-1 antitrypsin deficiency occurs in approximately 1 in 2000 people. Over 75 different protease inhibitor (P_i) alleles have been described. The P_iSZ and P_iZZ phenotypes can be associated with development of cirrhosis, but acute liver failure has not been described.

Glycogenic hepatopathy occurs due to glycogen deposition in the liver in patients with poorly controlled type 1 diabetes mellitus. It causes hepatomegaly, abdominal pain, and elevated liver enzymes, but it does not typically cause acute liver failure.

Rodriguez-Castro KI, Hevia-Urrutia FJ, Sturniolo GC. Wilson's disease: a review of what we have learned. *World J Hepatol.* 2015;7(29):2859–2870.

34. ANSWER: C. Vitamin E

Vitamin E deficiency, if severe, may result in abnormalities affecting the posterior columns, leading to ataxia, loss of proprioception, and areflexia. However, severe vitamin E deficiency occurs infrequently. Vitamin A deficiency may lead to diminished nocturnal visual acuity. Vitamin D deficiency may result in metabolic bone disease. Vitamin K deficiency may result in prolongation of prothrombin time and increased susceptibility to bleeding. Although neurologic symptoms can be associated with vitamin B_{12} deficiency, vitamin B_{12} is not a fat-soluble vitamin.

Pfeiffer RF. Neurologic manifestations of malabsorption syndrome. *Handb Clin Neurol.* 2014;120:621–632.

35. ANSWER: A. Refractory ascites in a patient with right heart failure

TIPS increases right-sided heart pressure due to the creation of a portosystemic shunt and is therefore contraindicated in patients with right heart failure. Acceptable indications for TIPS include management of acute refractory variceal bleeding, hemorrhage from inaccessible gastric or intestinal varices, bleeding from portal hypertensive gastropathy, recurrent severe variceal bleeding after endoscopic therapy, refractory hepatic hydrothorax, Budd-Chiari syndrome, and some other venoocclusive disorders.

Ascha M, Abuqayyas S, Hanouneh I, et al. Predictors of mortality after transjugular portosystemic shunt. *World J Hepatol.* 2016;8(11):520–529.

36. ANSWER: C. Positive anti–Scl-70 antibody

Systemic sclerosis (scleroderma) is characterized by thickened skin and internal organ involvement, including myocardial fibrosis (resulting in cardiomyopathy) and esophageal involvement. Patients often have heartburn and later develop dysphagia due to esophageal hypomotility and GERD, and they frequently develop reflux esophagitis and peptic strictures. Esophageal manometry shows low-amplitude contractions in the distal esophagus and incompetence of the lower esophageal sphincter (LES). The anti–Scl-70 antibody is often positive in systemic sclerosis.

Idiopathic achalasia, pseudoachalasia, and Chagas disease cause an achalasia-like picture, including distal "bird beak" narrowing seen on a barium esophagram. Achalasia does not typically have extraesophageal manifestations, and characteristic manometric findings are poor to absent esophageal peristalsis, incomplete relaxation of the LES, and elevated LES pressure. Older age (especially over age 60), weight loss, and a relatively short onset of symptoms (<6 months) raise concern for pseudoachalasia due to malignancy at the esophagogastric junction. Paraneoplastic manifestations of extraintestinal tumors such as pancreatic, lung, and lymphoma may result in symptoms of dysphagia. Chagas disease is caused by infection with *Trypanosoma cruzi* and occurs most commonly in people of South American or Central American origin. The chronic form of Chagas disease can cause both cardiac and gastrointestinal disease. However, the cardiac disease is typically not ischemic in nature, and the esophageal picture is similar to achalasia, and testing for Chagas disease is initially done with antibodies for *T. cruzi.*

Gyger G, Baron M. Systemic sclerosis: gastrointestinal disease and its management. *Rheum Dis Clin North Am.* 2015; 41(3):459–473.

37. ANSWER: D. Amitriptyline

This patient appears to have functional dyspepsia. In a patient with no improvement after 8 weeks of PPI therapy and no evidence of *H. pylori* disease, treatment with a tricyclic antidepressant should be considered. Low-dose amitriptyline or desipramine 10–25 mg at night is most commonly used. An H_2 blocker is less likely to be helpful if a PPI was ineffective. Promotility agents such as metoclopramide can be considered if there is a concern for gastroparesis, although this patient does not have any clearly predisposing conditions (such as diabetes) or nausea, and a gastric emptying study can be performed for further evaluation. There is currently no evidence to support a low-fat diet or probiotics in the treatment of functional dyspepsia.

Lu Y, Chen M, Huang Z, Tang C. Antidepressants in the treatment of functional dyspepsia: a systematic review and meta-analysis. *PLoS One.* 2016;11(6):e0157798.

38. ANSWER: E. Testing for *H. pylori* infection

The etiology of duodenal ulcers is most commonly related to aspirin, NSAIDs, and H. *pylori.* Even though he has a history of recent NSAID use, he should still be evaluated for *H. pylori* infection as a contributing factor. Patients with uncomplicated duodenal ulcers generally do not need follow-up EGD, owing to the low likelihood of malignancy. If a patient requires aspirin for a cardiac indication, interruption of aspirin therapy my increase the risk of adverse cardiac outcomes. However, if other noncritical medications, such as NSAIDs in this case, can be avoided, this is advisable. Sucralfate can help ulcer healing, but it is not generally recommended in addition to PPIs. Because the recent use of NSAIDs was the likely cause of his bleeding and can be stopped, he most likely does not need to be on lifelong proton pump inhibitor (PPI) therapy.

Satoh K, Yoshino J, Akamatsu T, et al. Evidence-based clinical practice guidelines for peptic ulcer disease 2015. *J Gastroenterol.* 2016;51(3):177–194.

39. ANSWER: A. No treatment at this time

This patient is a chronic carrier of hepatitis B who appears to have a precore mutant strain and low levels of viremia. Antiviral therapy is not indicated for HBeAg-negative patients with normal liver enzymes and hepatitis B viral load <2000 IU/mL, as in this case. This patient appears to have inactive disease and no evidence of chronic liver disease.

All newborns born to mothers who are carriers should receive passive-active immunization consisting of HBIG and hepatitis B vaccination, a strategy that has high protective efficacy (95%). Tenofovir is the drug of choice for pregnant patients requiring antiviral therapy. Pegylated interferon is not recommended during pregnancy. Lamivudine is associated with rapid virologic resistance and is considered a pregnancy class C drug (not recommended during pregnancy). Cesarean delivery does not reduce the risk of vertical transmission of hepatitis B. Mothers should be encouraged to follow up after childbirth to discuss treatment for hepatitis B.

Terrault NA, Bzo Wej NH, Chang KM, et al. AASLD guidelines for the treatment of chronic hepatitis B. *Hepatology.* 2016;63(1):261–283.

40. ANSWER: D. Increase prednisone to 20 mg/day and add azathioprine.

Mild to moderate ulcerative colitis is often initially treated with 5-aminosalicylates (5-ASA) for induction and then maintenance of remission. Short courses of steroids are sometimes needed to induce remission or manage flares, but they are not recommended for maintenance therapy, owing to the side effects. Immunomodulator therapy such as 6-mercaptopurine or azathioprine, or an anti–tumor necrosis factor (TNF) biologic therapy such as infliximab, should be considered for patients whose disease is not effectively controlled with 5-ASA therapy. Switching to another 5-ASA agent at this time is unlikely to improve her symptoms. A slow-release form of budesonide has been approved for ulcerative colitis, but it is used similarly to prednisone in this case to attempt to induce remission and not as a maintenance or steroid-sparing agent. Antibiotics have not been shown to be effective in the treatment of ulcerative colitis.

Chaparro M, Gisbert JP. Maintenance therapy option for ulcerative colitis. *Expert Opin Pharmacother.* 2016;17(10):1339–1349.

41. ANSWER: B. Supportive care

This patient has alcoholic hepatitis based on her history and consistent laboratory findings and should be advised to abstain from alcohol use. Her paracentesis is not suggestive of spontaneous bacterial peritonitis, so she should not receive cefotaxime at this time. Her Maddrey discriminant function is less than 32 based on her total bilirubin and INR, so she should not receive prednisolone or pentoxifylline this time. Alcoholic hepatitis can cause portal hypertension, but this will often reverse with cessation of alcohol. She does not have clear evidence of cirrhosis at this time and has not had an upper endoscopy to evaluate for varices. Nadolol is not routinely started in the acute setting of alcoholic hepatitis.

Singal AK, Kodali S, Vucovich LA, et al. Diagnosis and treatment of alcoholic hepatitis: a systematic review. *Alcohol Clin Exp Res.* 2016;40(7):1390–1402.

42. ANSWER: B. Enteral nutrition with a nasojejunal tube

Acute fluid collections are an early complication of acute pancreatitis. They generally do not require any treatment. The patient has not had any nutrition in 5 days and is not expected to be able to tolerate oral intake in the near future; thus, enteral nutrition with a nasojejunal feeding tube is recommended at this time. Enteral nutrition in acute pancreatitis has been shown to decrease infectious complications and disease severity compared with parenteral nutrition. Antibiotics may be indicated if there is concern for infected pancreatic fluid collections, but this patient does not have a fever or evidence of pancreatic necrosis based on CT imaging. Pancreatic debridement is indicated for management of infected necrosis. Interventional radiology drainage of fluid collections might be beneficial if there is a dominant collection that is causing gastric outlet or intestinal obstruction or if there is concern for a superinfected fluid collection, but neither of these is present at this time.

Lodewijkx PJ, Besselink MG, Witteman BJ, et al. Nutrition in acute pancreatitis: a critical review. *Expert Rev Gastroenterol Hepatol.* 2016;10(5):571–580.

43. ANSWER: A. Prednisone

Autoimmune pancreatitis is characterized by elevated serum IgG4 levels, characteristic imaging (most commonly a diffusely enlarged pancreas, although focal lesions and pancreatic duct strictures can also occur), and diagnostic histology (which often includes a lymphoplasmacytic infiltrate with IgG4-positive cells). IgG4-related disease can also involve the biliary tract and salivary glands and may cause lung nodules, autoimmune thyroiditis, and interstitial nephritis. Initial treatment of pancreatic and extrapancreatic manifestations is typically glucocorticoids (such as prednisone). Alcohol cessation or cholecystectomy would be helpful if she had a history of significant alcohol use or gallstones, respectively. Pancreaticoduodenectomy (Whipple procedure) may be performed if a patient has a pancreatic head lesion such as a mass or stricture that is causing acute pancreatitis. Fibrate therapy can be used to treat patients with hypertriglyceridemia to reduce the risk of recurrent acute pancreatitis.

Madhani K, Farrell JJ. Autoimmune pancreatitis: an update on diagnosis and management. *Gastroenterol Clin North Am.* 2016;45(1):29–43.

44. ANSWER: D. Urinary 5-hydroxyindoleacetic acid

This patient most likely has carcinoid syndrome on the basis of secretory diarrhea, flushing, and evidence of heart failure with right-sided valvular lesions. The most useful initial test for carcinoid syndrome is a 24-hour urine for 5-hydroxyindoleacetic acid (5-HIAA), although it is more useful for midgut carcinoid tumors than for foregut and hindgut tumors. Vasoactive intestinal peptide is elevated in VIPomas, which can also cause secretory diarrhea and flushing but are not associated with right-sided valvular lesions. Calcitonin is elevated in medullary cancer of the thyroid, and gastrin is elevated in gastrinomas, both of which can cause a secretory diarrhea. A fat pad biopsy with Congo red staining is performed to diagnose amyloid, which could cause diarrhea and heart failure with a low-amplitude QRS on an electrocardiogram but would not be expected to cause the tricuspid regurgitation and flushing.

Sarshekeh AM, Halperin DM, Dasari A. Update on management of midgut neuroendocrine tumors. *Int J Endocr Oncol.* 2016;3(2):175–189.

45. **ANSWER: C. Ceftriaxone**

This patient has upper gastrointestinal bleeding concerning for variceal bleeding in light of the history of cirrhosis with evidence of portal hypertension. Octreotide is the preferred pharmacologic treatment in the United States. Vasopressin can also be used in this setting, but it has more side effects and would not be administered concurrently with octreotide. Short-term (maximum 7 days) spontaneous bacterial peritonitis (SBP) antibiotic prophylaxis should be given to any patient with cirrhosis and gastrointestinal hemorrhage, especially those who have ascites. Intravenous ceftriaxone or ciprofloxacin is the preferred initial antibiotic prophylaxis. Penicillin is not recommended for SBP prophylaxis. Intravenous albumin is not generally given in the setting of gastrointestinal or variceal bleeding. *N*-acetylcysteine is used in acute liver failure due to acetaminophen toxicity but not for gastrointestinal or variceal bleeding.

Garcia-Tsao G. Current management of the complications of cirrhosis and portal hypertension: variceal bleeding, ascites and spontaneous bacterial peritonitis. *Dig Dis.* 2016; 34(4)382–386.

46. **ANSWER: C. Wireless capsule endoscopy**

This patient has obscure, occult gastrointestinal bleeding, given the negative upper endoscopy, colonoscopy, and small bowel imaging with CT enterography. A small bowel source, such as angiodysplasia, is the most likely cause. The next test would therefore be a wireless capsule endoscopy. CT angiography and a tagged red blood cell scan are not sensitive for detection of occult gastrointestinal bleeding. Double-balloon and push enteroscopy are generally performed for further diagnosis and treatment of a small bowel bleeding source identified on capsule endoscopy or another study.

Tanabe S. Diagnosis of obscure gastrointestinal bleeding. *Clin Endosc.* 2016;49(6):539–541.

47. **ANSWER: D. Small intestinal bacterial overgrowth**

Small intestinal bacterial overgrowth (SIBO) typically causes loose stools and bloating and can also result in vitamin B_{12} deficiency (bacteria consume vitamin B_{12}) and elevated serum folate (bacteria synthesize folate). Chronic pancreatitis and diabetes can predispose to SIBO due to stasis. Steatorrhea due to exocrine pancreatic insufficiency is possible but typically improves with increased enzyme supplementation and is not associated with increased folate levels. Crohn disease can result in similar symptoms, but colonoscopy to the terminal ileum and abdominal imaging are not suggestive of this. Celiac disease is more common in patients with diabetes, but the normal tissue transglutaminase IgA antibody (and serum IgA level), as well as the normal duodenal biopsies, makes this diagnosis highly unlikely. Irritable bowel syndrome would not explain the vitamin B_{12} deficiency, anemia, and nocturnal stools.

Quigley EM. Small intestinal bacterial overgrowth: what it is and what it is not. *Curr Opin Gastroenterol.* 2014;30(2): 141–146.

48. **ANSWER: B. Low-oxalate diet and continue the calcium supplementation**

Patients with small intestinal Crohn disease, especially those with small bowel resections, are predisposed to nephrolithiasis, particularly calcium oxalate stones. As a result of bile salt malabsorption, fat binds to calcium in the intestines, leaving oxalate free to be absorbed and deposited in the kidney, where it can form into stones. Spinach is a high–oxalate-containing food, and eating large amounts of this may have contributed to stone formation. In addition to maintaining adequate hydration, the treatment for calcium oxalate stones is generally to eat a low-oxalate diet and ensure adequate calcium intake. Calcium intake should not be reduced (unless it is excessive), because a decrease in free calcium in the intestines can lead to increased absorption of oxalate due to decreased binding of oxalate by calcium. Potassium citrate is sometimes used to treat calcium stones that are thought to form due to hypocitraturia, which is not thought to be a common mechanism for nephrolithiasis formation in Crohn disease.

Worcester EM. Stones from bowel disease. *Endocrinol Metab Clin North Am.* 2002;31(4):979–999.

49. **ANSWER: E. Endoscopic retrograde cholangiopancreatography**

This patient has acute pancreatitis most likely due to gallstones on the basis of elevated liver enzymes as well as the gallstones and dilated common bile duct seen on the ultrasound. The ultrasound did not identify gallstones in the common bile duct, but it has relatively poor sensitivity for detecting choledocholithiasis. The persistent pain, elevated bilirubin, and fever suggest that this patient has cholangitis and persistent biliary obstruction. The most appropriate treatment is endoscopic retrograde cholangiopancreatography (ERCP), which will provide both diagnostic and therapeutic benefit. ERCP should be performed within 24 hours of admission for patients with gallstone pancreatitis and cholangitis.

Abdominal CT scan and magnetic resonance cholangiopancreatography (MRCP) would show acute pancreatitis (but may still be too early to show pancreatic necrosis) and may detect choledocholithiasis but offer no therapy. An elective cholecystectomy should be considered in this patient who has a history of gallstone-induced complications. Ursodiol can dissolve small gallbladder stones, but it is not a suitable therapeutic option for treating choledocholithiasis.

da Costa DW, Schepers NJ, Römkens TE, et al. Endoscopic sphincterotomy and cholecystectomy in acute biliary pancreatitis. *Surgeon.* 2016;14(2):99–108.

50. ANSWER: C. Constipation-predominant irritable bowel syndrome

This patient meets the Rome IV criteria for irritable bowel syndrome (IBS), which are recurrent abdominal pain, on average, at least 1 day per week in the last 3 months and associated with two or more of the following: (1) defecation, (2) change in stool frequency, and/or (3) change in stool form. Symptom onset should be at least 6 months prior to the diagnosis of IBS. Alarm features such as weight loss and rectal bleeding are not typical of IBS. This patient likely has constipation-predominant IBS. Colonic inertia (or slow-transit constipation) and dyssynergic defecation (or pelvic floor dysfunction) are not typically associated with the abdominal pain symptoms and are typically associated with retention of radiopaque markers in the right side of the colon and rectum, respectively. Anorectal manometry can be performed to further differentiate between these two entities. Multiple sclerosis can cause chronic constipation, but this patient does not appear to have any other symptoms of this. Chronic intestinal pseudoobstruction typically causes obstructive symptoms (nausea, vomiting) and is associated with underlying neuropathic or myopathic diseases, which she does not appear to have.

Siah KT, Wong RK, Whitehead WE. Chronic constipation and constipation-predominant IBS: separate and distinct disorders or a spectrum of disease? *Gastroenterol Hepatol (N Y).* 2016;12(3):171–178.

8 Cardiovascular Disease

ANJU NOHRIA

1. A 32-year-old woman presents for evaluation of palpitations. She notes the intermittent sensation of her heart "flip-flopping" in her chest for the past month. Review of systems is notable for fatigue and subjectively decreased energy. On physical examination, she is well appearing. Her jugular venous pressure is 5 cm H_2O. She has a parasternal lift and a grade 2 of 6 midpeaking systolic murmur at the left upper sternal border. The second heart sound is widely split without respiratory variation, and the pulmonic component of the second heart sound is prominent. The extremities are warm without edema. An electrocardiogram demonstrates a rightward axis, narrow QRS complex, and incomplete right bundle branch block.

   What is the most likely diagnosis?
   A. Wolff-Parkinson-White syndrome
   B. Arrhythmogenic right ventricular cardiomyopathy
   C. Atrial septal defect
   D. Mitral stenosis
   E. Hyperthyroidism

2. A 42-year-old corporate executive presents to the emergency department with 2 hours of unrelenting chest pain. He has a salient medical history of tobacco use and dyslipidemia. The pain is severe and exacerbated by movement. On physical examination, the patient appears uncomfortable. The cardiopulmonary examination is normal. A bedside echocardiogram reveals normal left ventricular function, a trace pericardial effusion, and no wall motion abnormality. An electrocardiogram is shown in Fig. 8.1.

   What is the most appropriate next step in management?
   A. Aspirin and thrombolysis
   B. Aspirin, heparin, and clopidogrel
   C. Prednisone
   D. Ibuprofen
   E. Ativan and nitroglycerin

3. A 52-year-old man with hypertension, dyslipidemia, and a smoking history presents with 6 hours of severe,

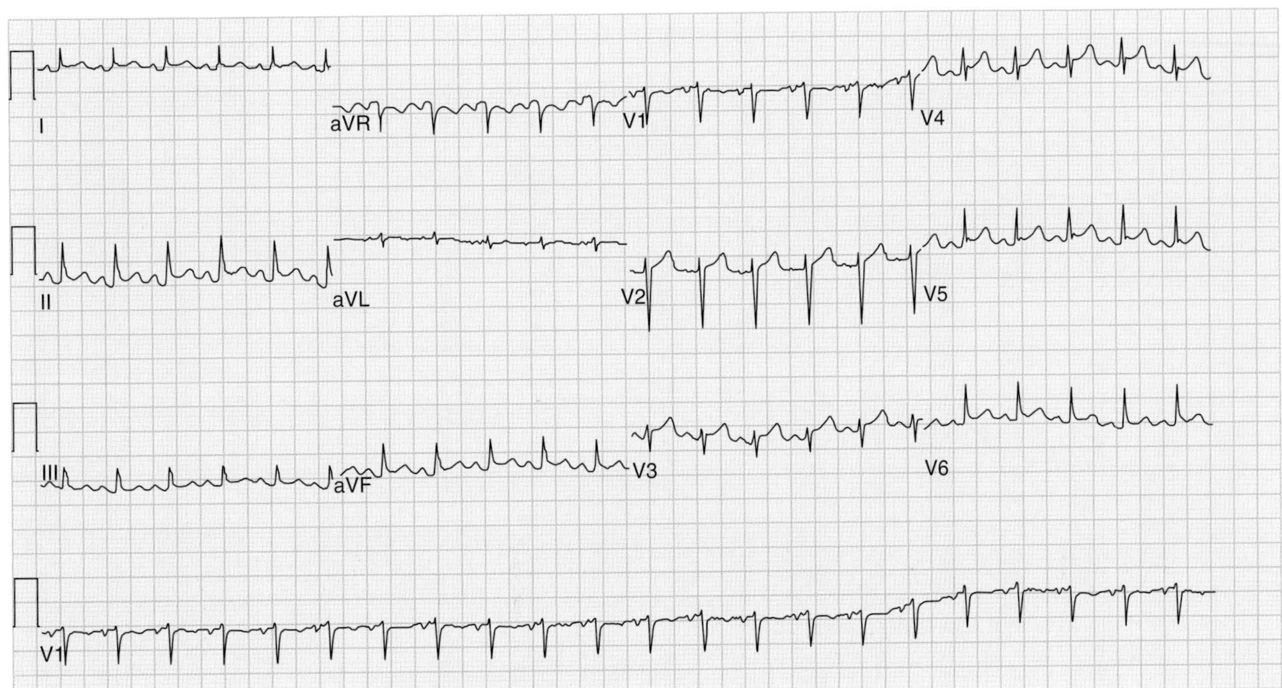

• **Fig. 8.1** Electrocardiogram for patient in Question 2.

unrelenting chest burning. On examination, his blood pressure is 88/66 mm Hg. His jugular venous pressure is 14 cm H_2O and increases with inspiration. His lungs are clear. Cardiac auscultation reveals normal first and second heart sounds without murmur. An electrocardiogram is shown in Fig. 8.2.

In addition to administering aspirin and activating the cardiac catheterization laboratory, the most appropriate management is:

A. Infusion of normal saline
B. Nitroglycerin infusion
C. Furosemide bolus
D. Phenylephrine
E. Esmolol infusion

4. A 36-year-old woman who is 22 weeks pregnant presents with dyspnea and palpitations. Her dyspnea began at 16 weeks of pregnancy but has progressed to the point where she is dyspneic at rest. She sleeps upright in a chair. On examination, her heart rate is 108 beats per minute with an irregularly irregular rhythm. Her blood pressure is 90/64 mm Hg. The first heart sound is louder than the second heart sound at the base. There is a high-pitched, snapping, discrete, early diastolic sound that follows the second heart sound. There is a diastolic rumbling murmur heard over the apex with the patient positioned in the left lateral decubitus position. Pulmonary auscultation reveals bibasilar wet rales. The patient's jugular venous pressure is 16 cm H_2O.

What is the most likely diagnosis?

A. Pregnancy-induced cardiomyopathy
B. Pulmonary embolism
C. Dyspnea secondary to normal progression of pregnancy
D. Thyroid storm
E. Mitral stenosis

5. A 64-year-old woman presents with increasing dyspnea and fatigue. She has a medical history notable for small cell lung cancer metastatic to the liver and bone and is currently undergoing chemotherapy. Her symptoms have been progressive over the past week; initially, she was dyspneic climbing stairs, and now she is dyspneic walking across the room. On examination, her heart rate is 128 beats per minute with a regular rhythm. The intensity and amplitude of the radial pulse are variable with respiration. The patient's blood pressure is 88/62 mm Hg. Her jugular venous pressure is 15 cm H_2O. Her heart sounds are quiet without murmur or gallop. Her lungs are clear. Her strength is 5 of 5 in both upper and lower extremities, and an electrocardiogram reveals sinus tachycardia with low voltage in the limb leads and precordial leads. A chest radiograph reveals a mass in the left upper lobe, which is increased in size compared with 2 weeks prior.

What is the most appropriate next diagnostic test?

A. Electromyography
B. Echocardiography
C. CT pulmonary angiography
D. Blood cultures
E. Whole-body FDG-PET/CT scan

6. A 67-year-old man presents for preoperative evaluation. He has a history of progressive osteoarthritis of the right knee, which has been refractory to medical treatment, and total knee replacement is planned. The remainder of the patient's medical

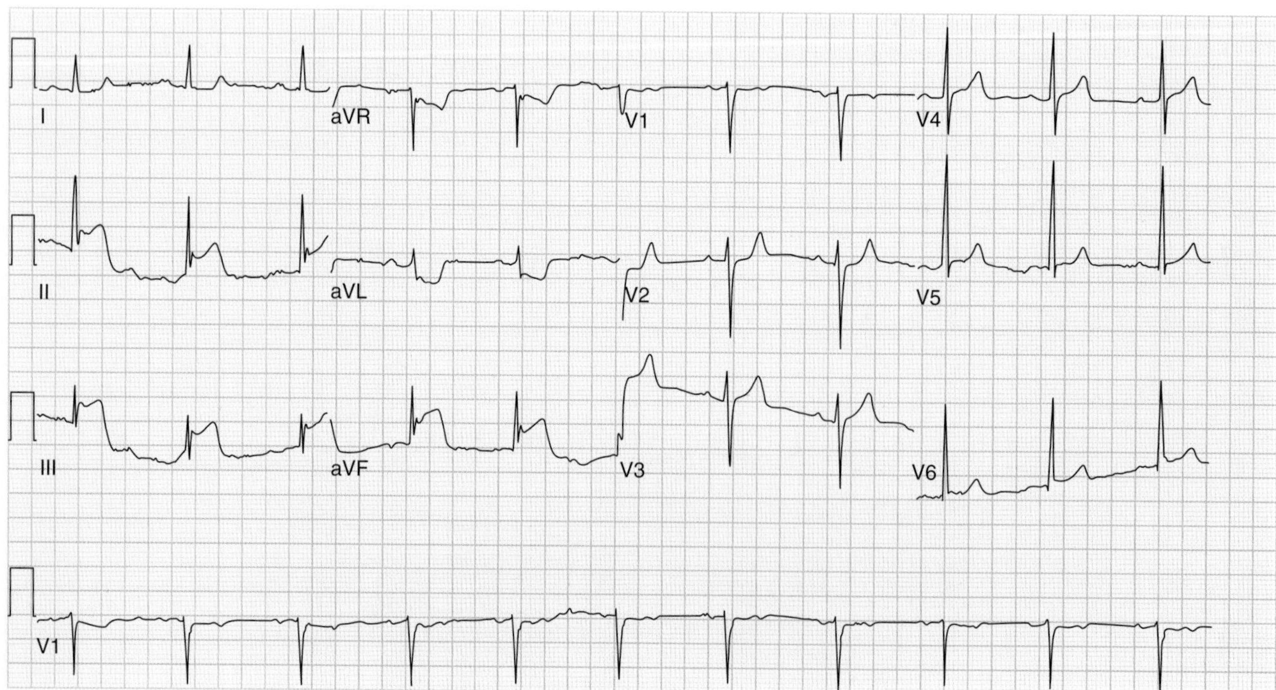

• **Fig. 8.2** Electrocardiogram for patient in Question 3.

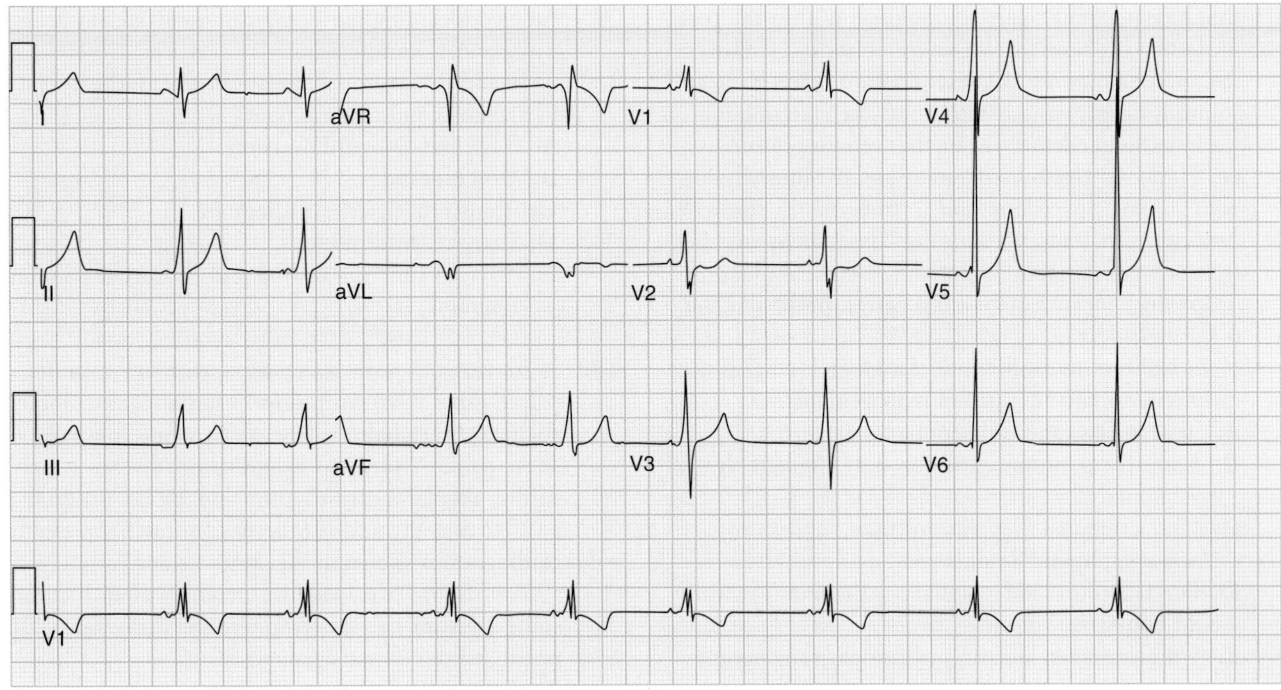

• **Fig. 8.3** Electrocardiogram for patient in Question 7.

history includes type 2 diabetes, for which he is maintained on insulin therapy; diabetic nephropathy with baseline creatinine of 2.5 mg/dL; hypertension; dyslipidemia; and ST segment elevation myocardial infarction 10 years prior, which had been treated successfully with thrombolytics. Knee pain limits his ability to ambulate, and he walks with a limp. He has no angina or symptoms of heart failure. His medications include aspirin, metoprolol, simvastatin, NPH insulin, glyburide, and lisinopril. A physical examination includes a heart rate of 88 beats per minute and blood pressure of 126/86 mm Hg and is otherwise normal.

What is the most appropriate recommendation?

A. Pharmacologic stress test prior to total knee replacement
B. Increase dosage of metoprolol for a goal heart rate of 55–65 beats per minute, then proceed with total knee replacement.
C. Echocardiogram prior to total knee replacement
D. Recommend against total knee replacement due to medical comorbidities.
E. Coronary angiography prior to total knee replacement

7. A 22-year-old collegiate cross-country runner presents with palpitations. Four times over the past month, he has noted the abrupt onset of a racing heartbeat and a sensation of pounding in the neck. Three of the episodes terminated after 1 minute, but the most recent episode lasted for 15 minutes before terminating. A physical examination reveals a thin, tall young man who is not distressed. The palate is slightly high arched. The arm span is normal. The first and second heart sounds are normal; there is a grade 1 of 6 systolic murmur at the left upper sternal border that diminishes with handgrip. The remainder of the examination is normal. The electrocardiogram is shown in Fig. 8.3.

What is the best next step?

A. Electrophysiologic study and mapping
B. Signal-averaged electrocardiogram
C. Exercise stress test
D. Holter monitor
E. CT coronary angiogram

8. A 52-year-old woman is referred to you by her dentist. She presented with multiple dental caries and is in need of several fillings. Her medical history is notable for hypertension and mitral valve prolapse. Other than tooth pain, she feels well. On examination, there is a midsystolic click and late systolic murmur heard over the apex.

What is the most appropriate next step?

A. Clindamycin
B. Amoxicillin
C. Repeat echocardiogram
D. Proceed with planned dental procedure.
E. Blood cultures

9. A 68-year-old man presents for evaluation of chest pain. He has a history of hypertension, diabetes, dyslipidemia, and cigarette smoking. Within the past 24 hours, he has had two severe episodes of substernal chest pain at rest. On examination, a fourth heart sound is noted without murmurs. The extremities are warm without edema. The jugular venous pressure is 5 cm H_2O. An electrocardiogram reveals sinus rhythm with T-wave inversions and 1 mm of ST segment depression in leads V5 and V6. The patient is pain-free and comfortable at the time of the evaluation. Troponin T measurement is 0.3 ng/mL (normal range, 0–0.1 ng/mL).

In addition to aspirin and clopidogrel, what is the most appropriate next step in management?

A. Tenecteplase and unfractionated heparin
B. Enoxaparin, nitrates, and coronary angiography in 72 hours
C. Unfractionated heparin, nitrates, and coronary angiography in 72 hours
D. Fondaparinux and coronary angiography within 24 hours
E. Unfractionated heparin and coronary angiography within 24 hours

10. A 67-year-old man with a history of cigarette smoking presents with accelerating anginal chest pain. On initial evaluation, his troponin T is elevated to 2.0 (0–0.1), and an electrocardiogram demonstrates T-wave inversions in leads I and aVL. He is referred for coronary angiography, whereupon a 60% stenosis in the middle right coronary artery and an 80% stenosis in a small first diagonal branch of the left anterior descending artery are demonstrated. Medical management in lieu of revascularization is advised. In addition to aspirin, beta blocker, statin therapy, and smoking cessation, you prescribe:

A. Fish oil
B. Ranolazine
C. Isosorbide mononitrate
D. Clopidogrel
E. Warfarin

11. A 63-year-old long-term patient of yours presents with worsening breathlessness and palpitations. He has a known history of mitral valve prolapse diagnosed years prior on the basis of auscultatory findings of a click–murmur complex and confirmed by echocardiogram. For the past 2 weeks, he describes progressive breathlessness, orthopnea, and palpitations. On examination, he appears uncomfortable and is dyspneic with conversation. His heart rate is approximately 100 beats per minute and irregular. His jugular venous pressure is 16 cm H_2O. He has a grade 4 of 6 pansystolic murmur with a thrill appreciated over the apex. The murmur is blowing in quality and is heard throughout the precordium with particular radiation toward the base of the heart. The apex beat is hyperdynamic. An electrocardiogram demonstrates atrial flutter with variable A-V conduction.

In addition to anticoagulation, what is the next step in diagnosis and management?

A. TEE and DC cardioversion
B. Beta blockade
C. Transthoracic echocardiogram
D. Exercise treadmill test
E. Thyroid function testing and nocturnal polysomnogram

12. A 32-year-old woman presents with 35 minutes of palpitations. Her symptoms began abruptly. She has slight lightheadedness but no syncope, dyspnea, or chest pain. A physical examination reveals a tachycardic, regular heart rhythm and blood pressure of 132/82 mm Hg and is otherwise normal. An electrocardiogram is shown in Fig. 8.4.

Performing the Valsalva maneuver and carotid sinus pressure fails to terminate the arrhythmia. The next best step in management is:

A. DC cardioversion
B. Adenosine
C. Amiodarone
D. Labetalol
E. Normal saline

13. A 45-year-old man with a heavy smoking history presents by ambulance with 3 hours of crushing substernal chest pain. On examination, he appears uncomfortable. His jugular venous pressure is 10 cm H_2O. The first and second heart sounds are normal. He has scant bibasilar rales. An electrocardiogram of the patient is shown in Fig. 8.5. A cardiac catheterization laboratory is 2.5 hours away, accounting for transfer time.

In addition to aspirin, clopidogrel, morphine, oxygen, and nitrate therapy, what is the most appropriate next step in management?

A. Transfer for primary percutaneous coronary angiography (PCI).
B. Administer tenecteplase and transfer to a PCI-capable facility.
C. Prescribe colchicine and aspirin.
D. Administer half-dose thrombolytics and transfer to a PCI-capable facility.
E. Administer intravenous metoprolol boluses for goal heart rate of 55 beats per minute.

14. A 48-year-old Caucasian woman presents for follow-up after a recent hospitalization for heart failure. She has a salient history of nonischemic cardiomyopathy with an ejection fraction of 25%. She presented with volume overload and dyspnea, which responded well to diuresis. Since discharge, however, she has remained dyspneic even climbing less than one flight

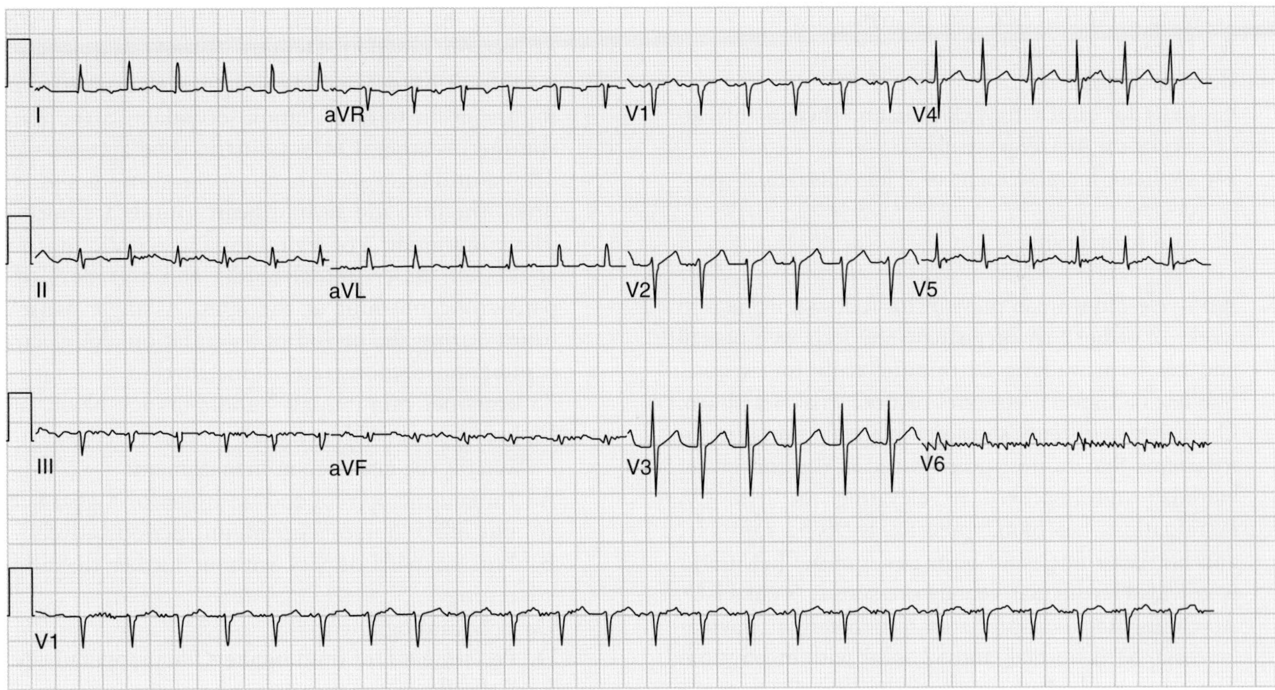

• **Fig. 8.4** Electrocardiogram for patient in Question 12.

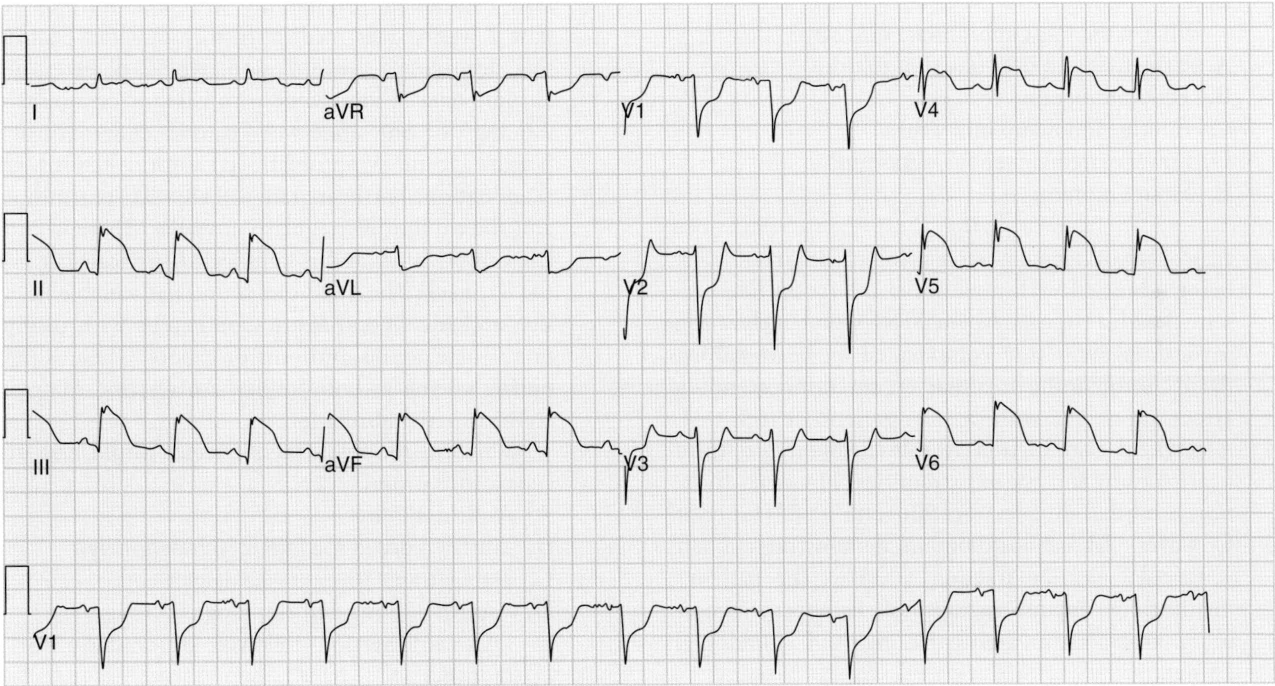

• **Fig. 8.5** Electrocardiogram for patient in Question 13.

of stairs. Her medications include lisinopril 40 mg daily, carvedilol 25 mg twice daily, spironolactone 25 mg daily, furosemide 40 mg twice daily, and potassium supplementation. On examination, she appears fatigued. Her heart rate is 68 beats per minute, and her blood pressure is 100/60 mm Hg. Her jugular venous pressure is 6 cm H_2O. The first and second heart sounds are normal, and a third heart sound is appreciated. She has scant bilateral pitting edema of the lower extremities. Her lungs are clear.

An electrocardiogram demonstrates left bundle branch block with QRS duration of 155 ms. Her serum creatinine level is 1.4 mg/dL, which is the baseline level.

What is the best next step in management?
A. Increase furosemide dose.
B. Add metolazone.
C. Refer for cardiac resynchronization therapy (biventricular pacemaker placement).
D. Evaluate for placement of a left ventricular assist device.
E. Add hydralazine.

15. A 34-year-old woman presents for follow-up. She is in week 32 of her first pregnancy. She feels well overall and has been walking 20 minutes daily for exercise. She has had several episodes of nocturnal heartburn. On review of systems, she notes bilateral lower extremity edema that is most pronounced at the end of her workday and improved by elevating the legs. On examination, her blood pressure is 96/52 mm Hg, and her heart rate is 88 beats per minute; her uterus is gravid. Her jugular venous pressure is 5 cm H_2O. A venous hum is appreciated over the right clavicular fossa. S1 is normal, and S2 splits with inspiration. There is a grade 2 of 6 midpeaking systolic murmur at the left upper sternal border. A third heart sound is appreciated. There is 1+ bilateral pitting edema at the ankle.
What is the most appropriate next step?
A. Urinalysis and liver function testing
B. Echocardiogram
C. Routine follow-up in 2 weeks
D. Lower extremity venous ultrasound
E. Holter monitor

16. A 48-year-old man is seen prior to discharge after being admitted with myocardial infarction. He presented with a large anterolateral ST segment elevation myocardial infarction complicated by heart failure. An occlusion of the proximal left anterior descending artery was treated with PCI. At present, he feels well. A physical examination reveals euvolemia, a third heart sound, and warm extremities. His renal function is normal. An electrocardiogram reveals anterior Q waves. An echocardiogram demonstrates a left ventricular ejection fraction of 35%. The patient's medications include metoprolol, lisinopril, furosemide, atorvastatin, aspirin 81 mg, and clopidogrel 75 mg.
What is the most optimal next step in management?
A. Increase aspirin from 81 to 325 mg daily.
B. Increase clopidogrel to 150 mg twice daily.
C. Ranolazine
D. Eplerenone
E. Metolazone

17. An 82-year-old man is referred for preoperative risk stratification prior to planned total hip replacement for severely painful, limiting osteoarthritis. His past medical history includes hypertension. A review of systems reveals he had an episode of syncope 3 months prior for which he did not seek care, attributing the event to dehydration secondary to the warm summer weather. On examination, he appears well. The carotid upstrokes are normal in contour and volume. The first and second heart sounds are normal. There is a grade 2 of 6 midpeaking systolic murmur at the left upper sternal border and a grade 1 of 6 pansystolic murmur at the apex. A single pause is heard during the period of auscultation. An electrocardiogram demonstrates sinus rhythm at a rate of 75 beats per minute, left bundle branch block, and Mobitz type II AV block.
What is the next step in management?
A. Initiate metoprolol and uptitrate for a goal heart rate of 55–65 beats per minute perioperatively.
B. Proceed with surgery without further diagnostic testing.
C. Echocardiogram
D. Prescribe 4 L of fluid intake daily preoperatively.
E. Refer for pacemaker placement prior to surgery.

18. A 76-year-old woman seeks care for palpitations. She notes sustained palpitations with exertion for the past 2 weeks. Her medical history includes obstructive sleep apnea, hypertension, type 2 diabetes, and chronic renal insufficiency with baseline creatinine of 2.6 mg/dL. She underwent carotid endarterectomy 8 years ago for symptomatic left carotid stenosis. On examination, her heart rate is 118 beats per minute, and the rhythm is irregularly irregular. There is a soft left carotid bruit and a well-healed surgical scar over the left neck. The first heart sound has variable intensity, and the second heart sound splits with inspiration. There are no murmurs or gallops. There is trace pitting edema at both ankles. An electrocardiogram confirms atrial fibrillation.
Which of the following strategies would best prevent future stroke?
A. Aspirin 325 mg
B. Warfarin dosed for INR 2–3 indefinitely
C. Dabigatran 150 mg twice daily
D. Aspirin 325 mg and clopidogrel 75 mg
E. DC cardioversion followed by warfarin for 1 month

19. A 35-year-old woman presents with 2 days of severe chest pain. She had an upper respiratory infection 1 week ago. Pain is worsened with deep inspiration and relieved by leaning forward. Review of systems is notable for cough. On examination, she appears uncomfortable. Her jugular venous pressure is less than 5 cm H_2O. There is a tricomponent friction rub heard at the left lower sternal border. An electrocardiogram reveals diffuse ST segment elevation, which is concave upward in morphology. An echocardiogram reveals a trace pericardial effusion and normal left ventricular function without wall motion abnormalities.

What is the most optimal management?

A. Aspirin and prednisone
B. Prednisone
C. Prednisone and ibuprofen
D. Aspirin
E. Ibuprofen and colchicine

20. A 16-year-old boy is evaluated for a preparticipation sports physical examination for swimming. He feels well. His family history is negative for sudden cardiac death; an uncle has aortic stenosis. On examination, he is tall and thin. The first heart sound is normal. There is an early systolic click and a grade 2 of 6 mid-peaking systolic murmur. There is a grade 1 of 6 diastolic murmur at the left upper sternal border. There is a harsh systolic bruit heard best over the posterior chest. There is slight radiofemoral pulse delay. The boy's blood pressure is 128/82 mm Hg in the right arm. An echocardiogram reveals a bicuspid aortic valve with no stenosis and mild regurgitation, normal aortic root diameter, normal left ventricular chamber size, and normal left ventricular function.

What is the next best step?

A. Refer for aortic valve replacement.
B. Proceed with sports participation with serial echocardiographic monitoring.
C. Aspirin 81 mg
D. Magnetic resonance angiography of the thoracic and abdominal aorta
E. Losartan

21. A 62-year-old man with diabetes and tobacco use presents with 6 hours of stuttering substernal chest pressure. On initial evaluation, there are ST segment depressions in leads V5 and V6 of the electrocardiogram with a troponin T of 1.0 (0–0.1) ng/mL. He is referred for coronary angiography, and a 95% stenosis of the first obtuse marginal coronary artery is treated with percutaneous coronary intervention. After the procedure, he feels well, and his chest pain has abated. He is prescribed metoprolol 25 mg, fluvastatin 10 mg daily, aspirin 81 mg daily, and prasugrel 10 mg.

Which of the following would you recommend?

A. Change prasugrel to clopidogrel.
B. Change fluvastatin to high-dose atorvastatin.
C. Increase aspirin 81 mg to 325 mg.
D. Add ranolazine.
E. Add isosorbide mononitrate.

22. A 64-year-old man is seen in consultation for preoperative risk assessment prior to cholecystectomy for biliary colic. He has a salient medical history of coronary artery disease presenting with non-ST-elevation myocardial infarction (NSTEMI) 3 years prior. At the time, he was treated with placement of a drug-eluting stent to a 90% stenosis of the right coronary artery. Since then, he has felt well without angina, dyspnea, or syncope. He plays singles tennis twice per week in a competitive league. His medications include metoprolol, aspirin, clopidogrel, and atorvastatin. The result of his physical examination is normal.

What is the next step in management?

A. Proceed with surgery, maintaining the current medication regimen.
B. Discontinue clopidogrel and proceed with surgery, continuing aspirin through the perioperative period.
C. Discontinue aspirin and clopidogrel prior to proceeding with surgery.
D. Discontinue clopidogrel and atorvastatin prior to proceeding with surgery.
E. Perform an exercise treadmill test prior to issuing a recommendation regarding the proposed surgery.

23. A 72-year-old man with a history of peripheral arterial disease requiring femoral-popliteal bypass and with a long-standing smoking history presents with substernal chest pain. Pain is evoked by walking four blocks briskly and abates readily with several minutes of rest. He has never had pain with activities of self-care or at rest. A coronary angiogram reveals a 60% stenosis in the middle right coronary artery (fractional flow reserve [FFR] = 0.92), a 70% stenosis in a small first diagonal branch of the left anterior descending artery, and a 40% stenosis in the middle left circumflex artery. Left ventriculography reveals normal left ventricular function. The patient's medications include metoprolol, aspirin, and atorvastatin. On examination, his heart rate is 60 beats per minute at rest, increasing to 80 with ambulation. His blood pressure is 132/82 mm Hg. The results of his cardiac and pulmonary examinations are normal.

What is the next step in management?

A. A PCI with stent placement of the first diagonal branch
B. Increase dosage of metoprolol.
C. Prescribe isosorbide mononitrate.
D. Prescribe ranolazine.
E. Prescribe clopidogrel.

24. A 42-year-old man with known cardiomyopathy presents for follow-up. His family history is notable for dilated cardiomyopathy in his father and one brother. A paternal uncle died suddenly at a young age of unknown cause. He presented 1 year prior with dyspnea on exertion; a transthoracic echocardiogram revealed a dilated left ventricle with an ejection fraction of 25%. The result of coronary angiography was normal, and no other reversible cause of cardiomyopathy was discovered.

Since then, he has been maintained on furosemide, lisinopril, carvedilol, spironolactone, and a multivitamin. He has one hospitalization for volume overload attributed to dietary indiscretion. He feels winded shoveling snow and working out on his exercise bicycle but otherwise has no current symptoms of heart failure. On examination, his blood pressure is 110/60 mm Hg, and his heart rate is 70 beats per minute. His jugular venous pressure is 5 cm H_2O. The first and second heart sounds are normal, and a third heart sound is noted. An electrocardiogram reveals sinus rhythm with a single premature ventricular beat. The QRS duration is 100 ms.

What is the best next step in management?

A. Refer for cardiac resynchronization therapy (CRT).
B. Add digoxin.
C. Refer for implantable cardioverter-defibrillator.
D. Add metolazone.
E. Refer for cardiac transplant evaluation.

25. A 48-year-old man presents with dyspnea and dizziness. He notes several months of progressive dyspnea, which has limited his ability to perform yard work. In addition, he notes pronounced dizziness and presyncope when moving from squatting to a standing position as he weeds his garden. His past medical history includes hypertension. His medications include amlodipine. On examination, he appears well. His jugular venous pressure is 8 cm H_2O. The first heart sound is normal, and the second heart sound splits with inspiration. A fourth heart sound is present. There is a grade 1 of 6 pansystolic murmur at the apex radiating to the back. There is a grade 2 of 6 harsh, late-peaking, diamond-shaped systolic murmur at the base with radiation to the clavicles and carotid arteries.

The murmur increases in intensity with the Valsalva maneuver and with squat-to-stand maneuvers. The patient's lungs are clear. His extremities are warm and well perfused.

What is the most likely diagnosis?

A. Dilated cardiomyopathy
B. Mitral stenosis
C. Aortic stenosis
D. Hypertrophic obstructive cardiomyopathy
E. Atrial septal defect

26. A 32-year-old woman presents with fever. She has a salient medical history of intravenous drug abuse. On examination, her temperature is 102°F. She has a grade 2 of 6 diastolic blowing murmur at the base. There are splinter hemorrhages in the nails. Blood cultures grow methicillin-sensitive *Staphylococcus aureus* (MSSA). An electrocardiogram reveals normal sinus rhythm. A transthoracic echocardiogram reveals moderate aortic regurgitation and an 8-mm vegetation on the aortic valve. She is hospitalized for evaluation and treatment and is initiated on nafcillin. On hospital day 3, her fevers persist. An electrocardiogram demonstrates a prolonged PR interval with periods of Mobitz II AV block.

What is the next step in diagnosis?

A. Electrophysiologic testing
B. Brain MRI
C. Transesophageal echocardiogram
D. Request blood cultures to be incubated for 14 days.
E. Serologies for *Coxiella burnetii*

27. A 65-year-old woman presents with chest and arm pain. Her pain is substernal with radiation to the right arm and is evoked by exertion but not predictably relieved with rest. She has a history of severe lumbar disc disease and osteoarthritis of the knee, which limit her functional capacity. In addition, she has hypertension and depression. A physical examination reveals a well-appearing, slightly overweight woman. The first and second heart sounds are normal, and the lungs are clear. An electrocardiogram demonstrates a left bundle branch block, which was noted on prior electrocardiograms obtained before treatment with antidepressant therapy.

What is the best next diagnostic step?

A. Exercise treadmill test
B. Exercise stress echocardiogram
C. Dobutamine stress echocardiogram
D. Nuclear stress test with regadenoson
E. Reassurance

28. A 76-year-old man with a significant smoking history presents with leg pain. He notes left-sided leg heaviness that occurs when he walks more than three blocks and resolves predictably with several minutes of rest, after which he can resume walking. He has no chest pain or dyspnea. On physical examination, there is a left femoral bruit and diminished left dorsalis pedis and posterior tibial pulses. The patient's ankle brachial index is 0.72 on the left and 0.9 on the right.

In addition to treating hypertension and dyslipidemia to target and prescribing aspirin, what is the best next step?

A. Supervised exercise program
B. Pentoxifylline
C. Lower extremity angiography and stenting
D. Peripheral arterial bypass surgery
E. Amlodipine

29. A 60-year-old woman with a bicuspid aortic valve and known aortic regurgitation presents for follow-up. She feels like she is slightly more limited in her activities of daily living than she was 1 year ago; she feels dyspneic playing with her 2-year-old grandchild. She has no chest pain, lower extremity edema, or paroxysmal nocturnal dyspnea. On examination, her blood pressure is 100/40 mm Hg, and her heart rate is 70 beats per minute. The carotid impulses are brisk with a rapid rise. The first heart sound is normal, and the second heart sound splits with inspiration. There is an early systolic click and a grade 2 of 6 midpeaking systolic murmur. There is a grade 2 of 4 early diastolic murmur with a blowing quality. The apex beat is laterally displaced. An echocardiogram demonstrates a left ventricular ejection fraction of 70%. The left ventricle is dilated with an end-diastolic diameter of 69 mm. The aortic valve is bicuspid with a wide jet of aortic insufficiency, which is graded as severe. There is systolic flow reversal noted in the descending thoracic aorta. The aortic root diameter is 30 mm.

What is the next step in management?

A. Prescribe losartan.
B. Aortic valve replacement
C. Echocardiogram in 6 months
D. Exercise treadmill testing
E. Carotid ultrasound

30. A 58-year-old man is seen in follow-up for management of hypertension. He has been maintained on pharmacotherapy for 8 months with persistently poor blood pressure control. He feels well and is asymptomatic. His past medical history includes osteoarthritis, for which he takes over-the-counter analgesics. His medications otherwise include amlodipine, hydrochlorothiazide, and lisinopril. On examination, he is an anxious-appearing, middle-aged man who is not distressed. His body mass index is 28 kg/m^2. His blood pressure in the right arm is 172/102 mm Hg. A fourth heart sound is appreciated. There are no murmurs and no peripheral bruits. There is no lower extremity edema.

What is the best next step in evaluation?

A. Twenty-four-hour urine free cortisol, serum renin, and aldosterone levels; thyroid function testing; and serum metanephrines
B. CT angiography of the renal and mesenteric arteries
C. Captopril renal scan
D. Obtain detailed over-the-counter medication use history.
E. Twenty-four-hour Holter monitor

31. A 66-year-old woman presents with arm pain and abdominal bloating that is evoked by climbing two flights of stairs. Her past medical history includes diabetes and hypertension. Her medications include simvastatin, aspirin, and losartan. She is referred for an exercise treadmill test, which demonstrates diffuse ST segment depressions of 2–3 mm at 70% of maximum predicted heart rate.

Coronary angiography demonstrates a 90% stenosis of the proximal right coronary artery, a 40% stenosis of a first obtuse marginal branch of the left circumflex artery, and an 80% stenosis of the proximal left anterior descending artery. A left ventriculogram demonstrates normal left ventricular function.

What is the optimal approach to management?

A. Add metoprolol and isosorbide mononitrate.
B. PCI with stent placement of the LAD artery
C. PCI with stent placement of the RCA and LAD artery
D. Refer for coronary artery bypass grafting of the LAD artery and RCA.
E. Myocardial viability study

32. A 77-year-old man with hypertension and a 60-pack-year smoking history presents for evaluation and routine follow-up. He feels well. His medications include lisinopril, aspirin, amlodipine, and atorvastatin. On examination, there is a soft bruit over the epigastrium, and the aortic pulsation is prominent. An abdominal ultrasound reveals an abdominal aortic aneurysm measuring 4.1 cm in transverse diameter.

In addition to smoking cessation counseling, what is the next step in management?

A. Refer for open surgical repair.
B. Refer for endovascular repair.
C. Urgent CT angiogram of the abdominal aorta
D. Repeat abdominal ultrasound in 6 months.
E. Exercise treadmill test

33. A 74-year-old man with hypertension, coronary artery disease, GERD, and osteoarthritis presents for follow-up. He had an ST segment myocardial infarction 2 years prior and underwent successful stenting of a complete LAD arterial occlusion. For the past 3 weeks, he has noted worsening dyspnea on light exertion coupled with lower extremity swelling. He has had no recurrent chest pain.

His medications include metoprolol, nifedipine, aspirin, and rosuvastatin. On examination, his blood pressure is 126/80 mm Hg. His heart rate is 70 beats per minute. His jugular venous pressure is 14 cm H_2O.

The first and second heart sounds are normal, and a third heart sound is appreciated. There is lower extremity edema to the knee bilaterally. A stress echocardiogram reveals mild anterior wall hypokinesis at rest, and all walls augment appropriately with stress. The left ventricular ejection fraction at rest is estimated at 40%.

In addition to diuresis and discontinuation of nifedipine, what is the most appropriate management?

A. Add hydralazine and isosorbide mononitrate.
B. Add clopidogrel.
C. Add lisinopril.
D. Add spironolactone.
E. Add digoxin.

34. A 48-year-old man presents with chest pressure. He has a history of diabetes, dyslipidemia, hypertension, and active tobacco use. For the past 3 weeks, he has noted substernal chest pressure that is evoked by climbing two flights of stairs briskly and relieved over several minutes with rest. His family history includes two brothers with myocardial infarction at ages 50 and 52, respectively. The result of his physical examination is normal. An electrocardiogram reveals normal sinus rhythm with no ischemic change and normal axis and intervals.

What is the best diagnostic step?

A. Cardiac MRI
B. Coronary artery calcium score
C. Exercise treadmill test
D. Coronary angiography
E. Pharmacologic stress myocardial perfusion imaging

35. A 78-year-old woman is seen in the office for a preoperative evaluation. She has a notable history of low back pain secondary to spinal stenosis, and it has been recommended that she undergo lumbar laminectomy. She is unable to ascend and descend stairs secondary to low back pain. Her medical history includes hypertension and diabetes leading to chronic kidney disease with baseline creatinine of 2.1 mg/dL. She had a transient ischemic attack 2 years prior. Her medications include aspirin, NPH insulin, rosuvastatin, and amlodipine. Her physical examination reveals a heart rate of 78 beats per minute, blood pressure of 138/68 mm Hg, and is otherwise normal. An electrocardiogram reveals sinus rhythm, left anterior fascicular block, and Q waves in leads V1 and V2.

What is the next step in diagnosis and management?

A. Exercise treadmill test
B. Dobutamine stress echocardiogram
C. Coronary CT angiogram
D. Proceed with surgery.
E. Prescribe metoprolol.

36. A 26-year-old medical student is seen in the office. In the midst of a workshop with his classmates, while learning to perform bedside cardiac ultrasound, an abnormality was appreciated. He feels entirely well, and the result of his physical examination is normal. A formal echocardiogram reveals a left atrial mass measuring 2.1 × 2.3 cm. The mass is pedunculated, mobile, and attached to the interatrial septum by a thin stalk. The remainder of the echocardiogram is normal.

What is the next step in management?

A. Echocardiography in 6 months
B. Two sets of blood cultures 12 hours apart
C. Anticoagulation with warfarin for goal INR of 2–3
D. Referral for surgical removal
E. PET-CT of the chest, abdomen, and pelvis

37. An 84-year-old woman presents with fatigue and dyspnea of 3 months' duration. Although previously active, she notes a decreased ability to garden, shop, and perform activities of daily living. She has no chest pain, orthopnea, or lower extremity edema. Her past medical history is unremarkable, and her only medication is a multivitamin. On examination, her heart rate is 42 beats per minute and regular. Her blood pressure is 128/70 mm Hg, and her oxygen saturation is 97% breathing room air. Her skin is warm and dry, venous pressure is low, and first and second heart sounds are normal. Her lungs are clear. An electrocardiogram reveals sinus bradycardia with a narrow QRS complex. With ambulation, her oxygen saturation is 96%, and her heart rate increases to 50 beats per minute. The result of thyroid function testing is normal.

What is the next step in management?

A. Forty-eight-hour Holter monitor
B. Thirty-day event monitor
C. Electrophysiologic study with measurement of sinus node recovery time
D. Serum Lyme titer
E. Referral for pacemaker placement

38. A 32-year-old man is seen in follow-up. He feels well. At a recent "health day event" at his office, his blood pressure was 120/60 mm Hg, and his total cholesterol was measured at 160 mg/dL. His past medical history is notable for tension headache well controlled with as-needed acetaminophen. On examination, his heart rate is 103 beats per minute, and his blood pressure 156/98 mm Hg. A funduscopic examination reveals a normal optic disc and normal retinal vessels. His thyroid gland is slightly full to palpation. His carotid arteries are normal in contour and volume. The first and second heart sounds are normal. There are no abdominal or flank bruits, and there is no radiofemoral pulse delay.

What is the best next diagnostic step?

A. Serum potassium and measurement of aldosterone-to-renin ratio
B. Renal artery Doppler ultrasound
C. Give the patient a home blood pressure diary, measure TSH, and repeat office blood pressure in 3 months.
D. Prescribe chlorthalidone.
E. Measure serum free metanephrines.

39. A 62-year-old man with diabetes and a tobacco use history presents for follow-up of chest pain. He initially presented with chest pain 5 months prior; coronary angiography demonstrated a 60% stenosis of the middle left anterior descending artery and an 80% stenosis of a moderate-sized obtuse marginal branch of the left circumflex. He was initiated on aspirin, metoprolol, and isosorbide mononitrate. For persistent chest pain with moderate exertion, ranolazine was added. He has undergone two courses of supervised cardiac rehabilitation, but his symptoms persist. Currently, he gets chest pain with moderate exertion, which precludes him from playing doubles tennis and bowling. His medications include metformin, metoprolol, rosuvastatin, isosorbide mononitrate, ranolazine, and lisinopril. On examination, his heart rate is 56 beats per minute, and his blood pressure is 100/60 mm Hg. The results of cardiopulmonary examinations are normal. His total cholesterol is 100 mg/dL, with HDL cholesterol of 38 mg/dL. His hemoglobin A1c is 6.2%.

What is the best next step in management?

A. Refer for coronary artery bypass surgery.
B. Refer for PCI of the obtuse marginal stenosis.
C. Increase metoprolol.
D. Increase isosorbide mononitrate.
E. Refer for cardiac rehabilitation.

40. A 65-year-old man presents for evaluation of worsening dyspnea on exertion. His past medical history is notable for Hodgkin lymphoma treated with mantle radiation, coronary artery disease status post-CABG, moderate restrictive lung disease, and stage 3 chronic kidney disease. His physical examination is notable for jugular venous distention, decreased carotid pulsation, normal S1, inaudible S2, late-peaking crescendo–decrescendo systolic murmur at the base radiating to both carotids, and a soft holosystolic murmur at the apex. An echocardiogram shows a left ventricular ejection fraction of 35%–40%, a severely calcified aortic valve with restricted opening (peak and mean transaortic gradients of 64 and 40 mm Hg, respectively; calculated aortic valve area, 0.7 cm^2), and a calcified mitral valve with mild to moderate regurgitation.

In addition to cautious diuresis, what is an appropriate next step in his management?

A. Continued medical management for heart failure
B. Aortic balloon valvuloplasty
C. Surgical aortic valve replacement
D. Transcatheter aortic valve replacement
E. Surgical aortic and mitral valve replacement

41. A 60-year-old woman presents to the emergency department with palpitations. Her past medical history is notable for well-controlled hypertension and mitral valve prolapse that were diagnosed when she was a teenager. On examination, her heart rate is 70 beats per minute with blood pressure 110/80 mm Hg. She has no evidence of jugular venous distention. Her cardiac examination shows regular rate and rhythm with normal S1 and S2. She has a holosystolic high-pitched blowing murmur at the apex that radiates to the left sternal border. An EKG shows normal sinus rhythm with occasional premature ventricular contractions. An echocardiogram shows normal left ventricular function (ejection fraction, 65%; left ventricular end-systolic dimension, 35 mm), thickened and redundant mitral leaflets with a flail posterior leaflet, dilated left atrium, 3–4+ mitral regurgitation with systolic flow reversal in the pulmonary veins, and estimated pulmonary artery systolic pressure of 36 mm Hg.

What is an appropriate next step in her management?

A. Referral for surgical mitral valve repair
B. Referral for surgical mitral valve replacement
C. Referral for MitraClip
D. Close follow-up with a transthoracic echocardiogram every 6–12 months
E. Vasodilators to reduce afterload

42. A 65-year-old woman with chronic systolic heart failure (left ventricular ejection fraction, 30%) comes for a routine clinic visit. She reports that she is dyspneic climbing one flight of stairs and uses two pillows to sleep at night. She has intermittent lower extremity edema, especially after eating a salty meal. Her medications include lisinopril 20 mg daily, carvedilol 25 mg twice daily, spironolactone 25 mg daily, and torsemide 40 mg daily. On examination, she has a heart rate of 70 beats per minute, blood pressure of 110/70 mm Hg, no jugular venous distention, normal heart sounds, a II/VI holosystolic murmur at the apex, and trace-1+ peripheral edema. Her laboratory values are notable for sodium 140 mEq/L, potassium 4.8 mEq/L, blood urea nitrogen 20 mg/dL, and creatinine 1.2 mg/dL.

What is the next most appropriate step in her management?

A. Continue her current medications.
B. Increase lisinopril to 30 mg daily.
C. Stop lisinopril and start sacubitril/valsartan 49/51 mg twice daily after 36-hour washout.
D. Increase torsemide to 60 mg daily.
E. Add digoxin 0.125 mg daily.

43. A 24-year-old woman with a history of nonischemic cardiomyopathy (left ventricular ejection fraction, 25%) comes for a postdischarge clinic visit after a recent hospitalization with heart failure. She reports postural lightheadedness and decreased exercise tolerance due to fatigue and dyspnea. Her medications include lisinopril 2.5 mg daily, metoprolol succinate 25 mg daily, spironolactone 12.5 mg daily, furosemide 20 mg daily, and warfarin. A physical examination reveals a heart rate of 100 beats per minute and blood pressure of 90/70 mm Hg. She has no jugular venous distention, her lungs are clear, her heart sounds are irregularly irregular with an audible S3. She has no peripheral edema. Her laboratory values are notable for sodium 136 mEq/L, potassium 4.2 mEq/L, blood urea nitrogen 16 mg/dL, and creatinine 1.0 mg/dL.

What is the next most appropriate step in her management?

A. Increase her furosemide dose.
B. Add digoxin.
C. Increase her metoprolol succinate dose.
D. Change lisinopril to sacubitril/valsartan.
E. Add ivabradine.

44. A 40-year-old man presents to the emergency department with sudden onset of tachypnea and chest pain after taking a trans-Atlantic flight. On examination, he has a heart rate of 120 beats per minute, blood pressure of 100/80 mm Hg, and room air oxygen saturation of 84%. Computed tomography of the chest shows an acute pulmonary embolus in the bilateral main pulmonary arteries. An echocardiogram shows a moderately enlarged right ventricle with reduced systolic function and an estimated right ventricular systolic pressure of 50 mm Hg. The result of a cardiac troponin test was negative.

What is the next best step in his management?

A. Systemic thrombolysis
B. Intravenous heparin
C. Emergent surgical thrombectomy
D. Catheter-directed thrombolysis
E. Placement of an inferior vena cava filter

45. A 70-year-old man with hypertension and diabetes presents with new-onset atrial fibrillation. His physical examination is notable for an irregularly irregular pulse of 120 beats per minute but is otherwise unremarkable. His laboratory test results are notable for a creatinine level of 1.3 mg/dL. In addition to starting him on metoprolol for rate control, you recommend anticoagulation with apixaban 5 mg twice daily. He inquires if he needs to make any dietary or medication changes with apixaban, similar to what he has heard with warfarin.

Which of the following drugs would be most likely to increase his risk of bleeding if combined with apixaban?

A. Sotalol
B. Amiodarone
C. Verapamil
D. Phenytoin
E. Ketoconazole

46. A 32-year-old woman who is 4 weeks postpartum presents with acute-onset chest pain and dyspnea. She has no prior cardiac risk factors or known cardiac disease. Her physical examination is notable for a heart rate of 120 beats per minute, BP 100/60 mm Hg, and room air oxygen saturation of 94%. She has evidence of jugular venous distention, bibasilar rales, and no peripheral edema. Her EKG shows sinus tachycardia with 2-mm ST elevation in leads V1–V4.

What is the most likely diagnosis?

A. Acute pulmonary embolism
B. Amniotic fluid embolism
C. Peripartum cardiomyopathy
D. Acute coronary dissection
E. Acute pericarditis

47. A 32-year-old recent immigrant from Haiti presents for her first clinic evaluation. When she was 12 years old, she had rheumatic fever that was treated with antibiotics. She is asymptomatic. Her physical examination shows a heart rate of 70 beats per minute with a blood pressure of 122/77 mm Hg. She has no jugular venous distention. Her lungs are clear. She has a regular rate and rhythm with a loud S1 and physiologically split S2. A soft early diastolic rumble is heard at the apex with an opening snap after S2. There is wide separation between A2 and the opening snap. No peripheral edema is present.

Which of the following is the most appropriate next recommendation for this patient?

A. Take antibiotics prior to dental procedures.
B. Start furosemide.
C. Start anticoagulation.
D. Start oral penicillin V 250 mg twice daily.
E. Start metoprolol.

48. A 70-year-old woman presents to your office for an annual health examination. She has no known cardiovascular risk factors or history of cardiovascular disease. She has never smoked and drinks alcohol socially. She leads an active lifestyle and is asymptomatic. Her physical examination is notable for a heart rate of 70 beats per minute and a blood pressure of 124/84 mm Hg. The rest of her physical examination is unremarkable. Her EKG is normal. She has a total cholesterol of 180 mg/dL and an HDL cholesterol of 50 mg/dL. Her Framingham risk score for cardiovascular disease is 8.6%. Her pooled cardiovascular risk score is 8.8%.

Which of the following is the most appropriate test?

A. Exercise stress test
B. Abdominal ultrasound
C. Ankle brachial index
D. Coronary artery calcium score
E. No further testing is needed.

49. A 28-year-old overweight woman presents for evaluation of recurrent headaches. She does not give a history of snoring and denies any daytime hypersomnolence, flushing, palpitations, or diaphoresis. She has no significant past medical history and is on no medications. Her physical examination is notable for a heart rate of

75 beats per minute and blood pressure of 180/100 mm Hg on the right and 178/98 mm Hg on the left. Her BMI is 28 kg/m^2. Her lungs are clear. Her cardiovascular examination is notable for an audible S4. Her extremities reveal no edema and have equal pulses without delay. Her electrolytes are normal, and her creatinine level is 1.0 mg/dL.

Which of the following tests is most likely to identify the cause of her hypertension?

A. Renal artery Doppler study
B. Polysomnography
C. Twenty-four-hour urine for metanephrines and catecholamines
D. Serum aldosterone and renin levels
E. Transthoracic echocardiogram

Chapter 8 Answers

1. **ANSWER: C. Atrial septal defect**

This patient presents with symptoms of palpitations, a common complaint. The physical examination in such cases should be focused on identifying underlying structural heart disease. The parasternal lift, widened second heart sound with a "fixed split," prominent pulmonic closure sound, and a pulmonary flow murmur are all classic findings of a secundum atrial septal defect (ASD). Assuming normal right and left ventricular compliance, ASDs cause left-to-right shunting of blood and chronic volume loading of the right atrium and ventricle, leading to progressive dilation and predisposing to arrhythmias, including atrial fibrillation, atrial tachycardia, and ventricular rhythms. The increased right-sided flow gives rise to the pulmonary valve murmur and fixed splitting of the second heart sound. The electrocardiographic findings of rightward axis and incomplete right bundle branch block are typical of a secundum ASD. Wolff-Parkinson-White syndrome would present with a short PR interval and delta waves on the electrocardiogram, whereas the electrocardiogram of patients with arrhythmogenic right ventricular cardiomyopathy classically demonstrates right ventricular conduction delay; low voltage; and T-wave inversions in the septal, anterior, and inferior leads. The diastolic rumbling murmur, loud S1, and opening snap of mitral stenosis are not appreciated. Finally, hyperthyroidism can present with arrhythmia and murmur related to the hyperdynamic state, but other findings of hyperthyroidism, including weight loss, stare, diaphoresis, and tremor, are not appreciated.

Geva T, Martins JD, Wald RM. Atrial septal defects. *Lancet.* 2014;383(9932):1921–1932.

2. **ANSWER: D. Ibuprofen**

This patient presents with chest pain and electrocardiographic findings of ST segment elevation; specifically, the electrocardiogram reveals sinus tachycardia and ST segment elevations of 1–3 mm in leads I, II, III, aVF, and V2–V6. There are PR segment depressions most prominent in leads I, II, and V6. The differential diagnosis for ST segment elevation on the electrocardiogram includes ST segment elevation, myocardial infarction, acute pericarditis, early repolarization, and left ventricular aneurysm. In this case, the diffuse nature of the ST segment elevation, the concave upward morphology of the ST segment, the lack of reciprocal ST segment depressions, and the PR segment depressions on the electrocardiogram are all most consistent with acute pericarditis rather than ST-elevation myocardial infarction (STEMI). Patients with acute pericarditis often assume a position of sitting up and leaning forward, which minimizes pericardial pain. Making the distinction between acute pericarditis and acute STEMI is sometimes difficult, and bedside echocardiography can be helpful. In this patient, the pericardial effusion and lack of a wall motion abnormality also favor pericarditis rather than STEMI. Nonsteroidal antiinflammatory agents, often coupled with colchicine, are the treatment of choice. Option A would be appropriate for a patient suspected of having STEMI, in which case urgent reperfusion therapy would be indicated. Option B would be appropriate for patients with high-risk non-ST elevation acute coronary syndromes. Prednisone, Option C, has been shown to increase the risk of recurrent disease when prescribed in patients with pericarditis and should be avoided. Option E is the management of choice for patients with cocaine-induced myocardial ischemia, which the history does not support in this case.

Imazio M, Gaita F, LeWinter M. Evaluation and treatment of pericarditis: a systematic review. *JAMA.* 2015;314(14):1498–1506.

3. **ANSWER: A. Infusion of normal saline**

This patient with multiple cardiac risk factors presents with an inferior ST segment myocardial infarction. Inferior STEMI can be due to occlusion of the right coronary or left circumflex coronary arteries; in this case, the ST segment elevation in lead III that is of greater magnitude than in lead II, coupled with the significant reciprocal depressions in lead aVL, suggests occlusion of the right coronary artery. The physical examination reveals a triad of hypotension, jugular venous distention with the Kussmaul sign, and clear lungs. This triad suggests a clinical diagnosis of right ventricular myocardial infarction. When the right coronary artery is occluded proximally, the acute RV marginal branches of the RCA receive no flow, leading to RV infarction. The hypocontractile, infarcted RV leads to elevated right atrial and jugular venous pressure, and the decreased right ventricular compliance gives rise to the Kussmaul sign. The right ventricle is unable to maintain left ventricular preload, leading to hypotension. The hypotension can be worsened markedly with nitrate therapy. Appropriate hemodynamic management includes judicious volume loading, often guided by a pulmonary artery catheter. The low left ventricular preload would be exacerbated by diuresis. Intravenous beta blockers should not be administered to patients in cardiogenic shock with acute myocardial infarction and would worsen hemodynamics in this case; esmolol can be a useful agent to control blood pressure in the management of acute aortic dissection. Finally, phenylephrine, an alpha agonist, causes increased afterload and can worsen myocardial performance in the setting of cardiogenic shock.

O'Gara PT, Kushner FG, Ascheim DD, et al. 2013 ACCF/AHA guideline for the management of ST-elevation myocardial infarction: a report of the American College of Cardiology Foundation/American Heart Association Task Force on Practice Guidelines. *J Am Coll Cardiol.* 2013;61(4):e78–e140.

4. **ANSWER: E. Mitral stenosis**

This patient who is 22 weeks pregnant presents with dyspnea; dyspnea is a common complaint in pregnancy and has myriad causes. Salient symptoms here include orthopnea, which is a historical feature with high specificity for elevated left heart filling pressures. The examination suggests atrial fibrillation with an irregularly irregular heart rhythm. The loud S1, opening snap, and diastolic murmur are all cardinal physical features of mitral stenosis. The state of pregnancy leads to significant hemodynamic changes even in normal cases, including decreased systemic vascular resistance, increased plasma volume, and increased cardiac output. These physiologic changes can lead to physical findings of systolic flow murmurs, a third heart sound, a venous hum, and a mammary souffle, which are normal findings in pregnancy. In patients with preexisting heart disease, however, the hemodynamic stressors can lead to significant decompensation. Stenotic valve lesions in particular tolerate pregnancy poorly, and it is often patients who had well-tolerated, asymptomatic occult mitral stenosis prior to pregnancy who present with symptoms as pregnancy progresses. Pregnancy-induced cardiomyopathy and pulmonary embolism are both important differential diagnoses for the pregnant patient with dyspnea, but the physical findings in this case are inconsistent with these diagnoses. Similarly, thyroid storm can present with new atrial arrhythmia and high-output heart failure, but it would not be associated with a systolic flow murmur rather than a diastolic rumble and opening snap. This patient's physical examination is not consistent with normal physical findings of pregnancy.

Carabello BA, Crawford FA Jr. Valvular heart disease. *N Engl J Med.* 1997;337(1):32–41.

5. **ANSWER: B. Echocardiography**

This patient with known malignancy presents with dyspnea. The differential diagnosis of a patient with cancer presenting with dyspnea includes hematologic abnormalities, pulmonary embolism, paraneoplastic syndromes, infection, and cardiac causes. Tachycardia, hypotension, and elevated jugular venous pressure are consistent with both pulmonary embolism and cardiac tamponade. The Kussmaul sign can be seen in both conditions. The low electrocardiogram voltage and quiet heart sounds, coupled with the aforementioned abnormalities, suggest cardiac tamponade as the cause of this patient's symptoms, which is best evaluated with an echocardiogram. EMG may be indicated to evaluate for neuromuscular paraneoplastic syndromes in the setting of small cell lung cancer, but there is no evidence of weakness on examination. Cardiac tamponade secondary to cancer can present insidiously with gradual onset of dyspnea, in contrast to the acute tamponade observed after cardiac surgery or intracardiac procedures. Cancers of the lung, breast, and kidney as well as hematologic malignancies, are the malignancies most likely to metastasize to the pericardium.

Spodick DH. Acute cardiac tamponade. *N Engl J Med.* 2003;349:684–690.

6. **ANSWER: B. Increase dosage of metoprolol for a goal heart rate of 55–65 beats per minute, then proceed with total knee replacement.**

This patient is referred for preoperative cardiac risk stratification prior to noncardiac surgery. The first step in assessing for operative risk is to assess whether the planned surgery is emergent and life-or-limb saving, in which case the surgical procedure should proceed without delay from further cardiovascular diagnostics or therapeutics. In this case, surgery is elective. Next, assess whether unstable cardiovascular conditions are present that should be addressed prior to elective surgery; these conditions would include unstable tachy- or bradyarrhythmias, unstable ischemic syndromes, decompensated heart failure, and critical symptomatic stenotic valvular disease. None of these syndromes are present. Next, assess the risk of the planned surgery. For low-risk procedures (endoscopy, dermatologic surgery, cataract surgery, and breast surgery), no further cardiovascular diagnostics or therapeutics are necessary prior to the procedure. Orthopedic procedures, intraabdominal surgery, and intrathoracic surgery are considered intermediate-risk procedures. Next, assess functional capacity. If a patient can achieve greater than 4 metabolic equivalents of activity (corresponding roughly to walking briskly up two flights of stairs) without cardiovascular limitation, the risk of perioperative cardiovascular events is low, and the planned operation can proceed. In this case, the functional capacity is limited by knee pain. Finally, the Revised Cardiac Risk Index (RCRI) can be calculated. This index assesses patient-specific risk factors for a cardiovascular event in the perioperative period. These include (1) history of heart failure, (2) history of stroke or transient ischemic attack, (3) history of ischemic heart disease (prior infarction, known coronary artery disease, or Q waves on the electrocardiogram, (4) serum creatinine greater than 2.0 mg/dL, and (5) diabetes requiring insulin. Depending on the RCRI and the risk of the planned procedure, no therapy, beta blockade, or rarely stress testing and possible revascularization could be considered. This patient has an RCRI of 3 (including coronary disease, diabetes, and renal insufficiency) and is already maintained on beta blockade therapy. The most optimal course of therapy is to uptitrate beta blockade over several weeks for a goal heart rate of 55–65 beats per minute and thereafter proceed with total knee replacement.

Fleisher LA, Fleischmann KE, Auerbach AD, et al. 2014 ACC/AHA guideline on perioperative cardiovascular evaluation and management of patients undergoing noncardiac surgery: a report of the American College of Cardiology/American Heart Association Task Force on Practice Guidelines. *J Am Coll Cardiol.* 2014;64:e77–e137.

7. ANSWER: A. Electrophysiologic study and mapping

This young athlete presents with palpitations. Historical features favoring a paroxysmal supraventricular tachycardia include abrupt onset and offset as well as the presence of neck pounding, which can be caused by retrograde atrial activation in the setting of AV nodal reentrant tachycardia (AVNRT) or AV reentrant tachycardia (AVRT). The electrocardiogram in this case is diagnostic, revealing sinus bradycardia with sinus arrhythmia that is a normal finding in a young, highly conditioned athlete. The PR interval is short, less than 120 ms, and there are delta waves visible as a broad, slurred initial portion of the QRS best seen in leads II, III, and aVF as well as leads V2 and V3. Lead aVL also has a short PR interval with a Q wave that represents a negative delta wave rather than evidence of prior infarction; this is a so-called pseudoinfarction pattern. A short PR interval and delta waves on the electrocardiogram, coupled with symptoms suggestive of arrhythmia, is diagnostic of the Wolff-Parkinson-White syndrome. First-line therapy for this condition is referral to electrophysiology for an EP study with mapping and ablation of the accessory pathway. This procedure is curative in the vast majority of cases. Signal-averaged electrocardiogram can be used in diagnosis of arrhythmogenic right ventricular cardiomyopathy, but the 12-lead electrocardiogram is inconsistent with this diagnosis. An exercise stress test or CT coronary angiogram could be helpful in diagnosing anomalous coronary or premature coronary obstruction. The Q wave on the electrocardiogram in lead aVL in this case is more consistent with a pseudoinfarct pattern from Wolff-Parkinson-White syndrome. A Holter monitor could document the presence of SVT; however, with symptoms and a 12-lead electrocardiogram consistent with Wolff-Parkinson-White syndrome, there are sufficient data to recommend an EP study as the initial step.

Cohen MI, Triedman JK, Cannon BC, et al. PACES/HRS expert consensus statement on the management of the asymptomatic young patient with a Wolff-Parkinson-White (WPW, ventricular preexcitation) electrocardiographic pattern. *Heart Rhythm.* 2012;9(6):1006–1024.

8. ANSWER: D. Proceed with planned dental procedure.

This patient has known valvular heart disease with mitral valve prolapse and is in need of dental work. For some patients with heart disease, the sequelae of infectious endocarditis mandate antibiotic prophylaxis before routine dental work. Patients with prior infectious endocarditis, prosthetic heart valves, cyanotic congenital heart disease that is unrepaired, or congenital heart disease repaired with prosthetic material and patient status post–cardiac transplant all mandate antibiotics prior to dental procedures that manipulate gingival tissue or involve the periapical area of the tooth. The patient in this case meets none of these criteria, and the optimal management is to proceed with planned dental work without antibiotic therapy. There is no indication for a repeat echocardiogram for mitral valve prolapse in the absence of a change in the physical examination or the development of interval cardiac symptoms. There is no indication for blood cultures, because there is no current evidence of infectious endocarditis.

Wilson W, Taubert KA, Gewitz M, et al. Prevention of infective endocarditis: guidelines from the American Heart Association: a guideline from the American Heart Association Rheumatic Fever, Endocarditis, and Kawasaki Disease Committee, Council on Cardiovascular Disease in the Young, and the Council on Clinical Cardiology, Council on Cardiovascular Surgery and Anesthesia, and the Quality of Care and Outcomes Research Interdisciplinary Working Group. *Circulation.* 2007;116(15):1736–1754.

9. ANSWER: E. Unfractionated heparin and coronary angiography within 24 hours

This patient presents with high-risk non-ST segment elevation myocardial infarction (NSTEMI). The non-ST segment acute coronary syndromes are comprised of unstable angina and non-ST segment myocardial infarction; serum biomarkers of myocardial necrosis (troponin in this case) are not present in unstable angina and are present in NSTEMI. It has been established that there is no benefit to thrombolysis in NSTEMI; in contrast to ST-elevation myocardial infarction (STEMI), the infarct-related artery is partially rather than completely occluded. A "selectively invasive" strategy consists of medical management of the patient with antiplatelet, antithrombin, and antiischemic therapy followed by noninvasive risk stratification with stress testing. An "early invasive" strategy includes aggressive medical therapy and coronary angiography with revascularization within 24–48 hours of hospitalization. It has been shown that patients with higher-risk non-ST-elevation acute coronary syndrome (NSTE-ACS) have proportionally more benefit from an "early invasive" strategy of management with angiography within this time frame. There are several validated scores available for risk stratification of patients with NSTE-ACS, including the GRACE score and TIMI score.

This patient's age, multiple risk factors, severe angina at rest, ST depression on the electrocardiogram, and positive troponin all place him at high risk, and an early invasive strategy of management would be favored. Fondaparinux is less favored as an antithrombin agent in patients going to the catheterization laboratory, due to risk of catheter-associated thrombus that is not present when unfractionated heparin is used.

Amsterdam EA, Wenger NK, Brindis RG, et al. 2014 AHA/ACC Guideline for the Management of Patients with Non-ST-Elevation Acute Coronary Syndromes: a report of the American College of Cardiology/American Heart Association Task Force on Practice Guidelines. *J Am Coll Cardiol.* 2014;64(24):e139–e228.

10. ANSWER: D. Clopidogrel

This patient with cardiac risk factors presents with a non-ST segment myocardial infarction; the single severe stenosis demonstrated on angiography was not amenable to percutaneous coronary intervention, and a course of medical management was undertaken. Aspirin, statin therapy, beta blockade, smoking cessation, and cardiac rehabilitation should be prescribed, and lipids and blood pressure should be treated to current goals. In addition, a large randomized controlled trial (The Clopidogrel in Unstable Angina to Prevent Recurrent Events Trial Investigators. Effects of clopidogrel in addition to aspirin in patients with acute coronary syndromes without ST-segment elevation. *N Engl J Med.* 2001;345:494–502.) demonstrated the additive benefit of thienopyridine therapy added to aspirin therapy in patients with NSTEMI. Clopidogrel therapy in addition to aspirin reduced a composite endpoint of cardiovascular death, nonfatal myocardial infarction, and stroke. Thus, for this patient with NSTEMI managed medically, clopidogrel should be added to aspirin therapy for 12 months, assuming there is not a high risk of bleeding. Ranolazine and isosorbide mononitrate are antiischemic therapies that can improve anginal symptoms but have no effect on cardiovascular mortality. There is no role for fish oil or warfarin in managing NSTEMI absent another indication for these therapies.

Amsterdam EA, Wenger NK, Brindis RG, et al. 2014 AHA/ACC Guideline for the Management of Patients with Non-ST-Elevation Acute Coronary Syndromes: a report of the American College of Cardiology/American Heart Association Task Force on Practice Guidelines. *J Am Coll Cardiol.* 2014;64(24):e139–e228.

11. ANSWER: C. Transthoracic echocardiogram

This patient has a history of mitral valve prolapse, which is a common cardiac valve lesion; myxomatous valve degeneration leads to redundant chordal tissue and billowing of the leaflets back into the left atrium during ventricular systole, causing the characteristic click–murmur complex. Consequences of mitral valve prolapse include progressive mitral regurgitation, an increased risk of infective endocarditis, and chordal rupture leading to subacute decline. This patient presents with new atrial arrhythmia, heart failure, and auscultatory findings of severe mitral regurgitation rather than the known click–murmur complex, all suggesting that he has experienced a ruptured chord, leading to subacute decompensation. An echocardiogram should be ordered to confirm the diagnosis, and it is likely that surgical correction will be necessary. A surgeon with experience in mitral valve repair should be consulted. In this circumstance, mitral valve repair is preferred over mitral valve replacement. Warfarin and DC cardioversion could be considered for new atrial fibrillation of recent onset; however, that would not address the underlying cause of dysrhythmia in this case. Similarly, thyroid testing and screening of sleep apnea are reasonable in an uncomplicated case of new atrial fibrillation or atrial flutter, but neither is the most likely diagnosis here. An exercise treadmill test is not recommended for a patient in decompensated heart failure. Beta blockade would not be indicated.

Stout KK, Verrier ED. Acute valvular regurgitation. *Circulation.* 2009;119(25):3232–3241.

12. ANSWER: B. Adenosine

This young patient presents with supraventricular tachycardia. The electrocardiogram demonstrates a narrow complex regular tachycardia at approximately 150 beats per minute. No clear atrial activity is seen, and the differential diagnosis includes AVRT, AVNRT, atrial flutter, and ectopic atrial tachycardia. Vagal maneuvers were an appropriate first step but were unsuccessful. Adenosine should be administered, which will be both diagnostic and possibly therapeutic by terminating AV node–dependent arrhythmias (AVNRT and AVRT) and unmasking occult atrial activity in atrial flutter, ectopic atrial rhythm, or sinus tachycardia. There is no need for DC cardioversion, because this patient is hemodynamically stable. Amiodarone is not indicated in this case. Normal saline would be prescribed if there were sinus tachycardia secondary to volume depletion. Labetalol is a drug better suited to hypertensive urgency than supraventricular tachycardia.

Page RL, Joglar JA, Caldwell MA, et al. 2015 ACC/AHA/HRS Guideline for the Management of Adult Patients With Supraventricular Tachycardia: a report of the American College of Cardiology/American Heart Association Task Force on Clinical Practice Guidelines and the Heart Rhythm Society. *J Am Coll Cardiol.* 2016;67(13):e27–e115.

13. ANSWER: B. Administer tenecteplase and transfer to a PCI-capable facility.

This patient is having an inferoposterolateral ST segment myocardial infarction. Timely reperfusion therapy is paramount—"time is muscle." The time standards for reperfusion in the setting of STEMI include a "door-to-needle time" of 30 minutes or less if thrombolytics are chosen as the reperfusion strategy and a "door-to-balloon time" of 90 minutes or less if primary PCI is chosen as the reperfusion strategy. Timely PCI has been demonstrated to be superior to timely lytic therapy with improved patency of the infarct-related artery, less reinfarction, and less hemorrhagic complications. If a patient with STEMI presents to a non-PCI center, transfer for PCI should be considered if the first medical contact to device time is less than 120 minutes. First medical contact is defined as the time at which the EMTs arrive at the bedside. In this case, there would be an unacceptable delay (2.5 hours) associated with transfer, and on-site full-dose tenecteplase should be administered. Recent guidelines recommend transfer to a PCI-capable facility even if on-site thrombolysis is successful, and not just for failure of lytic therapy or for early reocclusion. Intravenous beta blockers are no longer recommended acutely for myocardial infarction, owing to the potential to precipitate low cardiac output states. Half-dose thrombolytics prior to transfer for PCI (with or without a glycoprotein 2B/3A antagonist) is not recommended.

O'Gara PT, Kushner FG, Ascheim DD, et al. 2013 ACCF/AHA guideline for the management of ST-elevation myocardial infarction: a report of the American College of Cardiology Foundation/American Heart Association Task Force on Practice Guidelines. *J Am Coll Cardiol.* 2013;61(4):e78–e140.

14. ANSWER: C. Refer for cardiac resynchronization therapy (biventricular pacemaker placement).

This patient with cardiomyopathy has persistent symptoms of dyspnea despite optimal medical therapy. Using the New York Heart Association symptom scale, this patient would be categorized as NYHA class III. Patients with left bundle branch block have delayed depolarization of the lateral left ventricle, and this dyssynchrony can worsen symptoms of heart failure in patients with depressed ejection fraction. For patients with an ejection fraction <35%, a left bundle branch block with QRS duration >120 ms, and NYHA class III symptoms despite optimal medical therapy, a biventricular pacemaker should be placed for cardiac resynchronization. Of note, the trials of cardiac resynchronization therapy (CRT) enrolled patients with QRS duration >120 ms, but in subgroup analysis, the most profound benefit was seen in patients with QRS duration >150 ms. A recent trial demonstrated the benefit of CRT in patients with left bundle branch block and NHYA class II symptoms, but this indication has yet to be incorporated into guidelines. Augmentation of diuretic therapy in this patient is not indicated, because there are no stigmata of volume overload. Referral for LVAD placement would be premature.

Yancy CW, Jessup M, Bozkurt B, et al. 2013 ACCF/AHA guideline for the management of heart failure: a report of the American College of Cardiology Foundation/American Heart Association Task Force on Practice Guidelines. *J Am Coll Cardiol.* 2013;62(16):e147–e239.

15. ANSWER: C. Routine follow-up in 2 weeks

This pregnant patient presents with mild lower extremity edema, a venous hum and flow murmur, and a third heart sound. These are normal physical findings in pregnancy, and in the absence of symptoms or other signs of cardiovascular disease, no further testing is indicated. In normal pregnancy, circulating plasma volume nearly doubles, systemic vascular resistance decreases, and cardiac output increases. These changes lead to an exaggerated early diastolic filling phase in the cardiac cycle and increased outflow tract flow with attendant S3 and pulmonary flow murmur in many patients. Venous hums and mammary souffle murmurs are also benign findings.

Lower extremity venous pressure increases due to compression of the pelvic veins lead to edema. Urinalysis and liver function tests could be obtained if preeclampsia were suspected on the basis of significant edema, hypertension, and headache. An echocardiogram could be obtained if peripartum cardiomyopathy were suspected, but the patient's good functional capacity and low venous pressure make this less likely. Lower extremity ultrasound would be indicated to evaluate for deep vein thrombosis if leg pain or unilateral edema, warmth, and redness were present, because pregnancy is a hypercoagulable state. Finally, there is no indication of arrhythmia, and a Holter monitor would not be indicated.

May L. Cardiac physiology of pregnancy. *Compr Physiol.* 2015;5(3):1325–1344.

16. **ANSWER: D. Eplerenone**

This patient presented with a large myocardial infarction complicated by heart failure and depressed ejection fraction. The EPHESUS trial demonstrated the benefit of the addition of an aldosterone antagonist to such patients. Trial inclusion criteria included an ejection fraction of 40% or less and a syndrome of heart failure after myocardial infarction. Randomization occurred between 3 and 14 days after myocardial infarction, and there were reductions in total mortality and cardiovascular mortality as well as in sudden cardiac death in the eplerenone arm. Importantly, aldosterone antagonists increase the risk of hyperkalemia, so creatinine and potassium should be monitored closely. There is no evidence that aspirin 325 mg per day has superior efficacy to aspirin 81 mg per day in this setting, and there is an increased risk of bleeding with the higher dose. A higher dose of clopidogrel was tested in the OASIS-7 trial, which assessed whether a higher loading dose of clopidogrel followed by double-dose clopidogrel for 1 week was superior to standard dosing of 75 mg daily. The primary endpoint in this trial was negative; however, there may be a decreased risk of stent thrombosis with the increased dosing regimen. There is no indication for ranolazine in this patient, and given that he is euvolemic, there is no indication for augmented diuresis with metolazone.

Pitt B, Remme W, Zannad F, et al. Eplerenone, a selective aldosterone blocker, in patients with left ventricular dysfunction after myocardial infarction. *N Engl J Med.* 2003;348(14):1309–1321.

17. **ANSWER: E. Refer for pacemaker placement prior to surgery.**

This patient is planning elective noncardiac surgery. An important task in the perioperative medicine evaluation is an assessment for unstable cardiac conditions that mandate treatment prior to surgery. This patient presents with syncope and evidence of significant conduction system disease on the 12-lead electrocardiogram with left bundle branch block and type II AV block. He has a high risk of progression to complete heart block, and a pacemaker should be placed prior to elective surgery. Other unstable cardiac conditions that should be addressed prior to elective noncardiac surgery include unstable cardiac ischemic syndromes, including unstable and accelerating angina, STEMI, and NSTEMI; symptomatic bradycardia and supraventricular tachycardia; ventricular tachycardia; decompensated heart failure; and critical symptomatic stenotic valvular heart disease (aortic and mitral stenosis). Beta blockade is indicated to prevent perioperative events in patients at high risk but would be inappropriate in this patient with symptomatic heart block. An echocardiogram could be ordered if severe stenotic heart disease were suspected, but this patient's murmurs are not consistent with severe aortic or mitral stenosis. The syncope is likely due to heart block rather than to dehydration, so fluid loading would not address the underlying cause.

Epstein AE, DiMarco JP, Ellenbogen KA, et al. 2012 ACCF/AHA/HRS focused update incorporated into the ACCF/AHA/HRS 2008 guidelines for device-based therapy of cardiac rhythm abnormalities: a report of the American College of Cardiology Foundation/American Heart Association Task Force on Practice Guidelines and the Heart Rhythm Society. *J Am Coll Cardiol.* 2013;61(3):e6–e75.

18. **ANSWER: B. Warfarin dosed for INR 2–3 indefinitely**

This patient presents with atrial fibrillation. Atrial fibrillation is a common arrhythmia with aging; the main goals of treatment include prevention of stroke and control of symptoms. With regard to the latter, beta blockers and calcium channel blockers can be prescribed for rate control, and antiarrhythmic drugs and atrial fibrillation ablation can be used to maintain sinus rhythm. With regard to prevention of stroke, the first step in choosing a therapy is assessing the baseline risk of stroke. The CHADS2 score is a scoring system to determine stroke risk. One point is assigned for each of a history of congestive heart failure, hypertension, age >75 years, and diabetes, and 2 points are assigned for prior stroke or transient ischemic attack. Patients with a score of 0 can be maintained on aspirin or no anticoagulation. A score ≥2 would be an indication for warfarin therapy in the absence of a high risk of bleeding. A score of 1 is indeterminate, and a discussion should be had with the patient about the risks and benefits of anticoagulation. The CHADS2 score has been further refined with publication of the CHADS2-VASc score, which gives additional points for age between 65 and 75, female sex, and vascular disease. This patient's scores based on both scoring systems suggest that anticoagulation should be pursued. Warfarin is favored over dabigatran, given her age and renal insufficiency. Even if cardioversion were pursued, anticoagulation would need to be maintained indefinitely, given her high risk of stroke.

January CT, Wann LS, Alpert JS, et al. 2014 AHA/ACC/HRS guideline for the management of patients with atrial fibrillation: a report of the American College of Cardiology/American Heart Association Task Force on Practice Guidelines and the Heart Rhythm Society. *Circulation.* 2014;130(23):e199–e267.

19. **ANSWER: E. Ibuprofen and colchicine**

This patient presents with acute pericarditis on the basis of typical history, friction rub on physical examination, and characteristic electrocardiographic and echocardiographic findings. Coronary angiography is not needed in such typical cases, although it is reasonable in cases in which the distinction between pericarditis and ST segment myocardial infarction is unclear. The management of acute pericarditis should include both a nonsteroidal antiinflammatory agent and colchicine; the combination reduced recurrence of symptoms in the pivotal COPE trial and was superior to NSAIDs alone. Prednisone is effective for acute treatment but is associated with an increased risk of relapses and should not be used routinely.

Lilly LS. Treatment of acute and recurrent idiopathic pericarditis. *Circulation.* 2013;127(16):1723–1726.

20. ANSWER: D. Magnetic resonance angiography of the thoracic and abdominal aorta

This pediatric patient presents with a bicuspid aortic valve, a common congenital cardiac condition. Regarding the valve itself, there is only mild regurgitation and no stenosis, so no specific therapy is indicated for aortic valve disease. Aortic root dilation and aortic coarctation are both associated with bicuspid aortic valve disease. This patient's aortic root is normal in size; however, the presence of a posterior bruit and a radiofemoral pulse delay suggest that there may be concomitant coarctation. Magnetic resonance angiography would visualize the coarctation and enable quantification of severity. This should be performed prior to clearance for sports participation. Losartan has been shown to decrease aortic root diameter and aortic dilation associated with Marfan and Loeys-Dietz syndromes but is not indicated in this case.

Siu SC, Silversides CK. Bicuspid aortic valve disease. *J Am Coll Cardiol.* 2010;55(25):2789–2800.

21. ANSWER: B. Change fluvastatin to high-dose atorvastatin.

This patient with diabetes presents with NSTEMI and underwent successful PCI. Several medications have been shown to improve outcome in patients with diabetes and NSTEMI. Compared with clopidogrel, prasugrel has been shown to improve a composite endpoint of cardiovascular death and repeat myocardial infarction, with a greater benefit in patients with diabetes. There is no advantage to aspirin 325 mg per day over 81 mg per day at a higher cost of greater bleeding. Given that this patient has no residual angina, there is no role for isosorbide mononitrate or ranolazine. High-dose atorvastatin therapy has been shown to be superior to moderate-dose statin therapy when administered early to patients with acute coronary syndrome in the PROVE-IT trial. Patients receiving atorvastatin 80 mg had improvement in a composite endpoint, including myocardial infarction and all-cause mortality, with the initial improvements beginning within 24 hours of randomization. Hence, this patient should be transitioned from a low-potency statin to high-dose atorvastatin.

22. ANSWER: B. Discontinue clopidogrel and proceed with surgery, continuing aspirin through the perioperative period.

This patient with coronary artery disease and prior PCI presents prior to elective noncardiac surgery. He has been maintained on dual antiplatelet therapy with aspirin and clopidogrel since his PCI. Guidelines suggest that dual antiplatelet therapy be strictly maintained for 30 days after placement of a bare metal stent and for 1 year after placement of a drug-eluting stent to reduce the risk of acute stent thrombosis, a catastrophic and life-threatening event. Given that this patient's stent placement was 3 years prior, it is permissible to discontinue clopidogrel. Aspirin should be maintained perioperatively if possible, because the inflammatory milieu of the postsurgical state is prothrombotic. There is emerging data that statin therapy in high-risk patients can reduce perioperative events, and statins should be continued in patients already taking them. Given this patient's excellent functional status (playing competitive singles tennis), there is no role for exercise stress testing or other diagnostic testing prior to surgery.

Levine GN, Bates ER, Bittl JA, et al. 2016 ACC/AHA Guideline Focused Update on Duration of Dual Antiplatelet Therapy in Patients With Coronary Artery Disease: a report of the American College of Cardiology/American Heart Association Task Force on Clinical Practice Guidelines: An Update of the 2011 ACCF/AHA/SCAI Guideline for Percutaneous Coronary Intervention, 2011 ACCF/AHA Guideline for Coronary Artery Bypass Graft Surgery, 2012 ACC/AHA/ACP/AATS/PCNA/SCAI/STS Guideline for the Diagnosis and Management of Patients With Stable Ischemic Heart Disease, 2013 ACCF/AHA Guideline for the Management of ST-Elevation Myocardial Infarction, 2014 AHA/ACC Guideline for the Management of Patients With Non-ST-Elevation Acute Coronary Syndromes, and 2014 ACC/AHA Guideline on Perioperative Cardiovascular Evaluation and Management of Patients Undergoing Noncardiac Surgery. *Circulation.* 2016;134(10):e123–e155.

23. ANSWER: C. Prescribe isosorbide mononitrate.

This patient presents with typical angina that has a stable pattern; that is, the angina is predictably evoked by a stable level of exertion and readily relieved with rest. His angiogram reveals nonobstructive right coronary artery and left circumflex artery disease and a 70% stenosis in a small branch of the left anterior descending artery. In addition, FFR across the right coronary artery lesion indicates a non–ischemia-producing stenosis. Revascularization, either with PCI and stent placement or bypass surgery, in this circumstance does not provide any survival advantage over medical therapy, and as such, a trial of medical therapy should be attempted. Medical therapies for patients with stable angina should include agents to decrease myocardial oxygen demand, including beta blockers, nitrates, and calcium channel blockers. This patient's heart rate is well controlled, and increasing the dose of beta blockers is unlikely to be helpful. A long-acting nitrate would be a good choice to decrease myocardial oxygen consumption by decreasing preload and wall stress. Ranolazine can be considered as an antianginal agent but typically is added after nitrates, beta blockers, and calcium channel blockers are maximized. There is no indication for dual antiplatelet therapy with aspirin and clopidogrel in this patient.

Fihn SD, Blankenship JC, Alexander KP, et al. 2014 ACC/AHA/AATS/PCNA/SCAI/STS focused update of the guideline for the diagnosis and management of patients with stable ischemic heart disease: a report of the American College of Cardiology/American Heart Association Task Force on Practice Guidelines, and the American Association for Thoracic Surgery, Preventive Cardiovascular Nurses Association, Society for Cardiovascular Angiography and Interventions, and Society of Thoracic Surgeons. *J Am Coll Cardiol.* 2014;64(18):1929–1949.

24. ANSWER: C. Refer for implantable cardioverter-defibrillator.

This patient has nonischemic dilated cardiomyopathy, likely familial, and is doing well overall on appropriate medical therapy with good functional status. For patients with systolic dysfunction secondary to nonischemic cardiomyopathy, an ejection fraction less than 35% despite optimal medical therapy, and functional status that is New York Heart Association class II–III, placement of an implantable cardioverter-defibrillator is indicated for primary prevention of sudden cardiac death. The pivotal SCD-HeFT trial demonstrated benefit of an implantable cardioverter-defibrillator in such patients. This patient has a narrow QRS and as such has no indication for CRT, which could be considered if the QRS were prolonged with a left bundle branch block pattern. The venous pressure is low, and there would be no benefit to adding an additional diuretic metolazone. Given his good functional status, referral for transplant would be premature. Digoxin improves symptoms of heart failure without an effect on mortality and can be considered for patients with persistent symptoms despite optimal medical therapy.

Yancy CW, Jessup M, Bozkurt B, et al. 2013 ACCF/AHA guideline for the management of heart failure: a report of the American College of Cardiology Foundation/American Heart Association Task Force on Practice Guidelines. *J Am Coll Cardiol.* 2013;62(16):e147–e239.

25. ANSWER: D. Hypertrophic obstructive cardiomyopathy

This patient presents with dizziness evoked by squatting to standing and dyspnea. The examination reveals a harsh systolic murmur that becomes louder with maneuvers that decrease preload, a cardinal physical examination finding present in hypertrophic obstructive cardiomyopathy. In this condition, there is left ventricular outflow tract obstruction caused by a hypertrophied interventricular septum. Decreased preload decreases left ventricular cavity size and worsens obstruction with an attendant increase in the loudness of the murmur. The obstruction can cause a "Venturi effect," leading to systolic anterior motion of the mitral valve and mitral regurgitation, as is also appreciated in this patient. An echocardiogram should be ordered to confirm the diagnosis. Dilated cardiomyopathy can present with a third heart sound and murmurs of mitral and tricuspid regurgitation. Mitral stenosis presents with a diastolic rumbling murmur at the apex. The harsh systolic murmur of aortic stenosis would be expected to decrease with the Valsalva maneuver. An atrial septal defect presents with fixed splitting of the second heart sound and murmurs of tricuspid regurgitation as well as increased pulmonary artery flow.

Gersh BJ, Maron BJ, Bonow RO, et al. 2011 ACCF/AHA Guideline for the Diagnosis and Treatment of Hypertrophic Cardiomyopathy: a report of the American College of Cardiology Foundation/American Heart Association Task Force on Practice Guidelines. Developed in collaboration with the American Association for Thoracic Surgery, American Society of Echocardiography, American Society of Nuclear Cardiology, Heart Failure Society of America, Heart Rhythm Society, Society for Cardiovascular Angiography and Interventions, and Society of Thoracic Surgeons. *J Am Coll Cardiol.* 2011;58(25):e212–e260.

26. ANSWER: C. Transesophageal echocardiogram

This patient presents with *Staphylococcus aureus* bacteremia and a vegetation on the aortic valve consistent with bacterial endocarditis. Appropriate antibiotic therapy for MSSA was initiated with nafcillin. Vancomycin is appropriate therapy if MRSA is suspected; however, nafcillin has bactericidal activity against MSSA and is a preferred agent. Despite therapy, however, the patient develops evidence of new heart block. The aortic valve and aortic root are in close anatomic proximity to the bundle of His, and an aortic root abscess complicating bacterial endocarditis can progress to complete heart block. Serial monitoring of AV conduction in patients with bacterial endocarditis is mandatory to identify this complication early. Transesophageal echo should be performed to confirm the suspected aortic root abscess and provide anatomic information to guide surgical drainage. Surgical intervention for bacterial endocarditis is indicated for abscess formation, severe valvular destruction with heart failure, failure to clear the infection, and persistently positive blood cultures, as well as for large vegetation with significant risk for embolism. Blood cultures can be incubated for a prolonged period to increase yield if endocarditis associated with the fastidious HACEK organisms is suspected; similarly, serologies for *C. burnetii* can be requested if Q fever, a cause of culture-negative endocarditis, is suspected. Implantation of a pacemaker in this patient with active infection would not be the treatment of choice.

Baddour LM, Wilson WR, Bayer AS, et al. Infective endocarditis in adults: diagnosis, antimicrobial therapy, and management of complications: a scientific statement for healthcare professionals from the American Heart Association. *Circulation.* 2015;132(15):1435–1486.

27. ANSWER: D. Nuclear stress test with regadenoson

This woman presents with a chest pain syndrome. She has an intermediate pretest probability of coronary artery disease based on her age and the characteristics of her pain. Hence, a form of stress testing is appropriate rather than reassurance. Her severe knee osteoarthritis and lumbar disc disease make it unlikely that exercise as a stressor will yield diagnostic information; that is, it is unlikely she could exercise on a treadmill to reach her target heart rate. A dobutamine stress echocardiogram could be considered, but the presence of left bundle branch block makes image interpretation in this setting more difficult, although not impossible. Nuclear stress testing with exercise in patients with left bundle branch block can produce a perfusion abnormality in the septum, and therefore pharmacologic stress testing is preferred in these patients. The best diagnostic test for this patient who cannot exercise with a left bundle branch block is a pharmacologic nuclear stress test.

Wolk MJ, Bailey SR, Doherty JU, et al. ACCF/AHA/ASE/ASNC/HFSA/HRS/SCAI/SCCT/SCMR/STS 2013 multimodality appropriate use criteria for the detection and risk assessment of stable ischemic heart disease: a report of the American College of Cardiology Foundation Appropriate Use Criteria Task Force, American Heart Association, American Society of Echocardiography, American Society of Nuclear Cardiology, Heart Failure Society of America, Heart Rhythm Society, Society for Cardiovascular Angiography and Interventions, Society of Cardiovascular Computed Tomography, Society for Cardiovascular Magnetic Resonance, and Society of Thoracic Surgeons. *J Am Coll Cardiol.* 2014;63(4):380–406.

28. ANSWER: A. Supervised exercise program

This patient with tobacco use history presents with typical claudication and ankle-brachial index confirming moderate peripheral arterial disease (PAD). Patients with PAD are also at risk for atherosclerosis of other arterial beds, so an aggressive regimen of antihypertensive, antiplatelet, and lipid therapy is mandatory. To treat PAD that is moderate and not limb threatening, an exercise program has been demonstrated to increase pain-free walking distance and is an effective initial therapy. The data for efficacy of pentoxifylline are marginal; cilostazol can be effective in increasing walking distance, but it should be avoided in patients with heart failure. Cilostazol can be used in conjunction with an exercise program. Detailed anatomic imaging should be pursued if limb-threatening ischemia is present or if medical therapy fails and revascularization is being considered; referral for revascularization would be premature at this time.

Gerhard-Herman MD, Gornik HL, Barrett C, et al. 2016 AHA/ACC Guideline on the Management of Patients With Lower Extremity Peripheral Artery Disease: a report of the American College of Cardiology/American Heart Association Task Force on Clinical Practice Guidelines. *Circulation.* 2017;135(12):e726–e779.

29. ANSWER: B. Aortic valve replacement

This patient presents with bicuspid aortic valve and severe aortic regurgitation (AR). Patients with AR should be referred for surgery if symptoms are present, as in this case. If patients have asymptomatic severe AR, they should undergo valve replacement when the ejection fraction begins to fall or when the left ventricle begins to dilate; repair at this stage forestalls the eventual development of dilated cardiomyopathy associated with chronic volume loading of the left ventricle. Bicuspid valve can be associated with aortic root dilation that in some instances mandates concomitant aortic root repair, but the aortic root diameter in this case is normal. Trials of afterload reduction in aortic insufficiency have been negative, and medical therapy specifically for AR is not indicated. Serial echocardiography would not be appropriate in this patient with symptomatic severe AR. Finally, the brisk carotid impulses are an expected finding in severe AR and do not mandate a carotid imaging study.

Nishinura RA, Otto CM, Bonow RO, et al. 2017 AHA/ACC Focused Update of the 2014 AHA/ACC Guideline for the Management of Patients With Valvular Heart Disease: a report of the American College of Cardiology/American Heart Association Task Force on Clinical Practice Guidelines. *Circulation.* 2017;135(25):e1159–e1195.

30. ANSWER: D. Obtain detailed over-the-counter medication use history.

This patient presents with apparent resistant hypertension, defined as blood pressure that is uncontrolled despite use of three medications at good doses, one of which is a diuretic. The first step in management of resistant hypertension is to confirm the diagnosis, and a home blood pressure diary or 24-hour ambulatory blood pressure monitoring can be used for confirmation. Next, ensure good medication compliance because noncompliance is a frequent cause of apparently resistant hypertension. Medications that can contribute to hypertension, including possible NSAID use in this case as well as sympathomimetics, should be minimized. Alcohol intake and obstructive sleep apnea also can contribute to poorly controlled hypertension.

Secondary causes of hypertension can be evaluated, including Cushing syndrome, hyperaldosteronism, thyroid disease, and renal artery disease, although these conditions are less common than the aforementioned causes, which should be excluded first.

Braam B, Taler SJ, Rahman M, et al. Recognition and management of resistant hypertension. *Clin J Am Soc Nephrol.* 2017;12(3):524–535.

31. ANSWER: D. Refer for coronary artery bypass grafting of the LAD artery and RCA.

This patient with diabetes and normal left ventricular function presents with obstructive coronary stenoses in two vessels, one of which is the proximal left anterior descending artery. Coronary artery bypass grafting has been demonstrated to be superior to medical therapy in such patients and is a class I recommendation in current guidelines. PCI of one or both lesions could be considered if the patient were a poor candidate for surgery, in which case physiologic information, such as with stress myocardial perfusion imaging (MPI) or FFR, about the extent and anatomic distribution of ischemia may be helpful to guide revascularization. Regardless of the method of revascularization, aggressive medical therapy should be instituted with good control of blood pressure and lipids as well as antiplatelet therapy with aspirin. Other class I indications for coronary artery bypass surgery include patients with stenoses greater than 70% in three coronary vessels and those patients with left main coronary artery stenosis greater than 50%. In a subset of patients with anatomically amenable coronary artery disease who are at high risk for bypass surgery, PCI could be considered.

Hillis LD, Smith PK, Anderson JL, et al. 2011 ACCF/AHA guideline for coronary artery bypass graft surgery: executive summary: a report of the American College of Cardiology Foundation/American Heart Association Task Force on Practice Guidelines. *J Thorac Cardiovasc Surg.* 2012;143(1):4–34.

32. ANSWER: D. Repeat abdominal ultrasound in 6 months.

This patient presents with an asymptomatic abdominal aortic aneurysm (AAA) measuring 4.1 cm. AAA should be repaired electively when greater than 5.5 cm or when expanding greater than 0.5 cm in 6 months or 1.0 cm in 1 year. If repair is planned, detailed anatomic information should be obtained with an imaging study such as a CT angiogram, which can help guide the choice of endovascular versus open repair. Prior to repair, patients should be optimized medically, although stress testing should be recommended only if it would affect management and lead to preoperative coronary angiography and revascularization. AAA between 4 and 5.5 cm should be followed with an imaging study every 6–12 months; AAA smaller than 4 cm can be followed at a lesser interval, every 1–3 years unless new symptoms emerge. AAA is considered a coronary risk equivalent, and all patients should undergo aggressive therapy of hypertension and dyslipidemia as well as smoking cessation.

Rooke TW, Hirsch AT, Misra S, et al. 2011 ACCF/AHA Focused Update of the Guideline for the Management of Patients With Peripheral Artery Disease (updating the 2005 guideline): a report of the American College of Cardiology Foundation/American Heart Association Task Force on Practice Guidelines. *J Am Coll Cardiol.* 2011;58(19):2020–2045.

33. ANSWER: C. Add lisinopril.

This patient with prior myocardial infarction now presents with systolic heart failure. In addition to a diagnostic evaluation to determine underlying contributors to systolic dysfunction, appropriate pharmacotherapy should be provided. The calcium channel blocker may impair LV function and should be stopped. First-line therapy for patients with systolic dysfunction include blockade of the renin-angiotensin-aldosterone system with an angiotensin-converting enzyme (ACE) inhibitor or an angiotensin receptor blocker (ARB) coupled with a beta blocker (carvedilol, extended-release metoprolol, bisoprolol, and nebivolol are the agents that have been evaluated in randomized controlled trials for use in heart failure). This patient has been maintained on beta blockers for coronary disease, and lisinopril should be added and uptitrated as able while following blood pressure, serum potassium, and renal function. Hydralazine and nitrates can be used in patients intolerant of ACE and ARB and also have been shown to have incremental benefit in African American patients with heart failure, but they would not be a first-line therapy in this case. There is no indication for dual antiplatelet therapy with aspirin and clopidogrel. Spironolactone should be prescribed for patients with heart failure with NYHA class II or greater symptoms despite adequate doses of ACE inhibitors and beta blockers and normal potassium handing; there is a survival benefit with spironolactone treatment in this population. Digoxin can improve symptoms but offers no mortality benefit, and other agents should be optimized first.

Yancy CW, Jessup M, Bozkurt B, et al. 2013 ACCF/AHA guideline for the management of heart failure: a report of the American College of Cardiology Foundation/American Heart Association Task Force on Practice Guidelines. *J Am Coll Cardiol.* 2013;62(16):e147–e239.

34. ANSWER: C. Exercise treadmill test

This patient with multiple cardiac risk factors presents with substernal chest pain evoked by exertion and relieved with rest. In evaluation of the patient with chest pain, the pretest probability of coronary disease should be assessed. The patient's age and sex as well as the characteristics of the pain inform the pretest probability. In this case, the pretest probability of coronary artery disease is considered intermediate to high, and further evaluation with stress testing is appropriate. In patients where the pretest probability of coronary disease is low (<10%), a stress test that is positive likely represents a false-positive result. For patients with an intermediate pretest probability of coronary disease, stress testing is appropriate because the test characteristics meaningfully affect the posttest likelihood of disease. Research studies have yielded tools that can assist in estimating the pretest probability of coronary disease (Sox HC Jr, Hickam DH, Marton KI, et al. *Am J Med.* 1990;89:7–14). The coronary artery calcium score can be used to refine risk prediction in the primary prevention setting for patients at intermediate pretest risk of coronary disease, but at present it should not be used for patients with active cardiac symptoms. Proceeding directly to coronary angiography would be premature. Imaging with cardiac MRI can be useful in evaluation of pericardial disease of myopathic diseases; however, a stress test is more appropriate for this patient. Finally, an exercise test yields more hemodynamic data than a pharmacologic stress test and should be the first-line assessment in a patient who can exercise.

Wolk MJ, Bailey SR, Doherty JU, et al. ACCF/AHA/ASE/ASNC/HFSA/HRS/SCAI/SCCT/SCMR/STS 2013 multimodality appropriate use criteria for the detection and risk assessment of stable ischemic heart disease: a report of the American College of Cardiology Foundation Appropriate Use Criteria Task Force, American Heart Association, American Society of Echocardiography, American Society of Nuclear Cardiology, Heart Failure Society of America, Heart Rhythm Society, Society for Cardiovascular Angiography and Interventions, Society of Cardiovascular Computed Tomography, Society for Cardiovascular Magnetic Resonance, and Society of Thoracic Surgeons. *J Am Coll Cardiol.* 2014;63(4):380–406.

35. ANSWER: E. Prescribe metoprolol.

This patient presents for preoperative risk stratification prior to lumbar laminectomy, an intermediate-risk noncardiac surgical procedure. There is no evidence of unstable cardiac conditions such as acute coronary syndrome, tachy- or bradydysrhythmia, or severe stenotic valvular disease that would preclude surgery, and the surgery is not emergent. The patient's functional capacity is limited secondary to back pain. She has multiple risk factors for a perioperative coronary event, including creatinine >2.0 mg/dL, diabetes requiring insulin, and a history of cerebrovascular disease. Other risk factors include a history of heart failure and a history of coronary artery disease. Of note, when left anterior fascicular block is present, Q waves must be visualized from V1 through V3 to diagnose septal myocardial infarction. For patients with three of these risk factors, beta blockers should be prescribed and uptitrated over the weeks prior to the perioperative period for a goal heart rate of 55–65 beats per minute. Stress testing and coronary imaging should be pursued only as part of the preoperative evaluation if it would affect management—that is, if revascularization with coronary artery bypass grafting or PCI would follow if needed, and no trial to date has demonstrated the benefit of routine revascularization prior to noncardiac surgery. Given this patient's high risk, however, proceeding to surgery without beta blockade would not be appropriate.

36. ANSWER: D. Referral for surgical removal

This young patient presents with a cardiac mass that was incidentally discovered. Causes of intracardiac masses include thrombi, infectious and noninfectious vegetations, and cardiac tumors. Given lack of fever or other symptoms and lack of comorbidities, this is unlikely to represent a thrombus or vegetation. The description of a pedunculated mass attached to the interatrial septum by a thin stalk is consistent with atrial myxoma, which is the most common primary tumor of the heart. Myxomas should be removed surgically due to a risk of embolism; atrial myxomas can also secrete cytokines, leading to constitutional symptoms and paraimmune phenomena. Prognosis is good with surgical removal.

37. ANSWER: E. Referral for pacemaker placement

This patient presents with symptomatic sinus bradycardia and failure to augment the heart rate with exercise. Causes of sinus bradycardia include hypothyroidism, medications, and degenerative conduction system disease—the sick sinus syndrome. Given that thyroid function studies are normal and the patient is on no agents that would depress sinus node function, the most likely diagnosis is sick sinus syndrome with chronotropic incompetence. Pacemaker implantation is indicated for the symptomatic bradycardia. There is no indication for further confirmation and correlation of symptoms with arrhythmia using a 48-hour Holter monitor. Event monitors are best for diagnosis of paroxysmal symptoms hypothesized to be related to dysrhythmia. There are no symptoms to suggest Lyme disease. Sick sinus syndrome is a clinical diagnosis, and invasive measurement of the sinus node recovery time (a marker of sinus node function) is rarely performed.

38. ANSWER: C. Give the patient a home blood pressure diary, measure TSH, and repeat office blood pressure in 3 months.

This patient presents with a single elevated blood pressure reading in the office in the setting of a recent normal blood pressure reading outside the office. The funduscopic examination reveals no evidence of chronic hypertension; these facts should raise the question whether white coat hypertension is present. A home blood pressure diary, or ambulatory 24-hour blood pressure measurement if available, may help clarify whether sustained hypertension is present, and office blood pressure should be repeated at a follow-up visit. Given the abnormal thyroid on examination, hyperthyroidism as a cause of elevated blood pressure should be excluded. Patients with white coat hypertension have a risk of developing sustained hypertension and should be followed. There are no symptoms to suggest pheochromocytoma. White coat hypertension should be excluded before further evaluation for hyperaldosteronism and renal artery stenosis is undertaken. Empiric therapy is not indicated, given that only a single elevated blood pressure has been documented.

39. ANSWER: B. Refer for PCI of the obtuse marginal stenosis.

This patient presented originally with chest pain and was diagnosed with coronary disease with moderate middle LAD artery stenosis and obstructive disease in the left circumflex system. Despite aggressive medical therapy, lifestyle-limiting angina persists; because of refractory symptoms, revascularization should be pursued. Given that only a single vessel is affected with greater than 70% stenosis, PCI would be favored over bypass surgery. Increasing the dose of metoprolol would be limited by heart rate, and increase of nitrates would be limited by blood pressure.

Cardiac rehabilitation could be considered, but this patient is already fit and active, and conditioning is unlikely to lead to abatement of symptoms.

Fihn SD, Blankenship JC, Alexander KP, et al. 2014 ACC/AHA/AATS/PCNA/SCAI/STS focused update of the guideline for the diagnosis and management of patients with stable ischemic heart disease: a report of the American College of Cardiology/American Heart Association Task Force on Practice Guidelines, and the American Association for Thoracic Surgery, Preventive Cardiovascular Nurses Association, Society for Cardiovascular Angiography and Interventions, and Society of Thoracic Surgeons. *J Am Coll Cardiol.* 2014;64(18):1929–1949.

40. ANSWER: D. Transcatheter aortic valve replacement

This patient presents with radiation-induced severe symptomatic aortic stenosis. If left untreated, symptomatic aortic stenosis is associated with a high rate of death. He is at very high risk for adverse outcomes after surgery due to his prior chest radiation and prior cardiac surgery. Such high-risk patients with a "hostile chest" were enrolled in the inoperable arm of the PARTNER trial, which randomized patients to transcatheter aortic valve replacement (TAVR) or standard therapy. Compared with standard therapy, which often included balloon valvuloplasty, TAVR reduced the rates of death and hospitalization as well as improved symptoms and valvular hemodynamics over a follow-up period of 2 years.

Makkar RR, Fontana GP, Jilaihawi H, et al. Transcatheter aortic-valve replacement for inoperable severe aortic stenosis. *N Engl J Med.* 2012;366(18):1696–1704.

41. ANSWER: D. Close follow-up with a transthoracic echocardiogram every 6–12 months

The patient has severe mitral regurgitation secondary to mitral valve prolapse and a flail mitral leaflet. She is otherwise asymptomatic and has no evidence of heart failure on examination. Her echocardiogram shows preserved left ventricular function and dimensions. The class I indications for mitral valve surgery for primary severe mitral regurgitation include (1) symptomatic severe mitral regurgitation in patients with left ventricular ejection fraction >30% and (2) asymptomatic patients with severe mitral regurgitation and left ventricular dysfunction (ejection fraction 30%–60%, left ventricular end-systolic dimension ≥40 mm). This patient does not meet either of the criteria. Mitral valve repair is preferred to replacement for mitral valve prolapse. MitraClip is reserved for patients who have prohibitive surgical risk. Vasodilators are not indicated in the absence of elevated blood pressure. The most appropriate next step is close follow-up with referral for surgery once surgical criteria are met.

Nishinura RA, Otto CM, Bonow RO, et al. 2017 AHA/ACC Focused Update of the 2014 AHA/ACC Guideline for the Management of Patients With Valvular Heart Disease: a report of the American College of Cardiology/American Heart Association Task Force on Clinical Practice Guidelines. *Circulation.* 2017;135(25):e1159–e1195.

42. ANSWER: C. Stop lisinopril and start sacubitril/valsartan 49/51 mg twice daily after 36-hour washout.

The PARADIGM-HF trial randomized patients with symptomatic (NYHA class II-IV) heart failure and a left ventricular ejection fraction <40% to either the angiotensin receptor-neprilysin inhibitor (ARNI), sacubitril/valsartan, or enalapril in addition to recommended heart failure therapy. In this trial, sacubitril/valsartan reduced the composite endpoint of cardiovascular death and heart failure hospitalizations by 20% compared with enalapril alone over a median follow-up of 27 months. On the basis of these results, the

AHA/ACC/HFSA issued a guideline update recommending that in patients with symptomatic systolic heart failure who are able to tolerate an angiotensin-converting enzyme inhibitor or angiotensin receptor blocker, the angiotensin-converting enzyme inhibitor or angiotensin receptor blocker should be replaced with an angiotensin receptor-neprilysin inhibitor to reduce morbidity and mortality. Because of the risk of angioedema, patients should not start taking the angiotensin receptor-neprilysin inhibitor for at least 36 hours after their last dose of angiotensin-converting enzyme inhibitor or angiotensin receptor blocker. The patient is on a good dose of lisinopril and therefore would tolerate initiation of an ARNI, which is preferred to increasing lisinopril. The patient does not have increased intravascular volume, and therefore torsemide does not need to be increased. Digoxin has been associated with no mortality benefit in heart failure.

McMurray JJV, Packer M, Desai AS, et al. Angiotensin-neprilysin inhibition versus enalapril in heart failure. *N Engl J Med.* 2014;371(11):993–1004.

43. ANSWER: B. Add digoxin

The patient is complaining of postural lightheadedness and has borderline blood pressure and no evidence of jugular venous distention. Therefore increasing her furosemide dose does not seem appropriate. She is in atrial fibrillation, and improved rate control may help her symptoms. She does not have adequate blood pressure for uptitration of metoprolol, and therefore adding digoxin seems appropriate. In the PARADIGM-HF trial, patients had to tolerate a minimum dose of enalapril 10 mg daily prior to randomization, owing to the vasodilatory effects of sacubitril/valsartan. This patient is on a very low dose of lisinopril with marginal blood pressure and therefore would not be an ideal candidate to switch to sacubitril/valsartan. Ivabradine lowers the heart rate by inhibiting the funny channel in the sinoatrial node. In the SHIFT trial, patients with symptomatic heart failure and left ventricular ejection fraction ≤35% who were in sinus rhythm with a heart rate ≥70 beats per minute despite maximally tolerated beta blockers were randomized to receive ivabradine or placebo on top of guideline-based medical therapy. Ivabradine lowered heart rate and reduced heart failure hospitalizations compared with placebo. This patient is not a good candidate for ivabradine, because she is in atrial fibrillation.

Swedberg K, Komajda M, Böhm M, et al. Ivabradine and outcomes in chronic heart failure (SHIFT): a randomised placebo-controlled study. *Lancet.* 2010;376(9744):875–885.

44. ANSWER: B. Intravenous heparin

Patients who present with shock or persistent hypotension from massive pulmonary embolus are considered high risk and benefit from systemic thrombolytic therapy. Catheter-directed thrombolysis can be considered in patients with hemodynamic decompensation and high bleeding risk with systemic thrombolysis. Patients with submassive pulmonary embolus present with hemodynamic stability but with right ventricular dysfunction and positive biomarkers. Systemic thrombolysis has an unfavorable risk-to-benefit ratio in these patients. Patients with hemodynamic stability and negative biomarkers are considered low risk and should be treated with intravenous heparin followed by chronic anticoagulation with warfarin or direct oral anticoagulants for at least 3 months. Routine use of inferior vena cava filters is not recommended in patients who can receive anticoagulation.

Konstantinides SV, Barco S, Lankeit M, Meyer G. Management of pulmonary embolism: an update. *J Am Coll Cardiol.* 2016;67(8):976–990.

45. ANSWER: E. Ketoconazole

Absorption of apixaban is mediated by P-glycoprotein (P-gp). P-gp inhibitors can increase absorption of apixaban and thus apixaban levels. Metabolism of apixaban is mediated by CYP3A4. CYP3A4 inhibitors can decrease the metabolism of apixaban and increase levels. Drugs that are inhibitors of both P-gp and CYP3A4 are therefore more likely to interact with apixaban and increase the risk of bleeding than drugs that inhibit either P-gp or CYP3A4 alone. Ketoconazole is an inhibitor of P-gp and a strong inhibitor of CYP3A4. Sotalol is not metabolized and therefore does not interfere with either P-gp or CYP3A4. Amiodarone and verapamil are inhibitors of p-GP and moderate inhibitors of CYP3A4; they can be used with apixaban in patients with normal renal function with a mild increase in apixaban levels but should not be used in patients with creatinine clearance <30 ml/min, age >80, or body weight <60 kg. Phenytoin is an inducer of CYP3A4 and reduces apixaban levels.

Amin A, Deitelzweig S. A case-based approach to implementing guidelines for stroke prevention in patients with atrial fibrillation: balancing the risks and benefits. *Thromb J.* 2015;13:29.

46. ANSWER: D. Acute coronary dissection

Acute coronary dissection is a rare but well recognized complication of pregnancy that occurs most commonly in the third trimester or in the first 6 months after delivery. It occurs primarily in women >30 years of age and without traditional risk factors for atherosclerosis. Chest pain and shortness of breath are common symptoms, and the majority of patients present with an anterior ST elevation myocardial infarction. Acute coronary dissection is associated with a high rate of maternal and fetal mortality, and conservative management is favored in low-risk patients. Pregnancy is a hypercoagulable state, and the risk of acute pulmonary embolism is increased during pregnancy and in the postpartum period. This patient's EKG is not consistent with an acute pulmonary embolus. Amniotic fluid embolism is a life-threatening complication of pregnancy caused by the entry of amniotic fluid into the maternal circulation during labor or in the early postpartum period. It is characterized by cardiopulmonary collapse and disseminated intravascular coagulation (DIC) and is associated with increased maternal mortality. The patient's presentation is not consistent with amniotic fluid embolism. Peripartum cardiomyopathy is left ventricular dysfunction that occurs within the last month of pregnancy and the first 5 months after delivery, without any other identifiable cause. It is associated with shortness of breath but does not have ST elevations on an EKG. The most common pericardial complication in pregnancy is hydropericardium, which is characterized by a small, asymptomatic pericardial effusion that occurs in 40% of women in the third trimester of pregnancy. This patient's presentation and EKG are not consistent with acute pericarditis.

Havakuk O, Goland S, Mehra A, Elkayam U. Pregnancy and the risk of spontaneous coronary artery dissection: an analysis of 120 contemporary cases. *Circ Cardiovasc Interv.* 2017;10(3):e004941.

47. ANSWER: D. Start oral penicillin V 250 mg twice daily.

The patient's examination is consistent with rheumatic mitral stenosis. The severity of her mitral stenosis is mild based on her examination, and she is asymptomatic. The current guidelines recommend antibiotic prophylaxis for secondary prevention in patients with rheumatic fever and carditis. For patients with residual valvular disease, penicillin prophylaxis is recommended for 10 years from the last episode of acute rheumatic fever or until the age of 40. Antibiotic prophylaxis is no longer recommended for patients with mitral stenosis. Diuretic therapy is recommended for patients with symptoms of heart failure. Oral anticoagulation is indicated in the presence of atrial fibrillation or thromboembolic events. Beta blockers are recommended for rate control in patients with atrial fibrillation and can be considered in symptomatic patients with sinus rhythm to increase diastolic filling time and reduce left atrial pressures.

Gerber MA, Baltimore RS, Eaton CB, et al. Prevention of rheumatic fever and diagnosis and treatment of acute Streptococcal pharyngitis: a scientific statement from the American Heart Association Rheumatic Fever, Endocarditis, and Kawasaki Disease Committee of the Council on Cardiovascular Disease in the Young, the Interdisciplinary Council on Functional Genomics and Translational Biology, and the Interdisciplinary Council on Quality of Care and Outcomes Research: endorsed by the American Academy of Pediatrics. *Circulation.* 2009;119(11):1541–1551.

48. ANSWER: C. Ankle brachial index

The current guidelines recommend peripheral vascular disease screening for risk stratification, medical management, and reduction of cardiovascular events in asymptomatic high-risk patients (age ≥70 years, age ≥50 years with a history of smoking or diabetes, exertional leg symptoms, or nonhealing wounds). Screening for abdominal aortic aneurysms (AAAs) is recommended in men >60 years with a first-degree relative with an AAA or aged 65–75 years with a history of smoking. This patient is asymptomatic and at low risk for cardiovascular events (Framingham risk score <10%). Therefore routine exercise stress testing or coronary artery calcium scoring is not indicated. The patient's pooled cardiovascular risk score is >7.5%, and she would benefit from statin therapy for primary prevention of cardiovascular events.

Goff DC Jr, Lloyd-Jones DM, Bennett G, et al. 2013 ACC/AHA guideline on the assessment of cardiovascular risk: a report of the American College of Cardiology/American Heart Association Task Force on Practice Guidelines. *J Am Coll Cardiol.* 2014;63(25 Pt B):2935–2959.

49. ANSWER: A. Renal artery Doppler study

In a young patient with severe hypertension, one must evaluate secondary causes of hypertension. The most likely etiology in a young woman is fibromuscular dysplasia. Initial screening with renal Doppler can reveal increased velocities, and the next step would be evaluation with computed tomographic angiography or abdominal magnetic resonance angiography. Polysomnography can lead to the detection of obstructive sleep apnea, which can be a cause of hypertension, but this patient does not give a history that is consistent with obstructive sleep apnea. Pheochromocytoma is unlikely, given the lack of flushing, palpitations, or diaphoresis. Hyperaldosteronism is also unlikely, given normal electrolytes. A transthoracic echocardiogram may show left ventricular hypertrophy, but she is unlikely to have coarctation of the aorta, given the lack of a murmur and no delayed pulse in the lower extremities.

Vongpatanasin W. Resistant hypertension: a review of diagnosis and management. *JAMA.* 2014:311(21):2216–2224.

Acknowledgment

The author and editors gratefully acknowledge the contributions of the previous authors—Thomas S. Metkus Jr., Patrick O'Gara, and Donna M. Polk.

9 General Internal Medicine

LORI WIVIOTT TISHLER, SARAH P. HAMMOND, AND GALEN V. HENDERSON

1. A 55-year-old African American man comes for his first primary care office visit. He is without complaints but presents because his father had a myocardial infarction recently at age 75, and his mother is healthy at 74. He does not smoke. His blood pressure is 120/71 mm Hg on hydrochlorothiazide. His total cholesterol is 200 mg/dL, and his high-density lipoprotein (HDL) is 25 mg/dL. His 10-year risk for developing atherosclerotic cardiovascular disease, according to Pooled Cohort Equations, is 11.9%.

   Which of the following is the most appropriate management?
   - **A.** Recommend lifestyle change; follow up in 6 months.
   - **B.** Start a statin.
   - **C.** Obtain coronary calcium score.
   - **D.** Refer for cardiac stress test.
   - **E.** Refer for cardiac catheterization.

2. A 54-year-old woman with a remote history of migraines (but none in years) presents to her primary care physician with a new-onset headache. The pain is retroorbital on the right side only and has been progressive for 3 weeks with intermittent responsiveness to acetaminophen. She denies visual changes, fevers, chills, jaw claudication, or weakness. The result of her examination, including a thorough neurological examination, is normal.

   What is the most appropriate next step in management?
   - **A.** Prescribe oxycodone.
   - **B.** Order a head MRI/MRA.
   - **C.** Prescribe amitriptyline.
   - **D.** Prescribe sumatriptan.
   - **E.** Refer for physical therapy.

3. A 56-year-old woman with obesity who has not had a period for 5 years comes in for her routine Pap test. All of her Pap smears in the past have been normal and HPV negative. She is at low risk for cervical cancer and has been having screening Pap tests every 3–5 years with consistently negative HPV test results. Her cervical and vaginal examinations are entirely normal. Her Pap test result is notable for "benign endometrial cells." She has not had any vaginal bleeding.

   What is the best next step in management?
   - **A.** Nothing. The cells are benign; repeat at regular intervals until age 65.
   - **B.** Repeat in 6 months.
   - **C.** Refer for endometrial biopsy.
   - **D.** Repeat in 1 year.
   - **E.** Refer for colposcopy.

4. A 35-year-old woman presents to the clinic with her husband due to difficulty becoming pregnant. The couple has been trying to become pregnant for the last 6 months without success, despite having intercourse three times per week consistently. Her periods are usually regular on a 26-day cycle. Her partner had semen analysis, the result of which was normal. Her physical examination is unremarkable.

   What is the most appropriate next step in management?
   - **A.** Reassurance and workup in 6 months if still not pregnant
   - **B.** Day 20 serum progesterone
   - **C.** Hysterosalpingogram
   - **D.** Referral for in vitro fertilization
   - **E.** Day 20 luteinizing hormone (LH) and follicle-stimulating hormone (FSH)

5. A 30-year-old woman presents to the clinic complaining of bilateral breast pain. She states that the pain is worse toward the end of her menstrual cycle and also in the evening. She has had the pain for approximately 3 months and describes it as an aching, diffuse pain. Her examination is notable for a BMI of 28 kg/m^2 and pendulous breasts without erythema, masses, or discharge. She has no lymphadenopathy or skin changes. She is concerned that she may have cancer and tells you that her maternal grandmother had cancer at age 76.

   What is the best next step in management?
   - **A.** Bilateral mammography
   - **B.** Bilateral breast MRI

C. Bilateral breast ultrasound
D. BRCA testing
E. Reassurance and a more supportive bra

6. A 31-year-old man with a family history of Hashimoto thyroiditis presents to the clinic for evaluation of hair loss. He states that he noticed a small bald spot on his occiput several months ago. Hair did regrow in that area but was white instead of black. He now presents to the clinic because he has three well-circumscribed round areas of complete hair loss on his scalp as well as one in his beard. He otherwise denies any complaints. The result of a thyroid-stimulating hormone (TSH) laboratory test was within normal range.

What is the best next step in management?
A. Intradermal injection of triamcinolone
B. Minoxidil 2% solution applied twice a day
C. Biopsy of the bald area
D. Ketoconazole shampoo

7. A 36-year-old Ashkenazi Jewish woman comes to see you. She is concerned because her 45-year-old sister was diagnosed with premenopausal breast cancer. As you take her history, you learn that there are several other first-degree relatives who have had breast cancer or ovarian cancer. You use the Gail model to determine the patient's lifetime risk (based on your knowledge of when she had menarche, her family history, and absence of previous breast biopsies). You determine that she has a 25% lifetime risk of developing breast cancer. She and her family are considering genetic testing, and you refer her to a genetic counselor.

In the meantime, what is the best screening protocol for our patient?
A. Annual mammograms starting at age 40
B. Annual mammograms starting at age 45
C. Annual MRI starting now
D. Mammograms and MRI annually, ideally 6 months apart
E. MRI every 6 months

8. A 30-year-old man is evaluated in the emergency department (ED) for a 3-day history of confusion and visual loss, and he has a 4-day history of gradually increasing headache. One week ago, he had a bout of severe gastroenteritis with diarrhea. A review of his medical records shows that he has a heterozygous factor V Leiden mutation. His examination is remarkable for papilledema, a right pronator drift, right homonymous hemianopsia, and fluent aphasia. The results of a CT scan of the brain and laboratory studies are normal.

Which of the following is the most appropriate next diagnostic test for this patient?
A. Carotid ultrasonography
B. Electroencephalography (EEG)
C. Lumbar puncture (LP)
D. Magnetic resonance venography

9. A 69-year-old man is found to have an alkaline phosphatase level of 365 U/L. The results of radiographs and a radionuclide bone scan are consistent with Paget disease of the bone involving the left humerus, right ischium, and several vertebrae. The patient is asymptomatic.

What is the next best step in management at this time?
A. No further workup or treatment
B. Start an oral bisphosphonate.
C. Start an intravenous bisphosphonate.
D. Start calcitonin.
E. Refer for orthopedic surgery.

10. A 28-year-old woman calls the office with ongoing symptoms of dysuria, urgency, and frequency. She developed symptoms of a urinary tract infection 1 week ago that was treated with amoxicillin without resolution of her symptoms. Urine cultures were not sent at that time.

What is the next most appropriate step in management?
A. No further workup or treatment
B. Prescribe a 3-day course of levofloxacin.
C. Prescribe another 7-day course of amoxicillin.
D. Prescribe a 5-day course of nitrofurantoin.
E. Prescribe a 3-day course of ciprofloxacin.

11. A 62-year-old man with a history of gout who is taking allopurinol 300 mg presents after a recently inflamed first metatarsal joint. A joint aspiration showed monosodium urate crystals within neutrophils. He is currently asymptomatic, but this is his second gout flare in the last 3 months. He has a history of hypertension and is being treated with lisinopril. He states that he is taking all of his medications regularly. His serum creatinine is 0.9 mg/dL, and his serum uric acid is 8.3 mg/dL.

What is the next best step in management?
A. No further workup or treatment
B. Increase allopurinol with concurrent colchicine.
C. Colchicine alone
D. Switch allopurinol to febuxostat.
E. Switch allopurinol to probenecid.

12. A 37-year-old man presented to his primary care physician with epigastric discomfort and was found to be *Helicobacter pylori* positive. He did not have melena, weight loss, or any other concerning features. He was treated with omeprazole 20 mg twice daily, amoxicillin 1 g twice daily, and clarithromycin 500 mg twice daily for 14 days. He now represents with the same epigastric discomfort.

What is the next best step in management?

A. Empirically treat with the same regimen for 14 days.
B. Empirically treat with omeprazole 20 mg twice daily, bismuth subsalicylate two tabs four times per day, tetracycline 500 mg four times daily, and metronidazole 250 mg four times per day.
C. Order a repeat serology to confirm persistence of *H. pylori.*
D. Order a urea breath test to confirm persistence of *H. pylori.*

13. A 31-year-old monogamous woman with no past medical history presents for a routine Papanicolaou (Pap) smear. The cytological result is negative for intraepithelial lesion or malignancy. Reflex DNA testing for high-risk human papillomavirus (HPV) is performed, and the result is negative.

What is the next step in management?

A. Repeat cytology in 6 months.
B. Repeat cytology in 1 year.
C. Repeat cytology in 2 years.
D. Repeat cytology in 3 years.
E. Repeat cytology in 5 years.

14. A 22-year-old woman sustained a compound tibial fracture during a motor vehicle accident requiring surgery. Her hospital course was complicated by lower extremity deep venous thrombosis (DVT). She has no family history of pulmonary embolism or DVT, and the result of a hypercoagulability workup is negative. She is not taking any medication.

She is started on low-molecular-weight heparin followed by warfarin and achieves a target INR of 2.5.

How long should she be anticoagulated?

A. 1 months
B. 3 months
C. 6–12 months
D. Lifelong anticoagulation

15. A 19-year-old woman presents with 3 days of increasing vaginal discharge. She is sexually active with one partner. Her last menstrual period was 4 days ago. Physical examination reveals temperature 99°F, blood pressure 100/60 mm Hg, and heart rate of 90 beats per minute. Her pelvic examination shows copious mucopurulent discharge from a red, inflamed cervix. She has tenderness on palpation of the cervix but no adnexal or uterine tenderness. The result of a pregnancy test is negative, and you send a gonorrhea/chlamydia probe that returns positive for gonorrhea.

What is the next management step?

A. Ceftriaxone 125 mg intramuscular injection × 1
B. Ceftriaxone 250 mg intramuscular injection × 1
C. Ceftriaxone 125 mg intramuscular injection × 1 + azithromycin 1 g orally × 1
D. Ceftriaxone 250 mg intramuscular injection × 1 + azithromycin 1 g orally × 1
E. Doxycycline 100 mg orally twice daily × 7 days

16. A 35-year-old man presents to an urgent care facility with a 2-week history of worsening purulent rhinorrhea and right-sided maxillary sinus pain. His symptoms have persisted despite treatment with acetaminophen, fluticasone propionate, and saline irrigation. Examination is notable for a temperature of 101.5°F, copious rhinorrhea, and tenderness with percussion over the maxillary sinuses. The results of cardiac and pulmonary examinations are unremarkable.

He takes hydrochlorothiazide 25 mg daily and amlodipine 5 mg daily for hypertension. He has no known drug allergies.

What is the most appropriate next step in management?

A. Amoxicillin 500 mg three times daily × 5–7 days
B. Amoxicillin/clavulanate 500/125 mg three times daily × 5–7 days
C. Azithromycin 500 mg po × 1 then 250 mg po daily × 4 days
D. Doxycycline 200 mg once daily × 5–7 days
E. Levofloxacin 750 mg daily × 5–7 days

17. A 34-year-old woman is seen in the emergency department with confusion, malaise, and lower extremity rash. Her past medical history is notable for allergic rhinitis. Her medications include loratadine and fluticasone propionate nasal spray. The patient is alert and oriented to self only. Physical examination is notable for jaundice and bilateral lower extremity petechiae. Laboratory data are notable for a hemoglobin of 7 g/dL, reticulocyte count of 15%, and platelets of 45,000/μL. The patient's lactate dehydrogenase (LDH) level is 1500 mg/dL. The results of coagulation studies are normal. Her serum creatinine is 3.6 mg/dL. A peripheral smear is shown in Fig. 9.1.

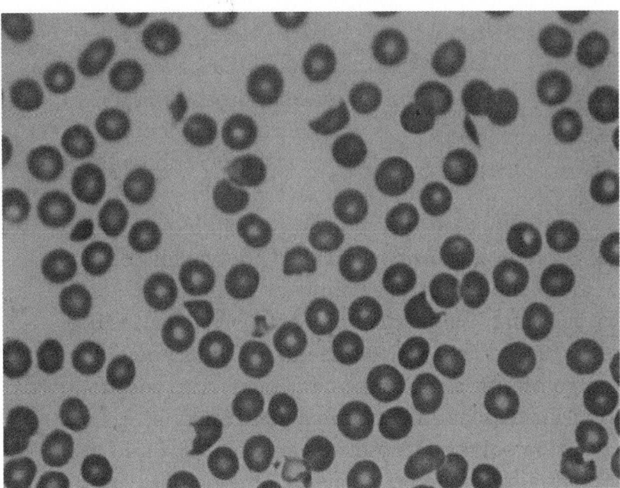

• **Fig. 9.1** Peripheral blood smear for patient in Question 17.

Which of the following is the best next step?
A. Intravenous immunoglobulin
B. Antinuclear antibody test
C. Plasma exchange
D. Transthoracic echocardiogram
E. Direct antiglobulin (Coombs) test

18. An 80-year-old man is reevaluated after a 5-mm left middle cerebral artery aneurysm is discovered incidentally on an MRI of the brain obtained because of headaches. The patient has no other relevant personal or family medical history and takes no medications. On physical examination, the patient's blood pressure is 140/80 mm Hg, and his pulse is 80 beats per minute. Results of his physical and neurological examinations are normal. An MRA scan shows an unruptured aneurysm but no additional intracranial aneurysms. No hemorrhage, infarction, mass, or mass effect is evident.

Which of the following is the most appropriate next step in the management of this patient's aneurysm?
A. Annual MRA
B. Endovascular coiling of the aneurysm
C. Nimodipine administration
D. Surgical clipping of the aneurysm

19. A 51-year-old man from western Massachusetts presents to his primary care physician with a fever and rash of 1 week's duration. He has no other symptoms. On examination, the rash is consistent with erythema migrans.

What is the next best step in management?
A. Doxycycline 200 mg × 1
B. Azithromycin 500 mg × 1 day, then 250 mg × 4 days
C. Amoxicillin-clavulanate 500/125 mg three times per day × 2 weeks
D. Doxycycline 100 mg twice daily × 2 weeks
E. Ceftriaxone 2 g IV daily × 3 weeks

20. A 68-year-old woman presents to her primary care doctor with parasthesias in her right foot, progressive right-sided foot drop, and erythematous rashes over both lower extremities. Five months ago, she had cough, sputum production, and a chest x-ray with patchy infiltrates, prompting treatment with antibiotics. She was diagnosed with asthma 2 years earlier. Laboratory data show a white blood cell count 9600/μL, hematocrit 36.2%, platelets 271,000/μL, with 58% neutrophils, 9% lymphocytes, and 31% eosinophils.

Which of the following diseases is most likely to be the cause of the patient's presentation?
A. Granulomatosis with polyangiitis (formerly Wegener granulomatosis)
B. Temporal arteritis
C. Schistosomiasis
D. Eosinophilic granulomatosis with polyangiitis
E. Hodgkin disease

21. An 18-year-old man presents for a physical examination prior to joining his college basketball team. A II/VI crescendo–decrescendo murmur without radiation is heard at the left lower sternal border on cardiac examination. The murmur increases with Valsalva maneuvers, and there is an extra heart sound preceding S1.

What is the most likely underlying etiology?
A. Congenital aortic stenosis
B. Marfan syndrome
C. Hypertrophic cardiomyopathy
D. Early-onset hypertension
E. Rheumatic heart disease

22. A 22-year-old male college football player without a significant past medical history presents to the emergency room with a small abscess on his neck. The collection is drained, and a Gram stain demonstrates gram-positive cocci in clusters.

What treatment would you prescribe?
A. Oral vancomycin
B. Dicloxacillin
C. Oral trimethoprim-sulfamethoxazole
D. Oral penicillin
E. Intravenous nafcillin

23. A 23-year-old man with a history of mild asthma presents for evaluation of intermittent dysphagia for solid foods. He denies heartburn. He has not lost weight. He reports that 1 year ago he underwent an upper endoscopy for removal of pieces of steak. He has taken 40 mg of omeprazole twice daily for the last month, but his symptoms have persisted.

His physical examination was unremarkable. An upper endoscopy reveals circular rings in the mid-esophagus. A biopsy shows a dense eosinophilic infiltrate.

Which of the following is the most appropriate first-line therapy?
A. Increase the omeprazole to 80 mg twice daily.
B. Esophageal dilation
C. Topical swallowed fluticasone
D. Oral nifedipine
E. Botulinum toxin injection into the lower esophageal sphincter

24. At a routine health review appointment, a 36-year-old man with type 1 diabetes blurts out, "This sweating thing is ruining my life." He goes on to explain that he has to change his clothes at work because of underarm sweating, tries not to shake hands, and has been missing out on getting together with friends. He notes that his wife is really upset by it. The sweating is not a lifelong problem. In fact, it has been notable that he has had it for only a couple of years. He is not particularly anxious and denies any symptoms of hypo- or hyperthyroidism. There does not seem to be a family history of this condition. It does not seem to be related to anxiety, to fluctuations in his blood sugar, to his hemoglobin A1c, or to any other conditions. He takes long- and short-acting human insulin, lisinopril, and atorvastatin.

What can you do for this distressed patient with hyperhidrosis?

A. Start an SSRI or SNRI; he is obviously too anxious.
B. Stop the lisinopril, and see if he improves.
C. Do a thorough evaluation for lymphoma, including blood tests and scans.
D. Check his TSH and liver function tests (LFTs). If they are normal, treat symptomatically.

25. A 35-year-old man presents to his primary care physician for a routine physical examination. His only medical history includes seasonal allergies, for which he uses intranasal fluticasone. He does not smoke cigarettes or drink alcohol. He has no family history of colorectal cancer, although his mother did have two adenomatous polyps at age 55.

When should he undergo his first screening colonoscopy?

A. Now
B. Age 40 years
C. Age 45 years
D. Age 50 years

26. A 70-year-old woman presents with pain in her hands and wrists of 9 months' duration. Her hands are stiff in the morning for 15 minutes. She has pain with sewing and typing. She has not noticed swelling or warmth. Her vital signs are normal. Her bilateral proximal interphalangeal joints are tender to palpation and have bony enlargements. The first carpometacarpal joints are also tender, and the palms appear "square" due to misalignment of the thumb base. The result of her metacarpal squeeze test is negative. The remainder of her examination is normal.

Which of the following studies should be done to establish the diagnosis?

A. ANA
B. Erythrocyte sedimentation rate
C. Bilateral x-rays of the hands
D. Anticitrullinated protein antibody
E. No additional studies are needed.

27. A 68-year-old man with a history of hypertension and gout presents for his routine annual examination. He has no complaints. He was a past smoker for 20 years but quit 30 years ago. He drinks one glass of red wine daily. He goes on long walks daily for exercise. He gets his flu shot annually, and he received his pneumococcal vaccine 3 years ago. He had a normal colonoscopy 7 years ago. He is on amlodipine and allopurinol. His vital signs are normal, and his physical examination is unremarkable.

Which of the following screening tests is most appropriate for this patient based on most evidence of benefit?

A. Coronary calcium CT imaging
B. Prostate-specific antigen
C. Thyroid-stimulating hormone
D. Abdominal ultrasound
E. Exercise treadmill test

28. An 80-year-old man is evaluated in the office for an episode of hesitancy in speech and word-finding difficulty, right facial weakness, and weak right arm. The episode occurred early yesterday, lasted 20 minutes, and was witnessed by his wife. The patient has a history of coronary artery disease, hypertension, and hyperlipidemia. His current medications are metoprolol, aspirin, hydrochlorothiazide, and lovastatin. On examination, his blood pressure is 150/80, and his heart rate is 70 beats per minute. The result of a neurological examination is normal.

Which of the following is the most appropriate next step in management?

A. Add clopidogrel.
B. Admit to the hospital.
C. Order outpatient diagnostic studies.
D. Schedule a follow-up visit in 1 week.

29. A 32-year-old man is evaluated for what he calls a "sinus headache." The headache occurs two or three times per month and is accompanied by facial pressure and occasional rhinorrhea; it worsens with movement. Resting in a dark, quiet room results in subjective improvement. The symptoms resolve in 1 or 2 days, regardless of treatment. He has tried multiple varieties of decongestants and antihistamines without success. Acetaminophen-aspirin-caffeine preparations offer minimal relief. He is currently symptomatic.

On examination, the patient is pale and moderately distressed. His temperature is 37.1°C (98.8°F), heart rate is 84 beats per minute, respiration rate is 16 breaths per minute, and blood pressure is 132/75 mm Hg. His face is tender on palpation.

What is the most likely diagnosis?

A. Cluster headache
B. Migraine without aura
C. Sinus headache
D. Tension headache

30. A 55-year-old obese (BMI, 35 kg/m^2) woman with a history of hyperlipidemia and hypertension presents for follow-up after a recent liver biopsy for

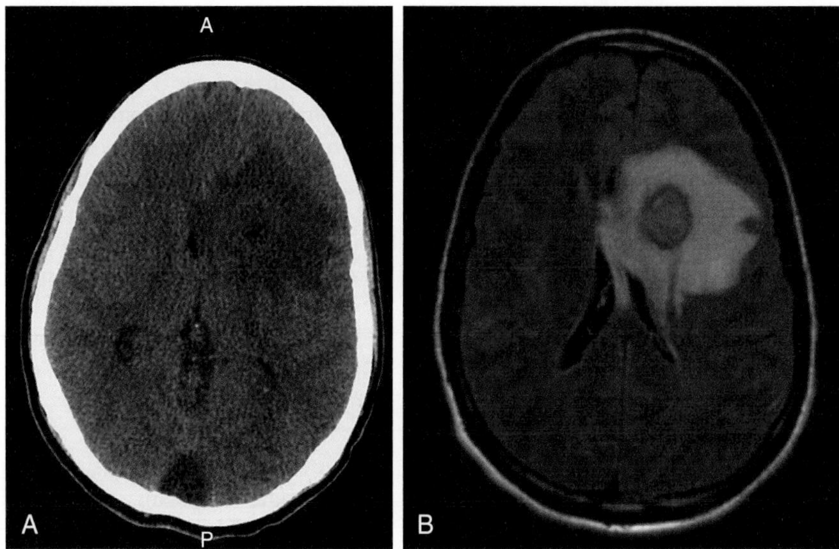

• **Fig. 9.2** (A) Noncontrast head computed tomography. (B) Axial T2-weighted FLAIR magnetic resonance imaging. Both images are from the patient described in Question 31.

evaluation of persistently abnormal aminotransferases. She has no history of heavy alcohol use. Her medications include atorvastatin and hydrochlorothiazide (HCTZ). Her alanine transaminase (ALT) was 85 U/L (reference range, 0–35 U/L), and her aspartate transaminase (AST) was 66 U/L (reference range, 0–35 U/L). The results of viral serologic testing and autoimmune markers were negative. An abdominal ultrasound revealed hepatic steatosis. She underwent a liver biopsy, which showed steatosis with inflammation consistent with steatohepatitis and stage 2 fibrosis.

In addition to weight loss, which of the following would you recommend?

A. Pioglitazone
B. Vitamin E
C. Metformin
D. No additional therapy

31. A 32-year-old man with no past medical history presents with low-grade fevers, anorexia, headache, and neck stiffness of 4 days' duration, which started shortly after a dental procedure. The night prior to presentation, he had one episode of emesis and a worsening posterior headache. This morning, his wife noticed that he seemed "not quite himself" and was "walking into walls," prompting her to bring him to the emergency department. In the emergency department, he undergoes head imaging, as shown in Fig. 9.2A, B.

What are the most likely diagnosis and best next management choice?

A. Meningitis: treatment with ceftazidime, vancomycin, and micafungin
B. Meningitis: treatment with ceftriaxone, vancomycin, and ampicillin
C. Brain abscess: treatment with ceftazidime, vancomycin, micafungin, and acyclovir
D. Ruptured brain abscess: treatment with ceftriaxone, vancomycin, and ampicillin, with neurosurgery consultation if symptoms do not improve with 24 hours of antibiotics
E. Ruptured brain abscess: treatment with ceftriaxone, vancomycin, and ampicillin, with emergency neurosurgery consultation

32. A 92-year-old community-dwelling senior comes to your office for follow-up of a fall. She was fortunate, and all that was actually wounded was her pride. You review her history. The fall occurred at home when she got up from a chair and headed for the bathroom. She lives alone, does not drive, and ignores her walker. She takes multiple medications, including atenolol, HCTZ, lisinopril, insulin, and metformin. At night, she takes amitriptyline for her diabetic neuropathy. She also drinks 6–8 oz of hard liquor daily, though she repeatedly denies this, and you have learned it only because her daughter told you.

Of the one-third of elderly people who fall every year, what percentage of them have multiple falls?

A. 20%
B. 30%
C. 40%
D. 50%
E. 60%

33. A 30-year-old woman with ulcerative colitis and autoimmune hepatitis complicated by cirrhosis, ascites, and esophageal varices presents with dyspnea and left-sided back pain. Abdominal ultrasound shows minimal ascites, and a chest x-ray is shown in Fig. 9.3.

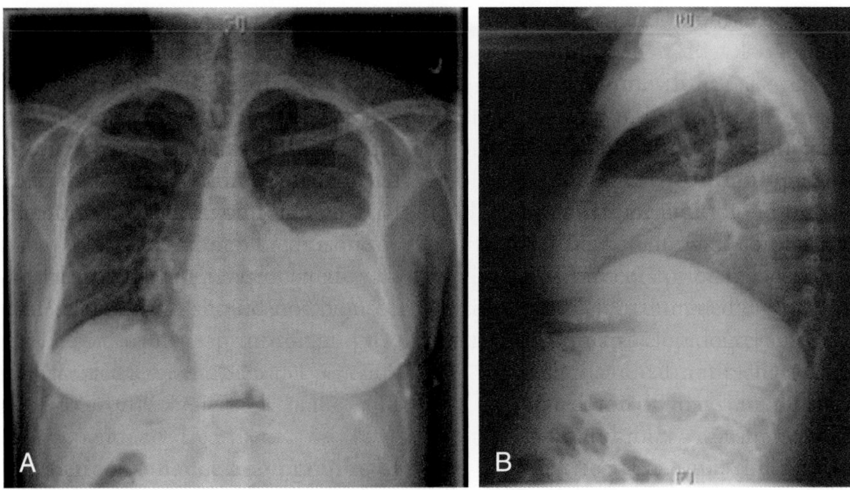

• **Fig. 9.3** (A–B) Chest x-ray for patient in Question 33.

Which of the following would be the next appropriate step?

A. Thoracentesis
B. Chest tube
C. Diuretics
D. TIPS (transjugular intrahepatic portosystemic shunt)
E. Evaluation for liver transplant

34. A 56-year-old woman with hypertension presents to the emergency room with abdominal pain in the left lower quadrant and no bowel movements for several days. Her medications include lisinopril and omeprazole. Her vital signs, including blood pressure, are normal. Her abdomen is soft, nontender, and nondistended. Abdominal CT suggests constipation but is otherwise normal. The CT also shows a 3.5-cm right adrenal lesion.

In addition to checking a dexamethasone suppression test and plasma metanephrines, which of the following tests is indicated to evaluate this adrenal lesion?

A. No additional tests necessary
B. Plasma aldosterone and renin
C. Fine-needle aspiration for cytology and culture
D. Cosyntropin stimulation test

35. A 42-year-old man with a history of morbid obesity status post–bariatric surgery with 75-pound weight loss presents for a follow-up visit. He complains of 5 years of progressive gait instability and numbness and weakness in his distal extremities. His family history is unremarkable. He takes high doses of vitamin supplements, including B complex and zinc.

On examination, he has an unsteady gait, Romberg sign, spasticity in the bilateral lower extremities, bilateral hyperreflexia, and Babinski sign. There is impaired vibration and position sense in the feet. Pain and temperature sensation in the lower extremities are normal. His laboratory test results reveal leukopenia, neutropenia, normocytic anemia, high serum zinc, and low ceruloplasmin; B_{12}, folate, homocysteine, and methylmalonic acid levels are normal.

Which of the following is the most likely cause of his condition?

A. Vitamin B_{12} deficiency
B. Paraneoplastic polyneuropathy
C. Copper deficiency
D. Vitamin B_6 toxicity
E. Lead toxicity

36. A 73-year-old woman is evaluated in the ED for sudden onset of explosive headache starting 8 hours ago. She initially rested in a dark room, but her condition was unchanged, so then she went to the ED. The patient has a history of hypertension controlled by lisinopril, and her family history is noncontributory. In the ED, she becomes nauseated, vomits, and then becomes rapidly more progressively weak; she eventually becomes obtunded and requires intubation and mechanical ventilation. On physical examination, she is afebrile, her blood pressure is 188/100 mm Hg, and her pulse is 120 beats per minute. The patient exhibits flaccid quadriplegia, and meningismus is present. Both pupils are 4 mm and nonreactive; the oculocephalic reflex is absent, and the corneal reflex is absent bilaterally. She has a depressed level of consciousness and a GCS score of 3. Subhyaloid hemorrhages are present bilaterally. The results of CBC and the remainder of the blood work are normal. CT of the head shows an extensive acute subarachnoid hemorrhage and mild prominence of the temporal tips of the lateral ventricles.

Which of the following neurologic complications is most likely to have caused this patient's rapid deterioration?

A. Hydrocephalus
B. Rebleeding
C. Syndrome of inappropriate antidiuretic hormone
D. Vasospasm

37. A 27-year-old woman presents for evaluation of secondary amenorrhea. She had onset of menarche at age 15 and had regular periods until a few years ago. She denies any other symptoms and states that she runs approximately 10–15 miles per day. There is no evidence of an eating disorder. Her pregnancy test result is negative, and her prolactin and TSH are normal. Her FSH, LH, and estradiol levels are in the low-normal range. Her BMI is 22 kg/m^2, and her examination is unremarkable. The female athlete triad is suspected, and a bone density test shows significant bone loss.

What is the best treatment for the patient?

A. Start oral contraceptive pills.
B. Start a bisphosphonate.
C. Encourage a decrease in exercise along with calcium and vitamin D.
D. Start leptin.

38. A 42-year-old man presents to the emergency department 1 week after developing chest pain. One week ago, he developed severe left-sided chest pain in the setting of cocaine use. The chest pain persisted for 1 day and then resolved. He has not had further chest pain. His EKG in the emergency department is shown in Fig. 9.4. Cardiac biomarkers are notable for a normal creatine kinase (CK) and CK-MB and an elevated troponin at 13.2 μg/L. The best next step in management is:

A. Echocardiogram
B. Anticoagulation with heparin
C. Urgent cardiac catheterization
D. Clopidogrel
E. Pharmacologic stress test

39. A 28-year-old woman with no past medical history presents with nausea and vomiting after completing her first marathon. She was able to complete the marathon and thereafter immediately rehydrated. She took four 200-mg ibuprofen tablets and was at a postmarathon party when she started to feel ill, saying unusual things to her friends such as "I made a terrible mistake" and "I am drowning." Her friends brought her to the emergency room. On physical examination, she appears tired and is mildly confused. She has an otherwise nonfocal neurological examination. Her jugular venous pressure is 6 cm H_2O.

What is the best next step in the workup and management of this patient?

A. Administration of 1 L of normal saline
B. Encouraging oral rehydration with an electrolyte replacement sports drink
C. Immediate electrolyte panel
D. Administration of hypertonic saline at a rate of 1 ml/kg/h
E. Checking an ibuprofen level

40. A 36-year-old woman with depression, mild asthma, and obesity presents with 2 weeks of a nonproductive cough. She also has paroxysms of coughing and post-tussive vomiting. She denies significant wheezing. She works at a day care. She received her vaccinations as a child. Vital signs, lung examination, complete metabolic panel, and chest x-ray are unremarkable.

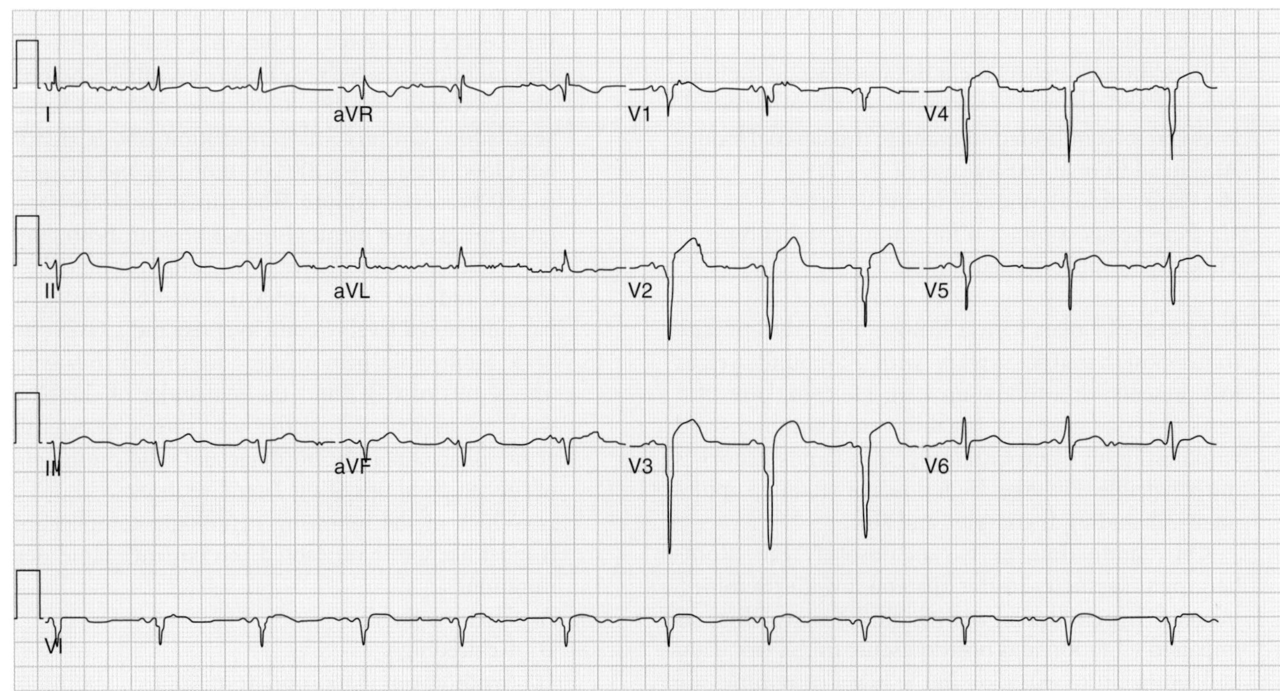

• **Fig. 9.4** Electrocardiogram for patient in Question 38.

The best treatment at this time would be:
A. Albuterol inhaler
B. Azithromycin
C. Prednisone
D. Antitussive agents
E. Admission to the hospital for IV antibiotics

41. A 36-year-old man calls your office with a complaint that he woke up and cannot hear out of his left ear very well. He has no history of ear problems and no recent infections. He did travel recently on an airplane and wonders if the plane trip is the cause. Your astute triage nurse had him hum, and the hum sound did not lateralize. He has no vertigo, but he has tinnitus and a little bit of ear pain.

What should be your next step?
A. Don't worry. It's the plane; take a decongestant, and let me know if not better.
B. Don't worry. See if you can come in this week, and we'll take out the wax.
C. Worry a little. Maybe he has otitis. See him later or tomorrow.
D. Worry. See him today or refer him to ENT.

42. A 38-year-old woman with a history of diffuse cutaneous systemic sclerosis presents with lower extremity edema of 1 week's duration. Her baseline blood pressures are 120–140/70–80 mm Hg. Her medications include nifedipine and omeprazole.

On examination, she is afebrile. Her heart rate is 98 beats per minute. Her blood pressure is 170/100 mm Hg. She has skin thickening over the face, hands, arms, chest, and abdomen. There are telangiectasias on her face and palms. Her cardiac examination is notable for an S4. Her lungs are clear bilaterally. She has 2+ lower extremity edema. Her laboratory test results reveal hemoglobin 9.8 g/dL, platelets 95,000/μL, BUN 40 mg/dL, creatinine 2.4 mg/dL, and albumin 3.4 g/dL, and urinalysis shows 2+ protein and 10 RBCs per high-power field. A blood smear shows 2+ schistocytes.

What is the most appropriate next step in management?
A. Increase the nifedipine dose.
B. Start captopril.
C. Start oral labetalol.
D. Begin IV methylprednisolone.
E. Start oral prednisone.

43. A 36-year-old man presented to his primary care physician with a weeklong history of severe pain in his left Achilles tendon. Over the past few days, he has also developed pain and swelling in his fingers and toes (Fig. 9.5A, B). He has been having difficulty walking and bearing weight. Of note, 2 weeks ago, he developed a weeklong course of diarrhea accompanied by chills and sweats following a weekend camping trip.

The most appropriate treatment is:
A. Ceftriaxone 1 g IV
B. Methylprednisolone 1000 mg IV
C. Prednisone 60 mg orally
D. Indomethacin 50 mg orally
E. Observation

44. A 39-year-old woman of Greek descent presents to the emergency room after experiencing a brief loss of consciousness while at work. Workup reveals a white blood cell count of 4000/μL, hematocrit 20%, and platelet count 207,000/μL.

She notes that she had a viral syndrome 1 week ago, which subsequently resolved. She has no history of bleeding. She moved into a new house 3 months ago. She notes that she has had a propensity to chew ice for the past 1 year. She has no family history of anemia.

Additional workup reveals:
- Mean corpuscular volume (MCV) 55 fL
- Iron less than assay, ferritin 1, total iron-binding capacity (TIBC) 400 μg/dL
- Erythrocyte sedimentation rate (ESR) 8 mm/h
- Normal haptoglobin, LDH, vitamin B_{12}, and folate levels

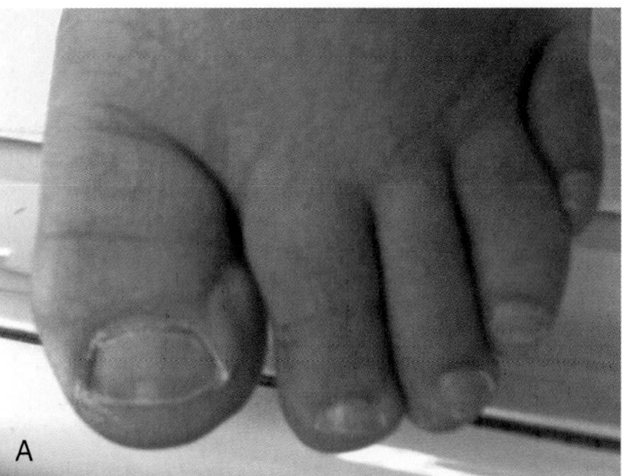

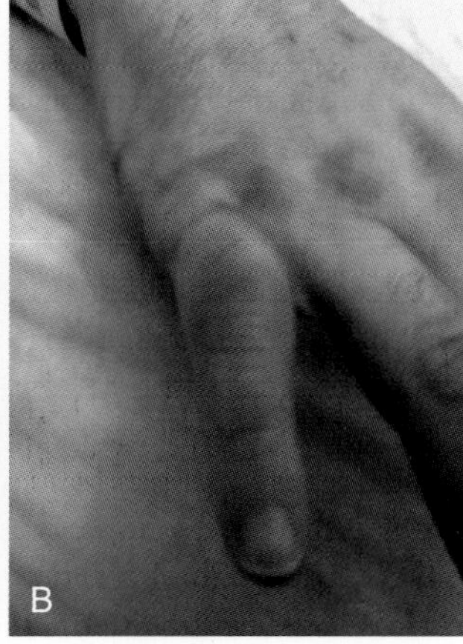

• **Fig. 9.5** Photograph of lower extremity (A) and upper extremity (B) for patient in Question 43.

A blood smear shows microcytic, hypochromic cells of varying shapes. Of note, a complete blood count 3 years ago showed a hematocrit of 28% with an MCV of 85 fL.

The most likely diagnosis is:

A. Thalassemia
B. Iron deficiency anemia
C. Lead toxicity
D. Hemolysis
E. Anemia of chronic disease

45. A 30-year-old woman comes to see you with wrist pain. She is having a really hard time, describing the pain as pain at the base of the wrist that is exacerbated by moving her thumb back and forth. She thinks it might be mildly swollen. Her past medical history is notable for a recent uncomplicated pregnancy and healthy delivery. Her baby is 6 weeks old. She has no personal or family history of autoimmune disease. She had a recent normal TSH. There are no sick contacts. She has sustained no trauma. On examination, you do not really appreciate the swelling she describes, but she is tender to palpation. It is particularly painful when you fold her fingers over her thumb and gently rotate her wrist in the ulnar direction.

What is the most likely cause of her wrist pain?

A. Carpal tunnel syndrome
B. De Quervain tenosynovitis
C. Ulnar nerve entrapment
D. Stress fracture of her first metacarpal
E. Ganglion cyst

46. A 37-year-old nurse presents to your office because a tuberculin skin test (TST) that was done before he could start a job at a new hospital was reactive. He was born in Portugal and thinks he was given the BCG vaccine during childhood. He grew up in New York City and most recently worked in a hospital with a large immigrant population. He does not recall taking care of anyone with tuberculosis (TB). He currently takes no medications. He is anxious about starting a long course of treatment. You look at the red patch on his arm but carefully measure the induration, finding that it is 22 mm across. A chest x-ray shows no abnormalities.

What do you advise him to do?

A. He does not need to be treated, because the TST result is positive due to his BCG vaccine.
B. Treat with weekly isoniazid and rifapentine for 12 weeks.
C. Offer to check a TB blood test because it is the "gold standard."
D. Treat with daily pyrazinamide and rifampin for 2 months.

47. A 22-year-old woman is evaluated for daily headaches that seemed to be initially worse in the supine position for 1–2 weeks but now have been present continuously for the last month. She previously had occasional headaches with photo- and phonophobia beginning at age 14 years. Therapy with triptans for her current headaches is only mildly effective; she is on no other medications. She has had intermittent blurred vision for the past month and notes a pulsatile sound in both ears when she lies in a quiet room.

Physical examination is significant only for obesity (BMI, 30 kg/m^2). Funduscopic examination reveals the presence of bilateral papilledema. No other abnormal findings are seen on neurologic examination. Magnetic resonance imaging (MRI) of the brain with contrast and magnetic resonance venography of the brain are normal.

Which of the following is the most appropriate next step in the management of this patient's headache?

A. Acetazolamide
B. Amitriptyline
C. Lumbar puncture
D. Neurosurgical consultation

48. A 27-year-old woman originally from Brazil who is 25 weeks pregnant (G1P0) presents with dyspnea, blood-tinged sputum, and pleuritic chest pain. Upon physical examination, her heart rate is 137 beats per minute, blood pressure is 96/53 mm Hg, and oxygen saturation is 82% on room air. Examination of the pulmonary and cardiac systems reveals diffuse rales in bilateral lung fields and a difficult-to-auscultate, low-pitched diastolic rumble at the apex. An electrocardiogram shows sinus tachycardia. A chest radiograph shows diffuse bilateral infiltrates. An echocardiogram reveals a normal ejection fraction, a diffusely thickened mitral valve, moderate to severe mitral stenosis, and elevated pulmonary artery systolic pressure. She is intubated for respiratory support. Fetal ultrasound was reassuring. The most appropriate regimen for medical management is:

A. Beta blockers and gentle diuresis
B. Digoxin
C. Dopamine
D. ACE inhibitors
E. Hydralazine and nitrates

49. A 29-year-old woman presents to the emergency department with sore throat, fever, and recurrent hematuria. She was in her usual state of health until 1 month ago, when she developed a sore throat and a fever of 101°F. The following day, she noticed frank blood in her urine and went to the emergency department. She was diagnosed with a presumed urinary tract infection and given a 7-day course of cephalexin. After several days of antibiotics, her fevers resolved, and her urine cleared. She remained in good health until 1 week ago, when she again developed fever, sore throat, and bloody urine, and she returned to the emergency department. She notes a similar episode about 3 years ago.

Urinalysis was notable for 3+ blood and 2+ protein. Urine sediment showed 493 dysmorphic red blood cells per high-power field. No casts were seen. Laboratory values were notable for a serum creatinine level of 3.4 mg/dL. Her complement component levels were normal. Renal ultrasound showed no evidence of obstruction, hydronephrosis, or perinephric fluid collections.

Which of the following is the most likely diagnosis?

A. Poststreptococcal glomerulonephritis
B. IgA nephropathy
C. Carcinoma of the bladder
D. Urinary tract infection
E. Nephrolithiasis

50. A 30-year-old woman with no past medical history was incidentally found to have a hyperpigmented linear lesion on her left arm following travel to Hawaii (Fig. 9.6).

Which activity mostly likely led to the development of this physical examination finding?

A. Handling fish in a saltwater tank
B. Squeezing limes while making mojitos
C. Applying sunscreen containing para-aminobenzoic acid (PABA)
D. Handling thorned roses
E. Injection drug use

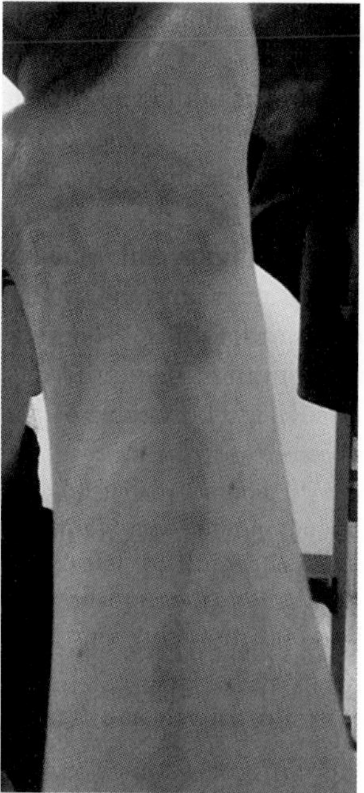

• **Fig. 9.6** Photograph of patient's left arm in Question 50.

Chapter 9 Answers

1. ANSWER: B. Start a statin.

The joint American College of Cardiology and American Heart Association guideline on the treatment of blood cholesterol identified four major groups of patients who would benefit from statin therapy: (1) those with clinical atherosclerotic cardiovascular disease (ASCVD), (2) those with LDL greater than or equal to 190 mg/dL, (3) diabetics aged 40–75 years old with an LDL >70 mg/dL, and (4) those with an estimated 10-year ASCVD risk greater than or equal to 7.5%. In patients with LDL <190 mg/dL, ASCVD risk is calculated on the basis of age, sex, race, total and HDL cholesterol, hypertension, and smoking status. (http://tools.acc.org/ASCVD-Risk-Estimator/). This patient has a 10-year ASCVD risk of 11.9% that would qualify for statin therapy. Lifestyle change should be encouraged but is insufficient to mitigate the patient's risk of ASCVD. A coronary calcium score is not necessary in this patient who already has an indication for statin therapy. Stress testing and catheterization are not indicated in this asymptomatic patient.

Stone NJ, Robinson JG, Lichtenstein AH, et al. 2013 ACC/AHA guideline on the treatment of blood cholesterol to reduce atherosclerotic cardiovascular risk in adults: a report of the American College of Cardiology/American Heart Association Task Force on Practice Guidelines. *Circulation.* 2014;129(25 Suppl 2):S1–S45.

2. ANSWER: B. Order a head MRI/MRA.

An MRI is indicated for this patient because she is presenting with a new headache after the age of 50 years. Imaging should be performed in those patients presenting with the following:

- "First or worst" headache
- Increased frequency and increased severity of headache
- New-onset headache after age 50
- New-onset headache with history of cancer or immunodeficiency
- Headache with mental status changes
- Headache with fever, neck stiffness, and meningeal signs
- Headache with focal neurologic deficits if not previously documented as a migraine with aura

Narcotics are generally not first-line therapy for headaches; amitriptyline can be used for chronic prophylaxis for migraines and tension headaches but should not be used prior to a proper evaluation.

Sumatriptan is a first-line therapy for migraines, but this patient does not seem to be experiencing a classic migraine. Physical therapy is not indicated.

3. **ANSWER: C. Refer for endometrial biopsy.**

In a postmenopausal woman, endometrial cells (even benign ones) on a Pap smear can be indicative of endometrial cancer. In this question, the patient's history of obesity may put her at increased risk for endometrial cancer as well. In this setting, endometrial cells are never normal, and the patient should be referred for endometrial biopsy. Some clinicians would also get an ultrasound to measure the patient's endometrial stripe. A decision not to biopsy based on the stripe is best made by the gynecologic consultant.

Massad LS, Einstein MH, Huh WK, et al. 2012 updated consensus guidelines for the management of abnormal cervical cancer screening tests and cancer precursors. *J Low Genit Tract Dis.* 2013;17(5 Suppl 1):S1–S27.

4. **ANSWER: B. Day 20 serum progesterone**

Reassurance is inappropriate because the patient is 35 years old, so evaluation should begin after 6 months of trying to become pregnant (or at 1 year if the patient is under 35 years old). A Day 20 or 21 serum progesterone can confirm the presence of ovulatory cycles and should be the first step in the workup of female infertility. Up to 40% of women with infertility have ovulatory dysfunction. Although a hysterosalpingogram is useful to confirm tubal patency, it should not precede assessing ovulation. IVF is inappropriate without completing a workup. LH and FSH can assess ovulatory reserve but would be checked on Day 3, not Day 20.

Practice Committee of the America Society for Reproductive Medicine. Diagnostic evaluation of the infertile female: a committee opinion. *Fertil Steril.* 2015;103(6):e44–e50.

5. **ANSWER: E. Reassurance and a more supportive bra**

The history is consistent with cyclic mastalgia, which may be due to Cooper ligament pain caused by inadequate support of her pendulous breasts. Imaging would be overly aggressive, as would BRCA testing.

Howard MB, Battaglia T, Prout M, Freund K. The effect of imaging on the clinical management of breast pain. *J Gen Intern Med.* 2012;27(7):817–824.

6. **ANSWER: A. Intradermal injection of triamcinolone**

The patient has alopecia areata, which typically presents before age 40, with 66% of patients presenting before 30. Alopecia areata causes rapid areas of well-circumscribed hair loss on the scalp but can involve any and all hair growth. Growth of white hair in the alopecic regions is a common occurrence. Intradermal injection of triamcinolone is the best studied and most effective treatment. Minoxidil has been used but is of limited benefit when used alone. Biopsy is unnecessary in this classic presentation.

7. **ANSWER: D. Mammograms and MRI annually, ideally 6 months apart**

This patient is at high risk for developing breast cancer. She has Ashkenazi Jewish heritage and several first-degree relatives with cancer. This makes it more likely that she may carry *BRCA1, BRCA2,* or other mutations that put her at increased risk. The current recommendations for women at high risk is annual screening with both MRI and mammography. The first two choices would not be correct even if she were not at markedly elevated risk. The age of her sister at diagnosis dictates that screening starting at age 35 (10 years younger than the index case) is important.

Bevers TB, Anderson BO, Bonaccio E, et al. NCCN clinical practice guidelines in oncology: breast cancer screening and diagnosis. *J Natl Compr Canc Netw.* 2009;7(10):1060–1096.

Bevers TB, Ward JH, Arun BK, et al. Breast cancer risk reduction, version 2.2015. *J Natl Compr Canc Netw.* 2015;13(7): 880–915.

8. **ANSWER: D. Magnetic resonance venography**

The patient should undergo a MR venogram. The most likely diagnosis is venous sinus thrombosis, given his known hypercoagulability, dehydration, and symptoms of mounting intracranial pressure and eventual focal deficits. Carotid ultrasound does not assist in the assessment of the intracranial vasculature. Seizures are a recognized complication of venous sinus thrombosis; however, EEG does not assist with the establishment of a preliminary diagnosis and should not be performed. An LP is contraindicated in this patient with evidence of elevated intracranial pressure.

Stam J. Thrombosis of the cerebral veins and sinuses. *N Engl J Med.* 2005;352(17):1791–1798.

9. **ANSWER: A. No further workup or treatment**

There is no reason to treat asymptomatic Paget disease of the bone. When symptomatic, bisphosphonates, orally or IV, can be effective in reducing pain due to bone turnover. Calcitonin may be effective but has less evidence than a bisphosphonate.

Ralston SH. Paget's disease of bone. *N Engl J Med.* 2013;368(7): 644–650.

10. **ANSWER: D. Prescribe a 5-day course of nitrofurantoin.**

This 28-year-old woman has uncomplicated cystitis and warrants treatment to relieve symptoms. The large majority of cases of uncomplicated cystitis in a premenopausal woman are caused by *Escherichia coli.* The Infectious Diseases Society of America guidelines for the treatment of uncomplicated cystitis recommend trimethoprim-sulfamethoxazole, fosfomycin, and nitrofurantoin as first-line treatment options. Neither quinolones (ciprofloxacin, levofloxacin) nor amoxicillin is recommended as a first-line agent. Quinolones and other broad-spectrum oral antibiotics are associated with "collateral damage," such as increased risk for colonization or infection with drug-resistant organisms, whereas amoxicillin is associated with high failure rates.

Gupta K, Hooton TM, Naber KG, et al. International Clinical Practice Guidelines for the Treatment of Acute Uncomplicated Cystitis and Pyelonephritis in Women: A 2010 Update by the Infectious Diseases Society of America and the European Society for Microbiology and Infectious Diseases. *Clin Infect Dis.* 2011;52(5):e103–e120.

11. ANSWER: B. Increase allopurinol with concurrent colchicine.

This 62-year-old man is having continued attacks of gout while on allopurinol, but his serum uric acid level is higher than the goal level. His allopurinol should be increased to bring his serum uric acid down to <6.0 mg/dL. He should be on colchicine or an NSAID while the allopurinol is increased. There is no reason to switch medications.

Neogi T. Gout. *N Engl J Med.* 2011;364(5):443–452.

12. ANSWER: D. Order a urea breath test to confirm persistence of *H. pylori.*

It is reasonable to use a test-and-treat strategy for *H. pylori* in patients with epigastric discomfort without any red-flag symptoms. Persistence of symptoms after treatment can be related to lack of cure or may be unrelated to *H. pylori.* Antibiotic resistance among patients with *H. pylori* has been increasing in the last decade. For this reason, 14-day treatment regimens are now recommended over shorter courses, and triple-therapy regimens such as this patient received (typically two antibiotics and a proton pump inhibitor) are recommended only in areas where treatment success rates are high and clarithromycin resistance is low; otherwise, treatment regimens that include four agents (typically two antibiotics, a proton pump inhibitor, and bismuth) are recommended. Testing for cure of *H. pylori* after therapy is now fairly standard practice, particularly if the patient has persistent symptoms. *H. pylori* serology will remain positive even with adequate treatment, thus a urea breath test or stool antigen must be used to confirm active infection. If found to be positive for *H. pylori,* quadruple therapy with alternative antibiotics given for 14 days would be appropriate.

Fallone CA. The Toronto Consensus for the Treatment of *Helicobacter pylori* Infection in Adults. *Gastroenterology.* 2016;151(1):51–69.

13. ANSWER: E. Repeat cytology in 5 years.

The U.S. Preventive Services Task Force (USPSTF) recommends cervical cancer screening every 3 years for women aged 21–65 with cytology (Papanicolaou). Women 30–65 years of age who desire longer screening intervals can be screened with a combination of cytology and HPV testing every 5 years. There is sufficient evidence that screening with HPV testing (alone or in combination with cytology) confers little to no benefit among women younger than 30 years of age.

Moyer VA. Screening for Cervical Cancer: U.S. Preventive Services Task Force Recommendation Statement. *Ann Intern Med.* 2012;156:880–891.

14. ANSWER: B. 3 months

For patients with a first episode of venous thromboembolism due to a reversible or time-limited risk factor (i.e., oral contraceptive use, surgery/prolonged immobilization, trauma, pregnancy), the treatment course is 3 months. Anticoagulation beyond 3 months is typically not required. Idiopathic or recurrent venous thromboembolism requires extended and/or lifelong therapy where the exact duration of therapy can vary on the basis of patient history and preference.

Kearon C, Akl EA, Ornelas J, et al. Antithrombotic Therapy for VTE Disease: CHEST Guideline and Expert Panel Report. *Chest.* 2016;149(2):315–352.

15. ANSWER: D. Ceftriaxone 250 mg intramuscular injection × 1 + azithromycin 1 g orally × 1

The 2015 CDC guidelines for the management of sexually transmitted infections introduced the recommendations to treat uncomplicated cervicitis and urethritis due to *Neisseria gonorrhea* with dual-antibiotic therapy due to emerging resistance among circulating *N. gonorrhea* internationally. The recommended first-line treatment regimen in the United States includes intramuscular ceftriaxone and a single high dose of oral azithromycin, which also treats for the possibility of *Chlamydia,* which is a common concurrent cause of infection. Note that because of the increased prevalence of *N. gonorrhea* resistance to doxycycline compared with azithromycin, azithromycin is the preferred agent for treatment of potential chlamydia infection.

Workowski KA, Bolan GA; Centers for Disease Control and Prevention. Sexually transmitted diseases treatment guidelines, 2015. *MMWR Recomm Rep.* 2015;64(RR-03):1–137.

16. ANSWER: B. Amoxicillin/clavulanate 500/125 mg three times daily × 5–7 days

Acute bacterial rhinosinusitis is characterized by at least one of the following three symptoms: persistent symptoms (≥7–10 days), severe symptoms (fever ≥102°F, purulent nasal discharge, or facial pain from onset lasting ≥3–4 days), or initial improvement followed by subsequent worsening of symptoms. The 2012 Infectious Diseases Society of America guidelines recommend amoxicillin-clavulanate as first-line therapy, instead of amoxicillin alone. Doxycycline is the recommended alternative for patients with a penicillin allergy but should be dosed at 100 mg by mouth twice daily. In 2016, the FDA issued a warning about the potential risk for serious and irreversible side effects with the use of fluoroquinolones such as levofloxacin and advised against using quinolones to treat uncomplicated acute bacterial sinusitis (and also uncomplicated urinary tract infections and acute bronchitis). Due to increasing rates of *Streptococcus pneumoniae* resistance to azithromycin, this drug is not recommended for the treatment of acute rhinosinusitis.

Chow AW, Benninger MS, Brook I, et al. IDSA clinical practice guideline for acute bacterial rhinosinusitis in children and adults. *Clin Infect Dis.* 2012;54(8):e72–e112.

U.S. Food and Drug Administration. FDA Drug Safety Communication: FDA updates warnings for oral and injectable fluoroquinolone antibiotics due to disabling side effects. https://www.fda.gov/Drugs/DrugSafety/ucm511530.htm; accessed 3/17/17.

17. ANSWER: C. Plasma exchange

This is a case of thrombotic thrombocytopenic purpura (TTP), also referred to as *ADAMTS13 deficiency–mediated thrombotic microangiopathy.* This syndrome is caused by a congenital or acquired deficiency of ADAMTS13, which is a protease that cleaves large multimers of von Willebrand factor. When the protease is deficient, accumulation of von Willebrand factor multimers leads to microvascular damage. The smear is microangiopathic, demonstrating schistocytes (>5/high-power field) and thrombocytopenia. The diagnosis of TTP is a clinical one; however, the presence of microangiopathic hemolytic anemia and thrombocytopenia without other clear cause is required for diagnosis and is sufficient, in this case, to make an initial diagnosis. The additional findings of renal failure, neurologic abnormalities, and fever constitute the remaining classical clinical and laboratory features of TTP. A low serum ADAMTS13 level supports the diagnosis. Plasma exchange is the treatment of choice for TTP, and early initiation is key to decreasing patient morbidity (see Fig. 9.1).

George JN, Nester CM. Syndromes of thrombotic microangiopathy. *N Engl J Med.* 2014;371(7):654–666.

18. ANSWER: A. Annual MRA

This patient should have an annual MRA or CT angiogram to monitor aneurysmal growth. For patients without a prior SAH, the lowest-risk aneurysms are those in the anterior circulation and <7 mm in diameter. The annual risk of rupture for an aneurysm of the size of this patient's is 0.05% annually. The risk of neurologic disability associated with intervention exceeds the potential benefit. After 3 successive years of annual monitoring, an MRA or CTA obtained once every 3 years will be sufficient.

Thompson BG, Brown RD Jr, Amin-Hanjani S, et al. Guidelines for the Management of Patients With Unruptured Intracranial Aneurysms: A Guideline for Healthcare Professionals From the American Heart Association/American Stroke Association. *Stroke.* 2015;46(8):2368–2400.

19. ANSWER: D. Doxycycline 100 mg twice daily × 2 weeks

The treatment of choice for early Lyme disease is doxycycline × 10–21 days because it will also treat anaplasmosis. Amoxicillin is an alternative in pregnant women and in children <8 years of age. Intravenous third-generation cephalosporins are required only in patients with advanced heart block, meningitis, neuritis, or other more advanced manifestations of this infection. In Europe, studies have shown azithromycin to be as effective as doxycycline. However, in the United States, studies have demonstrated azithromycin not to be as effective as amoxicillin (and presumably doxycycline) in the treatment of Lyme disease.

Wormser GP, Dattwyler RJ, Shapiro ED, et al. The clinical assessment, treatment, and prevention of Lyme disease, human granulocytic anaplasmosis, and babesiosis: clinical practice guidelines by the Infectious Diseases Society of America. *Clin Infect Dis.* 2006;43(9):1089–1134.

20. ANSWER: D. Eosinophilic granulomatosis with polyangiitis

This patient displays the classic triad of eosinophilic granulomatosis with polyangiitis: asthma, sinus disease, and peripheral eosinophilia. The diagnosis is made primarily by clinical features, including asthma (particularly of late onset), mononeuropathy (including multiplex), or polyneuropathy; skin disease with variable rash patterns seen in two-thirds of patients; paranasal sinus abnormalities (allergic rhinitis, recurrent sinusitis, nasal polyposis); eosinophilia with >10% or >1500 eosinophils/μL; and migratory or transient pulmonary opacities on x-ray.

Mouthon L, Dunogue B, Guillevin L. Diagnosis and classification of eosinophilic granulomatosis with polyangiitis (formerly named Churg-Strauss syndrome). *J Autoimmun.* 2014;48–49:99–103.

21. ANSWER: C. Hypertrophic cardiomyopathy

This murmur is characteristic of hypertrophic cardiomyopathy (HCM), specifically the increase with Valsalva maneuvers and lack of radiation to the carotids. HCM is an autosomal dominant disorder of the cardiac sarcomere and carries an increased risk of sudden cardiac death.

Aortic stenosis also has a crescendo–decrescendo murmur but decreases or does not change significantly with Valsalva maneuvers. The murmur associated with aortic stenosis also characteristically radiates to the carotids. Marfan syndrome can be associated with aortic insufficiency, which is a diastolic murmur. Rheumatic heart disease can cause systolic murmurs from aortic stenosis or mitral regurgitation. However, the murmur described in this case is not consistent with either of these valvular disorders.

22. ANSWER: C. Oral trimethoprim-sulfamethoxazole

Community-acquired MRSA (CA MRSA) is a common cause of skin and soft tissue infections. Outbreaks of CA MRSA have been seen in particular groups, such as athletes and intravenous drug users, but it should be considered in anyone presenting with a soft tissue infection. This patient has a characteristic presentation and appropriately had a Gram stain and culture performed.

CA MRSA is not susceptible to beta-lactam antibiotics such as nafcillin, penicillin, and dicloxacillin. Systemically ill-appearing patients with CA MRSA can be treated with intravenous vancomycin. There is no role for oral vancomycin to treat infections other than *Clostridium difficile* infections, because it is not absorbed. When treating suspected CA MRSA in an outpatient setting, oral antibiotic options include clindamycin, trimethoprim-sulfamethoxazole, or a long-acting tetracycline (e.g., minocycline or doxycycline).

Singer AJ, Talan DA. Management of skin abscesses in the era of methicillin-resistant *Staphylococcus aureus*. *N Engl J Med*. 2014;370(11):1039–1047.

Stevens DL, Bisno AL, Chambers HF, et al. Practice guidelines for the diagnosis and management of skin and soft tissue infections: 2014 update by the Infectious Diseases Society of America. *Clin Infect Dis*. 2014;59(2):e10–e52.

23. ANSWER: C. Topical swallowed fluticasone

The patient has eosinophilic esophagitis. The diagnostic criteria include clinical symptoms of esophageal dysfunction, biopsy showing >15 eosinophils/high-power field, lack of responsiveness to high-dose PPI, and normal pH monitoring in the distal esophagus. Men are affected more commonly than women. Adults with this disorder usually give a history of intermittent dysphagia and food impaction. First-line therapy includes topical corticosteroids. Fluticasone propionate at a dose of 440 µg twice daily administered for 4–6 weeks leads to clinical and histologic improvement. Other therapies include elimination diets, oral budesonide, and leukotriene receptor antagonists. Dilation is reserved for those patients with fixed strictures who do not respond to medical therapy, because there is a risk of esophageal tearing with dilation.

Furuta GT, Katzka DA. Eosinophilic esophagitis. *N Engl J Med*. 2015;373:1640–1648.

24. ANSWER: B. Stop the lisinopril, and see if he improves.

This patient has hyperhidrosis. A relatively common condition, it can be quite debilitating for patients, causing them to have a lot of social isolation and discomfort. Essential hyperhidrosis is a disorder of the eccrine glands. Sometimes it can be inherited. Secondary hyperhidrosis is suggested in this case because of its later onset, and it can be due to a host of medications. In this case, lisinopril may be the most likely culprit. If the patient improves after discontinuing the medicine, then it would be reasonable to consider other options.

Symptomatic treatment for patients can consist of using higher doses of aluminum chlorohydrate in a preparation such as aluminum chloride (Drysol, Hypercare), which can be used on the hands and feet as well as under the arms and in other areas. Some patients choose to undergo more invasive procedures for this condition.

25. ANSWER: B. Age 40 years

For average-risk persons, the preferred method of colon cancer screening is a colonoscopy beginning at age 50. Patients with a family history of adenomatous polyps in a first-degree relative should have a screening colonoscopy at age 40 or 10 years before the diagnosis of adenomatous polyps in the family member, whichever comes first.

Rex DK, Johnson DA, Anderson JC, et al. American College of Gastroenterology Guidelines for Colorectal Cancer Screening 2008. *Am J Gastroenterol*. 2009;104(3):739–750.

26. ANSWER: E. No additional studies are needed.

This patient has first carpometacarpal joint tenderness and squaring of the palm, consistent with osteoarthritis (OA). Although symmetric polyarticular arthritis is typical of rheumatoid arthritis (RA), the joints involved are not consistent with RA, and there are no signs of inflammation on exam. The distal interphalangeal joints are commonly involved in osteoarthritis of the hand and rarely involved in RA. Involvement of the first carpometacarpal joint is almost always a sign of osteoarthritis. Morning stiffness lasting <30 minutes indicates degenerative rather than inflammatory arthritis. Options A through D are part of the workup for inflammatory arthritis involving the hands. However, in this case, the diagnosis of OA in the hands can be made without additional testing (Option E).

Altman R, Alarcón G, Appelrouth D, et al. The American College of Rheumatology criteria for the classification and reporting of osteoarthritis of the hand. *Arthritis Rheum*. 1990;33:1601–1610.

27. ANSWER: D. Abdominal ultrasound

The U.S. Preventive Services Task Force (USPSTF) recommends that men between the ages of 65 and 75 with any current or past history of smoking undergo a one-time screening for abdominal aortic aneurysm (AAA) with abdominal ultrasound (Option D). Several studies have demonstrated a survival benefit to screening, including a population-based study of over 67,800 men aged between 65 and 74 who were randomized to AAA screening (with surgery for those found to have AAA >5.4 cm) or no screening. This study showed AAA-related mortality was reduced by an average of 42% (95% CI, 22%–58%) in the screened population compared with the unscreened population.

Several studies have shown no benefit in male nonsmokers and in women. There are insufficient data to determine whether the association of coronary calcium with coronary artery disease risk warrants coronary calcium CT screening (Option A) in asymptomatic men. Similarly, there are insufficient data to support the use of exercise treadmill testing (Option E) for screening asymptomatic patients. The utility of prostate cancer screening tests (Option B) to decrease mortality is uncertain. There is not enough evidence to recommend routine screening for thyroid disease (Option C).

LeFevre ML. U.S. Preventive Services Task Force. Screening for abdominal aortic aneurysm: U.S. Preventive Services Task Force recommendation statement. *Ann Intern Med.* 2014;161(4):281–290.

28. ANSWER: B. Admit to the hospital.

This patient should be admitted to the hospital. His history is consistent with transient ischemic attack (TIA). Risk for the development of stroke after a TIA can be estimated by the "ABCD2" score, which is a risk assessment tool that includes age, blood pressure, clinical features of the TIA, duration of the TIA, and diabetes. This patient has an elevated ABCD2 score of 5 based on his age over 60, systolic blood pressure above 140 mm Hg, and symptoms including focal weakness, which suggests his 2-day risk of stroke is 4.1% and that he would likely benefit from hospitalization for immediate further workup.

Johnston CS, Rothwell PM, Nguyen-Huynh MN, et al. Validation and refinement of scores to predict very early stroke risk after transient ischaemic attack. *Lancet.* 2007;369(9558): 283–292.

29. ANSWER: B. Migraine without aura

This patient presents with typical symptoms of migraine headache. The symptoms meeting criteria for migraine in this patient include worsening of the headache with movement, limitation of activities, and requiring absence of light and sound (dark, quiet room).

Although some autonomic features are present (congestion/rhinorrhea), the headache is not cluster type, because it lasts longer than 180 minutes (1–2 days in this patient's case). In addition, although not part of the absolute criteria for cluster headache, patients with cluster headache prefer to be mobile because resting causes worsening of the pain. On the basis of the lack of fever or discolored nasal discharge, the patient does not have the secondary headache of sinus infection. Although sinus symptoms are not part of the formal criteria for migraine, they are quite common and can complicate the diagnosis. Tension-type headache can be ruled out because of the disabling characteristic of the headache and the presence of both photo- and phonophobia.

Headache Classification Subcommittee of the International Headache Society. The International Classification of Headache Disorders: 2nd edition. *Cephalalgia.* 2004;24 Suppl 1:9–160.

30. ANSWER: B. Vitamin E

This patient has nonalcoholic fatty liver disease (NAFLD). A biopsy is recommended in patients with NAFLD and increased risk of steatohepatitis and advanced fibrosis. Patients with metabolic syndrome fall into this category. Weight loss is the mainstay of therapy for NAFLD. Vitamin E has been shown to improve liver histology in nondiabetic patients with biopsy-proven nonalcoholic steatohepatitis (NASH). Pioglitazone has been associated with improvement in some histologic changes of NASH. However, in a large placebo-controlled trial, it was not superior to placebo. Metformin has not been shown to affect liver histology or disease progression

Bariatric surgery is not currently used specifically to treat NASH. However, bariatric surgery is recommended for patients with obesity and a BMI >40 kg/m^2 or >35 kg/m^2 and serious medical comorbidities.

Chalasani N, Younossi Z, Lavine JE, et al. The diagnosis and management of non-alcoholic fatty liver disease: practice guideline by the American Association for the Study of Liver Diseases, American College of Gastroenterology, and the American Gastroenterological Association. *Hepatology.* 2012;55(6):2005–2023.

31. E. Ruptured brain abscess: treatment with ceftriaxone, vancomycin, and ampicillin, with emergency neurosurgical consultation

The patient's initial clinical syndrome of fevers, anorexia, headache, and neck stiffness is consistent with a diagnosis of meningitis. The abrupt change in symptomatology and focal neurological symptoms reported the night prior to presentation are an indication for emergent head imaging (noncontrast head CT). Upon imaging, head CT demonstrates a brain abscess with likely surrounding vasogenic edema, and magnetic resonance imaging (MRI) demonstrates pus within the ventricle, indicating rupture of the brain abscess. A ruptured brain abscess is considered a neurological emergency with a very high mortality rate.

Given the high mortality rate of ruptured brain abscesses with pus draining into the ventricles, broad-spectrum antibiotics as well as emergent neurosurgical consultation are indicated in this case (Option E).

32. ANSWER: D. 50%

Falls in the elderly are responsible for 70% of accidental deaths in people 75 and over. They increase with age, transcend ethnic groups, and cause significant morbidity, including decline of functional status and risk for hospitalization. Hip fracture occurs in 1%–2% of falls.

The following are risk factors for falls:

Intrinsic
- Muscle weakness
- Gait and balance dysfunction
- Visual impairment
- Cognitive impairment
- Orthostatic hypotension
- Medications (do not forget about alcohol)

Extrinsic
- Poor lighting
- Clutter
- Environmental obstacles
- Bad shoes

33. ANSWER: A. Thoracentesis

This patient most likely has pleural effusion due to cirrhosis and ascites (also called *hepatic hydrothorax*). It is due to a diaphragmatic defect, which can be microscopic. This occurs on the right side 85% of the time, on the left side 13% of the time, and bilaterally 2% of the time. Thoracentesis (Option A) should be the first intervention performed to assess for other possible etiologies of pleural effusion and to rule out infection. Diuretics (Option C) (and salt and fluid restriction) can be used to manage pleural effusion once the diagnosis is confirmed. A transjugular intrahepatic portosystemic shunt (TIPS) (Option D) is used to manage refractory effusion occurring in this setting. Patients with hepatic hydrothorax should be evaluated for liver transplant (Option E). A chest tube (Option B) should never be placed in patients with hepatic hydrothorax, because it can cause massive protein and electrolyte depletion, infection, renal failure, and bleeding.

Kumar S, Sarin SK. Paradigms in the management of hepatic hydrothorax: past, present, and future. *Hepatol Int.* 2013;7:80–87.

34. ANSWER: B. Plasma aldosterone and renin

This is an adrenal incidentaloma in a patient with a history of hypertension. Endocrinologic work to assess for autonomous secretion of cortisol, catecholamines, or aldosterone is indicated. The appropriate laboratory evaluation includes a dexamethasone suppression test to evaluate for Cushing disease in all patients, plasma metanephrines to evaluate for pheochromocytoma in all patients, and plasma aldosterone and renin if the patient has hypertension (as in this case). A cosyntropin stimulation test evaluates for adrenal insufficiency and is not a standard part of the workup for an adrenal incidentaloma. Fine-needle aspiration is not part of the first set of tests in the workup for an adrenal incidentaloma.

Young WF Jr. The incidentally discovered adrenal mass. *N Engl J Med.* 2007;356(6):601–610.

35. ANSWER: C. Copper deficiency

The patient has progressive upper motor neuron deficits. In a patient with a history of bariatric surgery, copper and vitamin B_{12} deficiency should be suspected. However, the vitamin B_{12} level (Option A) in this case is normal. Zinc competes with copper for absorption, and the patient is taking supplemental zinc, so this may be contributing. Copper deficiency (Option C) affects the corticospinal tract (hyperreflexia and Babinski sign) and posterior column (impaired vibration sensation).

Vitamin B_6 (Option D) toxicity causes peripheral neuropathy, not upper motor neuron signs. Lead toxicity (Option E) is more common in children. Adults with lead poisoning frequently have sleep disorders and may be hypersomnolent. A paraneoplastic polyneuropathy (Option B) would not explain all of his laboratory abnormalities.

Bal BS, Finelli FC, Shope TR, Koch TR. Nutritional deficiencies after bariatric surgery. *Nat Rev Endocrinol.* 2012;8(9):544–556.

36. ANSWER: B. Rebleeding

The most likely complication to have caused this patient's rapid deterioration is rebleeding. In the first few hours after an initial hemorrhage, up to 15% of affected patients have a sudden deterioration of consciousness, which strongly suggests rebleeding. In patients who survive the first day, the rebleeding risk is evenly distributed during the next 4 weeks, with a cumulative risk of 40% without surgical or endovascular interventions. Occlusion of the responsible aneurysm is thus the first aim in the management of the subarachnoid hemorrhage and is usually performed by coiling or clipping.

Connolly ES Jr, Rabinstein AA, Carhuapoma JR, et al. Guidelines for the management of aneurysmal subarachnoid hemorrhage: a guideline for healthcare professionals from the American Heart Association/American Stroke Association. *Stroke.* 2012;43(6):1711–1737.

37. ANSWER: C. Encourage a decrease in exercise along with calcium and vitamin D.

This patient has functional hypothalamic amenorrhea resulting from suppression of the hypothalamic-pituitary-ovarian axis due to energy imbalance. The best treatment for bone loss under these conditions is to treat the underlying energy imbalance by nutritional rehabilitation and decrease exercise along with calcium and vitamin D supplementation. Oral contraceptive pills will not correct the bone loss, though they would cause resumption of menses. Bisphosphonates would not be a good option in a young premenopausal woman who may desire pregnancy. Leptin has been shown to restore menses in functional hypothalamic amenorrhea, but its effects on bone health are unknown.

Weiss Kelly AK, Hecht S. Council on Sports Medicine and Fitness. The female athlete triad. *Pediatrics.* 2016;138(2):e20160922.

38. ANSWER: A. Echocardiogram

The clinical history of chest pain in the setting of cocaine use 1 week ago suggests a cocaine-induced myocardial infarction (MI). Following an MI, cardiac biomarkers peak at 18–24 hours. CK and CK-MB remain elevated for 48 hours, whereas troponins may remain elevated for 10 days. The pattern of biomarkers in this patient is consistent with an MI 1 week ago. The EKG demonstrates ST elevations in leads V1–V4, suggestive of an anterior ST-elevation MI. There are also Q waves in leads V1–V4. The presence of anterior Q waves plus persistent ST elevations with a clinical story of a cocaine-induced MI 1 week ago is most suggestive of a ventricular aneurysm. The differential diagnosis of chronic or persistent ST elevations includes early repolarization, ventricular aneurysm (when ST elevations occur with Q waves), a scar following a large anterior MI, and chronic pericarditis.

An echocardiogram (Option A) should be obtained to look for the presence of a ventricular aneurysm and ventricular thrombus. Ventricular aneurysms are a common complication of anterior MIs. They are treated with afterload reduction and anticoagulation.

Treatment with heparin (Option B) may be initiated if the patient has evidence of a ventricular aneurysm, but it would not be the next best step in management. Late catheterization of STEMI (after 24–48 hours) (Option C) should be done only for severe heart failure, electrical or hemodynamic instability, or persistent ischemia. A pharmacologic stress test (Option E) may be performed prior to discharge for risk stratification. Clopidogrel (Option D) and aspirin are indicated for secondary prevention after a STEMI.

Lange RA, Hillis LD. Cardiovascular complications of cocaine use. *N Engl J Med.* 2001;345(5):351–358.

39. ANSWER: C. Immediate electrolyte panel

This patient has symptoms associated with acute hyponatremia (confusion and altered mental status) caused by extreme hypotonic losses (through sweat) from exercise and replacement of the hypotonic fluid with free water. In the setting of euvolemia, as indicated by the normal to slightly high jugular venous pressure of 6 cm H_2O, rehydration with normal saline (Option A) and oral rehydration (Option B) is inadequate to correct hyponatremia and can result in worsening hyponatremia.

The first step in this emergency should be to obtain an immediate electrolyte panel (Option C) to confirm hyponatremia and to help guide further treatment. Empiric administration of hypertonic saline (Option D) should be avoided in a clinical setting where laboratory tests can be obtained rapidly, because overly hasty correction of hyponatremia can lead to an osmotic demyelination syndrome (also known as central pontine myelinolysis). The patient's signs and symptoms are inconsistent with ibuprofen overdose (Option E). Although her symptoms may be consistent with very severe acute kidney injury in the setting of potential hypovolemia and ingestion of ibuprofen as a second insult, this is much less likely.

Almond CSD, Shin AY, Fortescue EB, et al. Hyponatremia among runners in the Boston Marathon. *N Engl J Med.* 2005;352(15):1550–1556.

40. ANSWER: B. Azithromycin

The clinical presentation suggests pertussis, which can be a cause of persistent cough in adults, even those who received vaccinations as child. The paroxysms of coughing and posttussive vomiting are also features suggestive of pertussis. The clinical course is usually less severe than in children, but treatment is advised within 3 weeks of symptoms in nonpregnant patients and within 6 weeks of symptoms in pregnant patients in order to contain the spread of infection, which is especially important, given that she works at a daycare. Treatment options for pertussis include azithromycin (Option B), clarithromycin, erythromycin, and trimethoprim-sulfamethoxazole.

Albuterol inhaler (Option A) and prednisone (Option C) might be used for an asthma attack. Antitussive agents (Option D) may be helpful, but they will not treat the infection. There is no clinical indication for hospitalization or IV antibiotics for this patient (Option E).

Tiwari T, Murphy TV, Moran J. National Immunization Program, Centers for Disease Control and Prevention. Recommended antimicrobial agents for the treatment and postexposure prophylaxis of pertussis: 2005 CDC Guidelines. *MMWR Recomm Rep.* 2005;54(RR-14):1–16.

41. ANSWER: D. Worry. See him today or refer him to ENT.

This patient has sudden sensorineural hearing loss (SSNHL). It is characterized by rapid loss of hearing, often in one ear and often noticed in the morning. More than 90% of patients have tinnitus, and most have ear fullness as well. The etiologies include autoimmune, microvascular, or viral cochleitis. Most would evaluate for retrocochlear tumor (acoustic neuroma), which occurs in between 5% and 30% of studies. Most ENT doctors will treat patients with high-dose steroids, and a small subset of patients may do well with antivirals.

Rauch SD. Idiopathic sudden sensorineural hearing loss. *N Engl J Med.* 2008;359:833–840.

42. ANSWER: B. Start captopril.

The patient has scleroderma and newly elevated blood pressure, lower extremity edema, renal failure with proteinuria, and microangiopathy, consistent with scleroderma renal crisis. The drug of choice for scleroderma renal crisis is an angiotensin-converting enzyme inhibitor (Option B), which should be rapidly titrated to reduce blood pressure. ACE inhibitors help preserve or improve renal function in scleroderma renal crisis and have been shown to significantly reduce mortality in this setting.

There is no evidence that this is an inflammatory process; thus, glucocorticoids (Options D and E) are not indicated. In addition, high-dose glucocorticoids increase the risk of scleroderma renal crisis. Calcium channel blockers (Option A) may be used as additional treatment of resistant hypertension. Beta blockers (Option C) are usually avoided in patients with scleroderma because of the theoretical risk of worsening vasospasm.

Bose N, Chiesa-Vottero A, Chatterjee S. Scleroderma renal crisis. *Semin Arthritis Rheum.* 2015;44(6):687–694.

43. ANSWER: D. Indomethacin 50 mg orally

This is a presentation of reactive arthritis, which presents as an asymmetric mono-/oligoarthritis, predominantly of lower extremity joints. Classically, it also presents with enthesitis (inflammation of the insertion of ligaments, tendons, joint capsule, or fascia to bone—typically the Achilles tendon) and dactylitis ("sausage digits"). Extraarticular involvement may include urethritis, conjunctivitis, uveitis, oral ulcers, and rashes. Reactive arthritis may occur following GU or enteric infections caused by *Chlamydia trachomatis, Yersinia, Salmonella, Shigella, Campylobacter*, and possibly *Clostridium difficile.* Typically, there are a few days to a few weeks between infection and onset. Treatment is with NSAIDs such as indomethacin 50 mg three times daily for at least 2 weeks.

Gonococcal arthritis similarly may present with the abrupt onset of a mono- or oligoarthritis, but it typically does not cause sausage digits and frequently presents with a rash. Ceftriaxone (Option A) would be an appropriate initial treatment for this. IV (Option B) or oral (Option C) steroids may be used to treat numerous rheumatologic conditions, but they are not the treatment of choice for reactive arthritis. Observation (Option E) is not the best answer, given the severity of symptoms in this case.

44. ANSWER: B. Iron deficiency anemia

This is a case of profound iron deficiency anemia (Option B), as evidenced by microcytic anemia with very low iron levels. Causes of microcytic anemia include iron deficiency, thalassemia, and anemia of chronic disease. Rarer causes include copper deficiency, lead poisoning, and sideroblastic anemia. Iron deficiency may be subtle and insidious, with typical presenting symptoms including fatigue, weakness, exercise intolerance, headache, and irritability. Additional signs and symptoms include tongue pain, dry mouth, pica/pagophagia, and restless leg syndrome.

Thalassemia (Option A) typically presents with very low MCV, as in this case, but iron stores should be normal to increased. The prior MCV of 85 fL also makes thalassemia highly unlikely, because it is an inherited disorder. Family history is often positive.

Lead poisoning (Option C) may cause microcytic anemia. Basophilic stippling is often (but not always) evident on peripheral blood smear. Other manifestations include abdominal pain, joint and muscle aches, memory problems, and irritability

The normal haptoglobin and LDH make the diagnosis of hemolytic anemia (Option D) less likely. Hemolysis usually results in normocytic anemia.

Anemia of chronic disease (Option E) typically presents with low iron, low TIBC, and a normal to increased ferritin. The ESR would be expected to be elevated.

Camaschella C. Iron-deficiency anemia. *N Engl J Med.* 2015;372:1832–1843.

45. ANSWER: B. De Quervain tenosynovitis

This patient has the classic presentation of De Quervain tenosynovitis, which presents most commonly in women between 30 and 50 years old, with a significant subset of them being recently postpartum. It affects the abductor pollicis longus and extensor pollicis brevis in the first extensor compartment. Most people think that it is related to some sort of repetitive strain, though the etiology is unknown. It seems common in women with newborns because of the way that they hold and feed the baby. Treatment is generally conservative, and people do well with a thumb spica splint and nonsteroidals. Steroid injections can help if the pain continues.

46. ANSWER: B. Treat with weekly isoniazid and rifapentine for 12 weeks.

As a healthcare worker, our patient is at fairly high risk of converting to active TB. He was likely exposed to TB in the past few years on the basis of his history (conversion is highest in the first 2 years after exposure and drops off after more time). BCG vaccination should not play a role in the decision whether to treat additionally, on the basis of the large area of induration and how long ago he was vaccinated, BCG is unlikely to be contributing to the test result. Neither the skin test nor the blood test is a "gold standard"; both can have false-positive and false-negative results. This patient should be treated for latent TB with one of the regimens recommended by the Centers for Disease Control and Prevention. These include isoniazid for 9 months, rifampin for 4 months, or isoniazid and rifapentine given together weekly for 12 weeks. For patients who do not take other medications that interact with rifampin or rifapentine and who do not wish to take a long course of treatment, the isoniazid/rifapentine option is reasonable. Treatment of latent TB with rifampin and pyrazinamide for 4 months is no longer recommended by the CDC, owing to excess risk of hepatotoxicity. The CDC website provides updated information about diagnosis and management of latent tuberculosis (http://www.cdc.gov/tb/default.htm).

47. ANSWER: C. Lumbar puncture

This patient's symptoms and signs of headache, intermittent blurred vision, pulsatile tinnitus, and papilledema are most consistent with increased intracranial pressure. Her normal imaging studies exclude a mass lesion, hydrocephalus, or venous sinus thrombosis, leaving idiopathic intracranial hypertension (pseudotumor cerebri) as the most likely diagnosis. This condition is most commonly seen in obese women of childbearing age.

Because a mass lesion has been excluded by imaging, lumbar puncture is indicated to confirm increased cerebrospinal fluid pressure and to initiate treatment by removal of cerebrospinal fluid. Urgent ophthalmologic consultation also is important for formal assessment and subsequent monitoring of visual fields, because visual loss is a potential complication of this condition. Acetazolamide therapy to reduce cerebrospinal fluid production should be started only after lumbar puncture confirms the diagnosis. Amitriptyline therapy is not appropriate, because her current headaches are not consistent with migraine, and this therapy may cause increased weight gain. Neurosurgical consultation is not appropriate at this time, although patients with idiopathic intracranial hypertension who develop visual field loss despite medical management may require surgical intervention with optic nerve sheath fenestration or cerebrospinal fluid shunting procedures.

Friedman DI, Liu GT, Digre KB, et al. Revised diagnostic criteria for the pseudotumor cerebri syndrome in adults and children. *Neurology.* 2013;81(13):1159–1165.

48. ANSWER: A. Beta blockers and gentle diuresis

Given the epidemiologic features of being raised in Brazil, as well as the examination and echocardiographic features suggestive of mitral valve stenosis, this patient likely had rheumatic fever as a child, resulting in rheumatic heart disease and mitral stenosis, which was asymptomatic until her pregnancy.

Medical management of symptomatic mitral stenosis in pregnancy involves beta blockers (to slow the heart rate and improve diastolic filling) and gentle diuresis (Option A). If this is not adequate, percutaneous mitral valvuloplasty can be considered.

Inotropes such as digoxin (Option B) and dopamine (Option C) should be avoided in mitral stenosis. Vasodilators such as ACE inhibitors (Option D) and hydralazine/nitrates (Option E) are not first-line agents in the setting of decompensated mitral stenosis. The safety of medications during pregnancy should also be considered.

49. ANSWER: B. IgA nephropathy

IgA nephropathy (Option B) is the most common cause of primary glomerulonephritis in the developed world. It usually presents with recurrent gross hematuria, usually less than 5 days after a urinary tract infection or bacterial tonsillitis, though it may also present with microscopic hematuria and mild proteinuria.

Poststreptococcal glomerulonephritis (Option A) is an immune complex disease resulting from specific nephritogenic strains of group A streptococcus. It usually occurs 1–3 weeks after pharyngitis and 3–6 weeks after skin infection. Children ages 5–12 and adults >60 are at highest risk. The most common presenting symptoms are edema, gross hematuria, and hypertension, though the presentation ranges from asymptomatic to microscopic hematuria to full-blown acute nephritic syndrome. Complement components are usually decreased, and this may persist for 4–8 weeks. Renal function resolves within 3–4 weeks; hematuria may persist for 3–6 months. Unlike IgA nephropathy, it rarely recurs.

Proteinuria and dysmorphic red cells suggest glomerular (rather than extraglomerular) bleeding, making the remaining choices unlikely. Carcinoma of the bladder (Option C) typically affects older patients, with a mean age at diagnosis of around 70 years. Urinary tract infections (Option D) and nephrolithiasis (Option E) would be expected to present with additional signs and symptoms and without dysmorphic red blood cells in the urine.

Wyatt RJ, Julian BA. IgA nephropathy. *N Engl J Med.* 2013;368:2402–2414.

50. ANSWER: B. Squeezing limes while making mojitos

This strange, often bizarre, well-demarcated rash (phytophotodermatitis) is the result of a cutaneous phototoxic eruption that results from contact with light-sensitizing substances and exposure to UVA radiation (Option B). Symptoms typically begin within 24 hours of exposure, peak at 48–72 hours, and may take weeks to resolve. Manifestation can range from hyperpigmentation (as seen in Fig. 9.6) to bullous eruptions. The most frequently reported sensitizing agents are lime juice, mangoes, celery, occasionally roses/grasses, and bergamot oils in perfumes with essential oils. The treatment for this condition is watchful waiting.

Given the linear pattern on the arm, lymphangitis is also in the differential diagnosis, but in the absence of systemic symptoms, this is highly unlikely. Lymphangitis can be caused by various organisms, such as the following:

- *Mycobacterium marinum*—common in saltwater fish tanks (Option A)
- *Sporothrix* spp.—classically contracted through a rosebush thorn puncture (Option D)
- *Streptococcus pyogenes*—contracted through injection drug use (Option E)

A reaction to sunscreen would not be expected to have such a linear pattern (Option C).

Acknowledgment

The authors and editors gratefully acknowledge the contributions of the previous authors—Nikhil Wagle, Christopher Gibson, Ami Bhatt, Molly L. Perencevich, William Martinez, Jason Ojeda, Rose Kakoza, and Lindsay King.

Index

Page numbers followed by f indicate figures and t indicate tables.

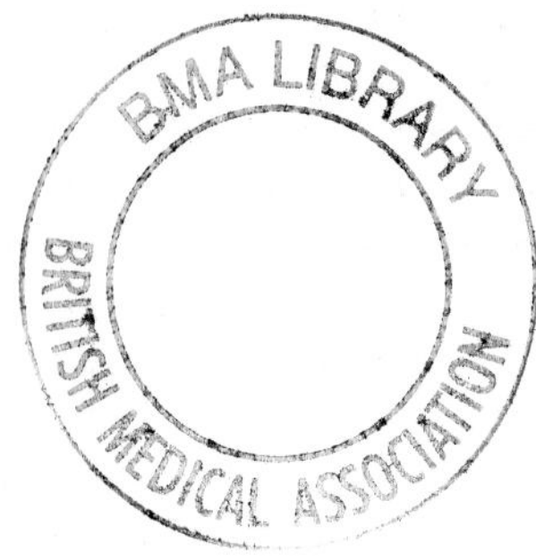
BMA LIBRARY
BRITISH MEDICAL ASSOCIATION